Hypertension Handbook for Clinicians and Students

Pathophysiology, Diagnosis, Clinical Trials,
Non Drug and Drug Treatments

First Edition

Mark C. Houston, MD, MSc, FACP, FAHA
Clinical Professor of Medicine
Vanderbilt University School of Medicine
ASH Specialist in Clinical Hypertension
Director, Hypertension Institute and Vascular Biology, Nashville
Section Chief, Division of Nutrition and Clinical Research
Staff Physician, Vascular Institute
Saint Thomas Hospital
Nashville, Tennessee

Ralph Hawkins, MD, LLM, FRCPC
Assistant Clinical Professor of Medicine
Vanderbilt University School of Medicine
ASH Specialist in Clinical Hypertension
Section Chief of Clinical Research and Nephrology
Hypertension Institute, Nashville
Staff Physician, Vascular Institute
Saint Thomas Hospital
Nashville, Tennessee

ANA Publishing, Birmingham, Alabama

ANA Publishing
5120 Selkirk Drive, Suite 100
Birmingham, AL 35252
(205) 980-5710   FAX (205) 991-9302
Website: www.hypertensionhandbook.com

Hypertension Handbook for Clinicians and Students, 1st Edition
ISBN 0-9753730-0-5

Printed in the United States of America

10 9 8 7 6 5 4 3 2

Mark C. Houston, MD, MSc, FACP, FAHA

Mark C. Houston, MD, MSc, FACP, FAHA graduated from Vanderbilt Medical School, completed his medical internship and residency at the University of California, San Francisco, then returned to Vanderbilt Medical Center as chief resident in medicine. Dr. Houston remained on the full time internal medicine faculty at Vanderbilt University medical school for 12 years where he served as Medical Director of the Executive Physical Program, of the Medical Director of the Cooperative Care Center, Co-Director of Medical Intensive Care Unit, Chief Clinical Section of the Division of General Internal Medicine and then Associate Professor of Medicine. He is board certified by the American Board of Internal Medicine, the American Society of Hypertension (ASH) as a specialist in clinical hypertension (SCH) and the American Board of Anti-Aging Medicine (ABAAM). He has a Masters of Science degree in clinical human nutrition from the University of Bridgeport, Connecticut. He is Editor-in-Chief for the *Journal of the American Nutraceutical Association (JANA)*. He has published over 130 articles and scientific abstracts in peer reviewed medical journals as well as textbook chapters, handbooks and films, and completed over 60 clinical research studies in hypertension, hyperlipidemia and cardiovascular disease. Dr. Houston has authored three best selling books entitled, *Handbook of Antihypertensive Therapy, Vascular Biology for the Clinician* and *What Your Doctor May Not Tell You About Hypertension.* His specialities include hypertension, lipid disorders, prevention and treatment of cardiovascular diseases, nutrition, clinical age management and general internal medicine. He has an active clinical and research practice as well as teaching responsibilities for Vanderbilt medical students, interns and residents. He is presently Clinical Professor of Medicine, Vanderbilt University School of Medicine, and Director of the Hypertension Institute, Vascular Biology and the Life Extension Institute of Nashville and practices at Saint Thomas Medical Group, Saint Thomas Hospital and Health Services in Nashville, Tennessee. He is also Medical Director of Clinical Research, Section Chief of the Division of Nutrition and Director of CME in the Hypertension Institute in Nashville. He is a staff physician of the Vascular Institute of Saint Thomas Hospital. He is a member of the AHA Council on Atherosclerosis, Thrombosis and Vascular Biology, and the ASH nominating committee, and serves on the editorial board and as an editorial consultant for numerous medical journals.

Ralph Hawkins, MD, LLM, FRCPC

Ralph Hawkins, MD received his medical degree in 1981 from the University of Saskatchewan in Saskatoon (Canada) and completed fellowships in Internal Medicine and Nephrology at the University of Calgary. He is the recipient of several medical and academic awards and has held many clinical positions in Western Canada. He moved to Tennessee in 2000 as an Associate Professor of Medicine at the University of Tennessee Health Center in Memphis. He joined the St. Thomas Medical Group and the Hypertension Institute in Nashville in January 2003. Dr. Hawkins is board certified both by the American Board of Internal Medicine and by the Royal College of Physicians and Surgeons of Canada in Internal Medicine and Nephrology, and is also certified as a specialist in Clinical Hypertension by the Board of American Society of Hypertension. His clinical and research interests are the epidemiology and prevention of kidney diseases associated with high blood pressure and diabetes. Dr. Hawkins also received a masters of Laws degree (LLM) in Medical Law from the University of Northumbria at Newcastle in 2002, and is experienced in the clinical application of medical ethics principles.

Contents

Contents

vii

Abbreviations

Ang-II	angiotensin II
ACE	angiotensin-converting enzyme
AV	atrioventricular
ARB	angiotensin II receptor blocker
BP	blood pressure
BB	beta-blocker
BUN	blood urea nitrogen
CHD	coronary heart disease
CHF	congestive heart failure
CO	cardiac output
CRF	chronic renal failure
CVA	cerebrovascular accident
D	diuretic
DBP	diastolic blood pressure
DHEAS	dehydroepiandrosterone sulfate
DHP	dihydropyridine
EPI	epinephrine
GFR	glomerular filtration rate
GITS	gastrointestinal therapeutic system
HCTZ	hydrochlorothiazide
HDL	high-density lipoprotein
HR	heart rate
IBW	ideal body weight
IGCP	intraglomerular capillary pressure
ISA	intrinsic sympathomimetic activity
IVP	intravenous pyelogram (pyelography)
LDL	low-density lipoprotein
Lp(a)	lipoprotein A
LVFP	left ventricular filling pressure
LVH	left ventricular hypertrophy
MAO	monoamine oxidase
MAP	mean arterial pressure
MI	myocardial infarction
MIBG	metaiodobenzylguanidine
MRI	magnetic resonance imaging
MSA	membrane-stabilizing activity
NE	norepinephrine

NPI	neuro-peptidase inhibitors
NSAIDs	nonsteroidal anti-inflammatory drugs
PET	positron emission tomography
PFTs	pulmonary function tests
PIH	pregnancy-induced hypertension
PRA	plasma renin activity
PWP	pulmonary wedge pressure
RAAS	renin-angiotensin-aldosterone
RBC	red blood cell
RBF	renal blood flow
RPF	renal plasma flow
RVR	renal vascular resistance
SBP	systolic blood pressure
SNS	sympathetic nervous system
SV	stroke volume
SVR	systemic vascular resistance
TPA	tissue plasminogen activator
UTI	urinary tract infection
VLDL	very-low-density lipoprotein
VMA	vanillylmandelic acid

General Introduction

The clinician seeking optimal antihypertensive drug therapy must recognize a myriad of new challenges and concepts. *Individualization of treatment* is recommended based on the *subsets of hypertension approach.*[5] An essential component of individualized treatment is a logical and tailored selection of drug therapies based on:

1. Pathophysiology and vascular biology
2. Hemodynamics
3. Risk factor reduction and end-organ damage reduction
4. Concomitant medical diseases or problems
5. Demographics
6. Quality of life and adverse effects of treatment
7. Compliance with therapy
8. Total health care cost

This first edition of *Hypertension Handbook for Clinicians and Students* includes these new concepts, changes in philosophy, clinical information, clinical trials, new antihypertensive drugs, drug delivery systems and nonpharmacological treatment. Large-scale clinical trials comparing the older antihypertensive drug regimens with newer agents have been completed and many others are in progress. The recently published studies include ALLHAT, INSIGHT, NORDIL, LIFE, AASK, RENAAL, IDNT, IRMA, CONVINCE, ANBP-2 and VALUE and MOSES. The Systolic Hypertension Trial in Europe (SYST-EUR), Shanghai Trial of Nifedipine in the Elderly (STONE), Systolic Hypertension in China (SYST-CHINA), Hypertension Optimal Treatment (HOT), and the Chen-Du Nifedipine Trial, INSIGHT, NORDIL, NIC-EH, CONVINCE, PREVENT, VHAS, GLANT, PATE, STOP-2, VALUE, and ALLHAT, have documented significant reductions in cardiovascular and cerebrovascular morbidity and mortality with calcium channel blockers. The Captopril Prevention Project (CAPPP) and ANBP-2 showed that angiotensin-converting enzyme inhibitors reduce cardiovascular morbidity and mortality in hypertensive patients equal to or better than conventional diuretic and beta-blocker therapy. The Heart Outcomes Evaluation (HOPE) and EU-ROPA studies showed that ACEIs reduced cardiovascular death in a high-risk nonhypertensive population. The treatment of the hypertensive patient with diabetes mellitus with proteinuria has now been shown in SYST-EUR, CAPPP, RENAAL, IDNT, IRMA and LIFE to be better with ACEIs, ARBs, and CCBs than with conventional diuretic or beta-blocker therapy in reducing cardiovascular morbidity and mortality. The Swedish Trial in Old Patients–2 (STOP-2) showed that calcium blockers and ACEIs are equal to conventional therapy in reducing cardiovascular morbidity and mortality and superior in reducing CVA and equal BP levels. The PROGRESS trial, STOP-2, MICROHOPE, QUIET, SCAT, AASK, ABCD, ALLHAT, FACET, GLANT, ANBP-2, and PATE have proven significant reductions in CV morbidity and mortality with ACEIs. New data on beta-blockers, SARAs, angiotensin-converting enzyme inhibitors and angiotensin receptor blockers in cardiac disease (congestive heart failure, myocardial infarction) are positive as well. ARBs (Losartan) significantly reduced cerebrovascular and cardiovascular morbidity and mortality in the LIFE tial. Valsartan reduced CV morbidity and mortality in the VALUE trial. Eprosartan reduced CV morbidity and mortality in the MOSES trial. No single antihypertensive drug can meet every need in all hypertensive patients. Fortunately, the armamentarium is large and rapidly growing.

Mark C. Houston, MD, MSc, FACP, FAHA
Ralph G. Hawkins MD, LLM, FRCPC

Acknowledgement: Some of the material presented in this first edition of *Hypertension Handbook for Clinicians and Students* has been adapted from the *Handbook of Antihypertensive Therapy* (edition #1–#10) by Houston, Meador and Schipani published between 1986 and 2000 (ISBN 1-56053-422-2)

Introduction

Hypertension is one of the major risk factors for coronary heart disease (CHD), cerebrovascular accident (CVA), chronic renal failure (CRF), and congestive heart failure (CHF) in the United States. CHD is the leading cause of death in the United States, accounting for more than 800,000 deaths per year (more than one death per minute), and CVA is the 4th leading cause of death in the U.S. The annual expenditure for CHD is over 200 billion dollars.[1–3]

Hypertension is part of a heterogeneous condition that is best described as an *atherosclerotic syndrome* or *hypertension syndrome* with genetic and acquired structural and metabolic disorders, including the following:[4,5,147]

1. Dyslipidemia
2. Insulin resistance and impaired glucose tolerance
3. Central obesity (android or portal obesity)
4. Endocrine changes (SNS, RAAS)
5. Renal function abnormalities (sodium, water, uric acid, protein load excretion, microalbuminuria)
6. Abnormalities of vascular and cardiac smooth muscle structure and function (arterial compliance) (LVH)
7. Membranopathy and abnormal cellular cation transport (Ca^{++}, Mg^{+}, Na^{+}, K^{+})
8. Abnormalities of coagulation (Prothrombotic)
9. Endothelial dysfunction
10. Vascular inflammation (HS-CRP)

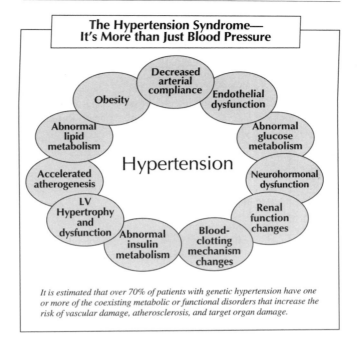

**The Hypertension Syndrome—
It's More than Just Blood Pressure**

Hypertension

- Decreased arterial compliance
- Endothelial dysfunction
- Abnormal glucose metabolism
- Neurohormonal dysfunction
- Renal function changes
- Blood-clotting mechanism changes
- Abnormal insulin metabolism
- LV Hypertrophy and dysfunction
- Accelerated atherogenesis
- Abnormal lipid metabolism
- Obesity

It is estimated that over 70% of patients with genetic hypertension have one or more of the coexisting metabolic or functional disorders that increase the risk of vascular damage, atherosclerosis, and target organ damage.

The goals in the treatment of hypertension are to reduce intra-arterial pressure, improve vascular biology, vascular health, treat the hypertension syndrome optimally and reduce target organ damage. Ideally the optimal treatment should maximize reduction in *all* end-organ damage, including CHF, CHD, CVA, CRF, left ventricular hypertrophy (LVH), and myocardial infarction (MI), as well as total mortality.

Recent advances in our understanding of the physiology and pathophysiology of the blood vessel show that endothelial function, inflamation and arterial compliance play an important role in end-organ damage. Attention must be directed at promoting **VASCULAR HEALTH** in order to achieve optimal reduction in end-organ damage. The accurate assessment of global CV risk is required in each patient in order to select the optimal antihypertensive regimen.

Re-think Treatment
Hypertension is a Disease of Blood Vessels

↓

Vascular Biology is Altered
(Structural and Functional)

↓

Target the Vasculature
- Risk Factors (Traditional)
- Risk Factors (Nontraditional—Vascular Biology)

↓

Target Organs—Optimal Treatment

The Blood Vessel is an Organ
- Largest Organ in the Body
- 5 x Heart in Mass
- 6 Tennis Courts in Area

The vessel wall is an active, integrated organ composed of endothelial, smooth muscle and fibroblast cells coupled to each other in a complex autocrine-paracrine set of interactions.

The Vascular System Regulates Vascular Health and Tone Through Chronic Active Balance Between:

| Vasoconstrictors | Vasodilators |
| Growth Promoters | Growth Inhibitors |

$$\Delta$$

↓

Vascular Tone
Vascular Health (Damage)

Blood Vessel Structure

The Blood Vessel Structure

■ Serosa ■ Muscularis ■ Endothelium

Structural and functional changes may cause dysfunction leading to vascular damage and target organ damage.

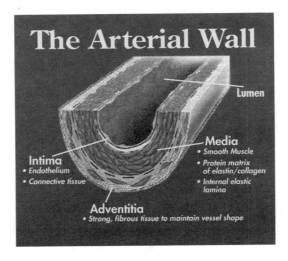

(Modified from Ross R: Atherosclerosis – an inflammatory disease. N Engl J Med 1999; 340:115-126, and Mulvany MJ, Aalkjaer C: Structure and function of small arteries. Physiol Rev 1990; 70:921-961).

The walls of the artery consist of the intima, media, and adventitia. The intima, the smooth inner lining of the vessel, comprises the endothelium and underlying connective tissue. Metabolically active endothelial cells line the lumen.

The middle layer, the media or muscularis, comprises smooth muscle cells (SMCs) that are surrounded by an extracellular protein matrix containing collagen, elastin fibers, fibroblasts, and an internal elastic lamina. Small arteries contain greater proportions of smooth muscles than large arteries. The media of large arteries (e.g., the aorta) has a relatively large amount of elastic tissue.

The adventitia, or outer layer of the arterial wall, comprises connective tissue that acts to maintain the shape of the vessel and limit distention. The structural heterogeneity in large vs. intermediate vs. small vessels is potentially important in terms of disease processes and therapeutic responsiveness.

Endothelial Dysfunction:

1. Vasospasm (vasoconstriction vs. vasodilation)
2. Thrombosis (procoagulant vs. anticoagulant)
3. Atherosclerosis (proinflammatory vs. anti-inflammatory)
4. Restenosis (growth promotion vs. inhibition)

Structural Dysfunction:

1. Vascular hypertrophy
2. Vascular hyperplasia
3. Vascular polyploidy

Vascular Endothelium: Strategic Anatomical Position

CIRCULATING BLOOD

Modulates
- Platelet Function
- Coagulation
- Monocyte and Leukocyte Adhesion
- Inflammation

ENDOTHELIUM *Strategic Location*

Modulates
- Permeability
- Contractile State
- Proliferative Response (Growth)
- Migratory Response
- Redox State

Vascular Smooth Muscle Cells (VSMC)

Vascular Biology in Clinical Practice, Oct. 2000; Mark C. Houston, MD

Functional Endothelium

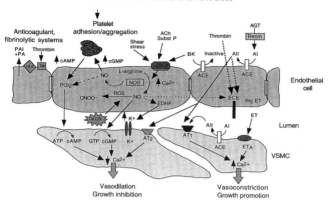

The diagram above illustrates the complexity of the processes mediated by the endothelium in carrying out its various regulatory functions. The vasorelaxant substances nitric oxide (NO), prostacyclin, and endothelium-derived hyperpolarizing factor (EDHF) released by the endothelium promote vasodilation and inhibit growth of vascular smooth muscle cells. Angiotensin II and endothelin are potent vasoconstrictors and growth-promoting factors released from the endothelium. Bradykinin, through a receptor-mediated mechanism, stimulates release of NO. Increased expression of ACE in the endothelium escalates production of angiotensin II and degradation of bradykinin, leading to decreased synthesis/release of NO from the endothelium. NO prevents platelet adhesion/aggregation and mediates synthesis of tissue plasminogen activator (t-PA), whereas angiotensin II promotes platelet aggregation and formation of plasminogen activator inhibitor (PAI-1).

Vascular Functions of Endothelium

- Maintain tone and structure
- Regulate cell growth
- Regulate thrombotic and fibrinolytic properties
- Mediate inflammatory and immune mechanisms
- Regulate leukocyte and platelet adhesion to surface of endothelium
- Modulate oxidation (metabolic activity)
- Regulate permeability

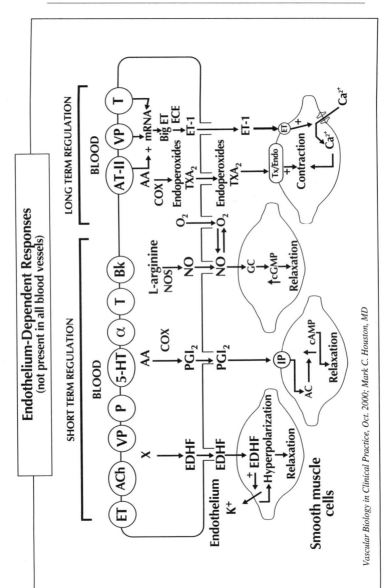

Endothelium-Dependent Responses
(not present in all blood vessels)

Vascular Biology in Clinical Practice, Oct. 2000; Mark C. Houston, MD

Endothelial Dysfunction

Definition*

- Injury or activation of the endothelial cell leads to altered endothelial function that may promote disease.
- The dysfunctional state may be characterized by numerous features such as an imbalance between endothelium-derived relaxing and contracting factors or growth-promoting factors.

Pathophysiologic Consequences*

Macromolecular barrier disruption

↓

Increased vessel permeability

↓

Physiologic clearance mechanisms overwhelmed

↓

LDL oxidation and initiation of atherosclerosis

Hypothesis

- Normal endothelium maintains balance between relaxant and constrictive factors.

- Endothelial dysfunction promotes vasoactive substance imbalance.
  ↓ NO (Nitric Oxide)
  ↑ tissue ACE
  ↑ Ang-II

From Lüscher TF: J Myocard Ischemia 7 (Suppl 1):15–20, 1995.

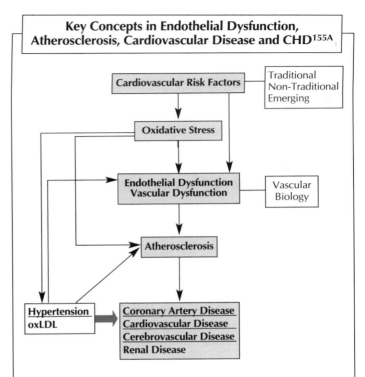

Key Concepts in Endothelial Dysfunction, Atherosclerosis, Cardiovascular Disease and CHD[155A]

Oxidative Stress to the blood vessels plays a major role in directly inducing endothelial dysfunction, vascular smooth muscle dysfunction, and atherosclerosis. Thus, oxidative stress is the mediator between cardiovascular risk factors and target organ damage.

Vascular Biology in Clinical Practice, Oct. 2002; Mark C. Houston, MD

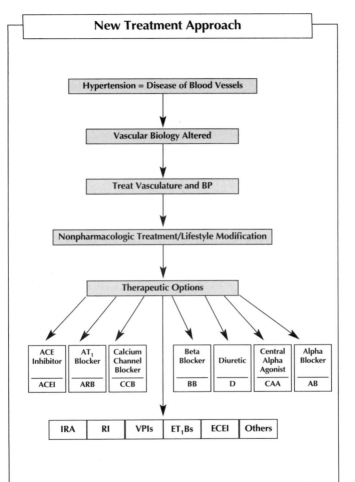

New Treatment Approach

Hypertension = Disease of Blood Vessels

Vascular Biology Altered

Treat Vasculature and BP

Nonpharmacologic Treatment/Lifestyle Modification

Therapeutic Options

| ACE Inhibitor | AT₁ Blocker | Calcium Channel Blocker | Beta Blocker | Diuretic | Central Alpha Agonist | Alpha Blocker |
| ACEI | ARB | CCB | BB | D | CAA | AB |

| IRA | RI | VPIs | ET₁Bs | ECEI | Others |

IRA – Imidazolindine receptor antagonist; RI – renin inhibitor; VPI – vasopeptidase inhibitor; ET1B – endothelin receptor blocker type B; ECEI– endothelin-converting enzyme inhibitor.

Treatment of Impaired Endothelial Function

- Cholesterol lowering (statins) (fibrates, niacin)
- Antioxidant therapy
- Weight reduction
- L-Arginine supplementation, folate
- ACE inhibition (ACEI)
- Angiotensin I blockade
- Calcium channel blocker therapy
- Omega-3 fatty acid supplementation
- Exercise training (shear stress)
- Improve insulin resistance
  (diet, TZDs, metformin)
- Low dose aspirin
- Non pharmacologic/lifestyle change

Endothelial Dysfunction and Atherosclerotic Vascular Disease (Clinical Events)

- Endothelial dysfunction
- ↑ Permeability

- ↓ Antithrombotic and fibrinolytic activity
- Induction of adhesion molecules
- ↓ Vasodilator function
- Inactivation of EDRF (oxygen free radicals)

- Vascular/atherosclerotic effects
- LDL or blood-borne mitogen penetration to subendothelium

- ↑ Thrombosis
- ↓ Fibrinolysis
- Recruit macrophages into vascular wall
- ↓ Antiproliferative activity and ↑BP
- ↑ Smooth muscle cell proliferation (LVH)

Estrogens and Vascular Function

- Receptor mediated
  - ↑ Endothelial NO
  - ↑ Vasodilation
  - ↓ LDL penetration
- Antioxidant nonreceptor effect

Oral therapy may result in different effects than transdermal therapy.

Hypothesis: Essential Hypertension and End-Organ Damage

The primary goal in the treatment of essential hypertension is to prevent and reduce *all* end-organ damage by reducing blood pressure (BP), improving the various components of the hypertension syndrome and promoting optimal vascular health or vascular biology (endothelial function and vascular smooth muscle function and structure). Hypertension is associated with an increased risk of cerebrovascular, cardiovascular, and renal morbidity and mortality. Pharmacologic therapy has partially reduced some, but not all, of these complications. To achieve optimal decreases in morbidity and mortality in hypertensive related diseases, the overall impact of antihypertensive drug therapy on vascular risk factors, risk markers, vascular biology and the pathogenesis of damage to each end organ must be considered.

Although a higher percentage of deaths occurs in patients with diastolic blood pressure (DBP) ≥105 mm Hg, patients with DBP ≤ 105 mm Hg account for more deaths. The majority of patients with hypertension have the mild form. The risks of therapy versus the benefits of therapy are particularly critical in this group. Pharmacologic therapy of mild to moderate hypertension (DBP ≤110 mm Hg) has reduced the complications of most pressure-related (arteriolar) damage, such as CVA, CHF, and some cases of CRF, but the atherosclerotic complications (CHD, angina, MI, and sudden death) have not been reduced to the extent predicted by the degree of BP reduction in those prospective clinical trials in which diuretics and beta-blockers were the primary antihypertensive drugs used.[4] The only exception, to date, for this statement, is the ALLHAT trial, in which the fatal and non-fatal CHD primary endpoint was equivalent among the chlorthalidone, amlodipine and lisinopril treated subjects. It should be noted, however, that this was a high risk elderly population (average age of 67 years) prospective clinical trial.[150] Systolic hypertension has emerged as an equal or more sensitive predictor of CV risk in most age groups (especially after age 50). Selection of initial and combination antihypertensive drug therapy is a com-

1

plex decision based on numerous factors such as goal BP, concomitant risk factors, renal function, age, gender, race, metabolic and hemodynamic parameters, pathophysiology, vascular biology, adverse effects, compliance, economics and finally, clinically proven ability to reduce target organ damage. The role of beta-blocker monotherapy in reducing CHD in the elderly has been questioned.[130] In addition, the indiscriminate use of some diuretics (HCTZ, chorthalidone, and thiazide-like diuretics, but not indapamide), in hypertensives may be associated with a higher incidence of insulin resistance, glucose intolerance, new onset of type 2 diabetes mellitus, renal cell carcinoma and progressive renal insufficiency.[90,148]

There is even a suggestion in many clinical trials of intrapatient superiority of some antihypertensive drugs in reducing specific target organ damage (i.e. CCB for CVA; ACEI, ARB for CRI; ACET, ARB or diuretic for CHF; CCB, ACEI, ARB for CHD and MI).

A more sophisticated and pathophysiologically oriented pharmacologic approach based on our knowledge of vascular biology, endothelial dysfunction, and the complex interplay of the components of the hypertension/atherosclerotic syndrome is reviewed in this *Hypertension Handbook for Clinicians and Students.*

Hypertension in the United States and Classification

1. Approximately 50–60 million people in the United States have hypertension—BP reading greater than 140/90 mm Hg.[6] Only 27% of this population controls their hypertension according to NHANES III, and only 31% in NHANES IV (see table 1, pg. 4).

2. JNC 7 Guidelines: [213] Classification and Management of Blood Pressure for Adults Aged 18 Years or Older (see table 1, page 5).

3. Prevalence rates: highest in African-Americans, men, and the elderly. African-Americans have the greatest morbidity and mortality.[4]

4. Hypertension occurs in approximately 60% of non-Hispanic whites, 70% of non-Hispanic blacks, and 61% of Mexican-Americans aged 60 years or older[6] (see figure 1, page 7).

5. A large proportion (60%) of the excess mortality, disability, and morbidity attributable to hypertension occurs among those with stage 1 of the disease.[6]

6. Hypertension is the most common medical problem seen by U.S. physicians, accounting for more office visits and prescriptions than any other disease.[4] The annual cost is over 10 billion dollars.

7. In the United States and other industrialized societies, BP increases with age,[4] especially SBP.

8. SBP and wide pulse pressure (PP) correlate with target organ damage (TOD) better than DBP, in most age groups except younger patients (< 50 years of age). The higher the BP the greater the TOD.

Trends in the Prevalence, Awareness, Treatment, and Control of High Blood Pressure in Adults
in the U.S. 1976–1994*

Percent	NHANES II 1976–1980	NHANES II (Phase 1) 1988–1991	NHANES III (Phase 2) 1991–1994	NHANES IV (Phase 3) 1994-2000
Awareness	51	73	68	68.9
Treated	31	55	53	58.4
Controlled	10	29	27	31

*Adults with hypertension (SBP > 140 mm Hg or DBP > 90 mm Hg) or taking antihypertensive medication. Age 18–74 years.
NHANES = National Health and Nutritional Examination Survey.
From Arch Intern Med 157: 2414, 1997, with permission. JAMA 2003; 290: 203.

Table 1.

Joint National Committee (JNC-7)
Classification and Management of Blood Pressure for Adults Aged 18 Years or Older

BP Classification	Systolic BP, mm Hg*		Diastolic BP, mm Hg*	Lifestyle Modification	Management* Without Compelling Indications	Management* With Compelling Indications†
Normal	<120	and	<80	Encourage		
Prehypertension	120-139	or	80-89	Yes	No antihypertensive drug indicated	Drug(s) for the compelling indications‡
Stage 1 hypertension	140-159	or	90-99	Yes	Thiazide-type diuretics for most; may consider ACE inhibitor, ARB, β-blocker, CCB, or combination	Drug(s) for the compelling indications Other antihypertensive drugs (diuretics, ACE inhibitor, ARB, β-blocker, CCB) as needed
Stage 2 hypertension	≥160	or	≥100	Yes	2-Drug combination for most (usually thiazide-type diuretic and ACE inhibitor or ARB or β-blocker or CCB)§	Drug(s) for the compelling indications Other antihypertensive drugs (diuretics, ACE inhibitor, ARB, β-blocker, CCB) as needed

* Treatment determined by highest BP category.
† See Table 6
‡ Treat patients with chronic kidney disease or diabetes to BP goal of less than 130/80 mm Hg
§ Initial combined therapy should be used cautiously in those at risk for orthostatic hypotension.

Abbreviations:
ACE–Angiotensin-Converting Enzyme;
ARB–Angiotensin-Receptor Blocker;
BP–Blood pressure;
CCB–Calcium Channel Blocker.

JAMA, May 21, 2003—Vol. 289, No. 19

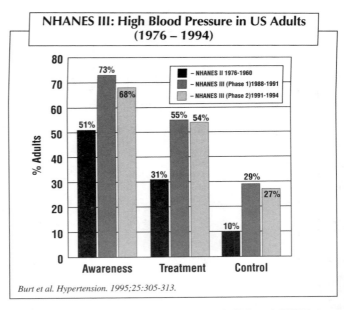

NHANES III: High Blood Pressure in US Adults (1976 – 1994)

Burt et al. Hypertension. 1995;25:305-313.

Despite reduction in BP, the incidence of CRI and ESRD is increasing (see figure).

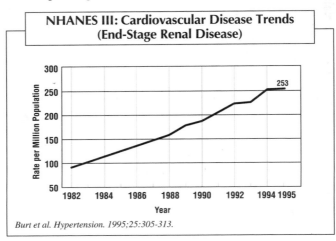

NHANES III: Cardiovascular Disease Trends (End-Stage Renal Disease)

Burt et al. Hypertension. 1995;25:305-313.

NHANES-IV: [217]

Key findings:

- Hypertension (HTN) prevalence in the US increased from 25% in 1988 to 28.7% of the population in 2000 (p=0.5).

- HTN awareness remained unchanged in 2000 compared to 1988 (68.9% in 2000 vs 69.2% in 1988) (p=.58).

- HTN treatment has increased since 1988 from 52.4% to 58.4% (p=.007).

- HTN control overall has increased from 24.6% in 1988 to 31% in 2000 (p=0.05).

- BP control among hypertensive diabetics has not improved since 1988 (28.5% achieving contemporary target in 1988, 25.4% achieving target BP in 2000) (p=.70).

Conclusion: HTN prevalence in the US is increasing and control rates are unacceptably low.

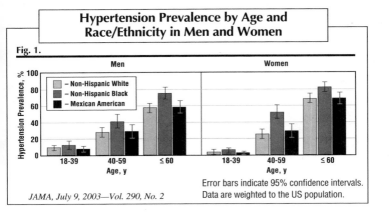

Hypertension Prevalence by Age and Race/Ethnicity in Men and Women

Fig. 1.

Error bars indicate 95% confidence intervals.
Data are weighted to the US population.

JAMA, July 9, 2003—Vol. 290, No. 2

Age-Specific and Age-Adjusted Prevalence of Hypertension by Sex and Race/Ethnicity[217]

Table 3. In the US Population, 1988-2000*

Characteristics	Prevalence, % (SE)			Change, 1988 to 2000	
	1988-1991	1991-1994	1999-2000	% (95% CI)	P Value
Age-Specific Data					
Age, y					
18-39	5.1 (0.6)†	6.1 (0.6)†	7.2(1.1)†	2.1(-0.3 to 4.5)	.05
40-59	27.0 (1.4)†	24.3 (2.2)†	30.1 (1.8)†	3.1 (-1.4to7.6)	.09
>60	57.9 (2.0)	60.1 (1.1)	65.4 (1.6)	7.5 (2.4 to 12.5)	.002
Age-Adjusted (to 2000 US Population) Data					
Overall	25.0(1.5)	25.0(1.7)	28.7(1.8)	3.7(0 to 8.3)	.02
Sex					
Men	24.9 (2.1)	23.9 (2.6)	27.1 (2.7)	2.2 (-4.5 to 8.9)	.26
Women	24.5 (1.7)	26.0(1.8)	30.1 (2.4)	5.6(0 to 11.4)	.03
Race/ethnicity					
Non-Hispanic white	25.9(1.8)	25.6 (2.1)	28.9 (2.3)	3.1 (-2.7 to 8.7)	.14
Non-Hispanic black	28.9 (2.2)	32.5 (2.1)‡	33.5 (3.2)‡	4.6 (-3 to 12.2)	.12
Mexican American	17.2(1.6)†	17.8 (2.0)†	20.7 (2.7)†	3.5 (-2.7 to 9.7)	.13
Sex and race/ethnicity					
Men					
Non-Hispanic white	26.7 (2.7)	24.4 (2.4)	27.7 (3.4)	1.0 (-7.5 to 9.6)	.41
Non-Hispanic black	29.1 (3.3)	29.5 (2.9)	30.9 (4.9)§	1.8 (-9.8 to 13.4)	NA
Mexican American	17,9(2.6)	17.8(1.8)	20.6 (3.9)§	2.7 (-6.5 to 11.9)	NA
Women					
Non-Hispanic white	25.1 (2.1)	26.8 (2.3)	30.2 (3.1)	5.1 (-2.2 to 12.4)	.09
Non-Hispanic black	28.6 (2.7)	35.0 (2.7)	35.8 (4.2)§	7.2 (-2.6 to 17.0)	NA
Mexican American	16.5(2.2)§	17.9(2.1)§	20.7 (3.4)	4.2 (-3.8 to 12.2)	NA

Abbreviations: CI–Confidence Interval; NA–Not Applicable due to unreliable data.

*Data are weighted to the US population.

† P< .001 for the difference among racial/ethnic groups, with non-Hispanic whites as referent, or for the difference among 3 age groups, with >60 years as referent.

‡ P< .01 for the difference among racial/ethnic groups, with non-Hispanic whites as referent, or for the difference among 3 age groups, with >60 years as referent.

§ Estimates are unreliable because of National Health and Nutrition Examination Survey minimum sample size criteria or coefficient of variation of at least 0.30.

Multiple Regression Analysis[217]

Table 4. Association Between Hypertension Prevalence, Demographic Factors and BMI

Factors	Regression Coefficient (SE)		
	1988-1991	1991-1994	1999-2000
Age (per 1-y increase)	1.2 (0.04)*	1.2 (0.03)*	1.3 (0.04)*
Sex (referent: women)	3.5 (1.3)	0.03 (0.7)	1.4 (1.5)
Race/ethnicity (referent Mexican American)			
Non-Hispanic white	-1.1 (0.9)	-0.2 (1)	0.6 (1.4)
Non-Hispanic black	7.0 (1.4)*	10 (0.1)*	8.2 (1.7)*
BMI			
(per 1 unit of increase)†	1.3 (0.07)*	1.3 (0.1)*	1.2 (0.1)*
R2	0.30	0.30	0.31

* $P < .001$ for the independent association between hypertension prevalence and each factor after adjusting for the remaining factors.

† Body mass index (BMI) was calculated as weight in kilograms divided by the square of height in meters.

JAMA, July 9, 2003—Vol. 290, No. 2: 203

Awareness, Treatment, and Control Among Participants with Hypertension[217]

Table 5. U.S. Population, 1988–2000.*

Characteristics	Prevalence, % (SE)			Change, 1988 to 2000	
	1988-1991 (n = 3045)	1991-1994 (n = 3045)	1999-2000 (n = 1565)	% (95% CI)	P Value
Awareness	69.2 (1.3)	67.8 (1.8)	68.9 (1.5)	-0.3 (-4.2 to 3.6)	.58
Treatment	52.4 (1.4)	52.0 (1.0)	58.4 (2.0)	6.0 (1.2 to 10.8)	.007
Control Among those treated	46.9 (2.2)	43.6 (1.7)	53.1 (2.4)	6.2 (0 to 12.6)	.03
Among all with hypertension	24.6 (1.4)	22.7 (1.1)	31.0 (2.0)	6.4 (1.6 to 11.2)	.004
< 140/90 mm Hg (Among treated hypertensive diabetic individuals)	53.1 (4.5)	41.6 (5.8)†	46.9 (4.7)	-6.2 (-19.0 to 6.6)	.83
< 130/85 mm Hg (Among treated hypertensive diabetic individuals)	28.5 (4.2)	17.2 (4.2)†	25.4 (4.0)	-3.1 (-14.5 to 8.3)	.70

Abbreviation: CI– Confidence Interval.

* Data are weighted to the US population.

† Estimates are unreliable because of National Health and Nutrition Examination Survey minimum sample size criteria or coefficient of variation of at least 0.30.

JAMA, July 9, 2003—Vol. 290, No. 2: 203

Hypertension Guidelines

JNC-7[213] Key Recommendations:

1. In people >50, SBP is a more important risk factor for CVD than DBP.

2. CVD risk doubles with each 20/10 mm Hg blood pressure increment above 115/75 mm Hg.

3. People with SBP 120 to 139 or DBP 80 to 89 mm Hg should be considered pre-hypertensive and require lifestyle modifications to prevent CVD.

4. Thiazide-type diuretics should be used either alone or in combination for most patients with uncomplicated HTN. Note: We do not agree with this recommendation or its validity (authors). Certain high-risk conditions are compelling indications for use of other agents as first line therapy (ACE-I, ARB, CCB, β-blockers).

5. Most patients require 2 or more drugs to achieve goal BP (< 140/90, or < 130/80 mm Hg for patients with diabetes or chronic kidney disease).

6. If BP is more than 20/10 mm Hg above target level, consider initiating therapy with 2 agents one of which should be a thiazide-type diuretic. Note: We do agree with this recommendation to use thiazide diuretics as initial or second drug therapy in most patients (authors).

7. **Clinician empathy builds trust and motivates patients to comply with therapy.**

Canadian Hypertension Society

2003 Canadian Hypertension Education Program Recommendations: [214]

" Based on ALLHAT, is it fair to conclude that diuretics should be recommended as sole "first line" therapy in the management of hypertension in patients "without other compelling indications?" Considering the evidence to date, the answer would have to be "No."

Quoted from CHEP 2003 Recommendation Summary, page 4.

Canadian Hypertension Society: [214]

Table 4. Considerations in the Individualization of Antihypertensive Therapy

	Initial Therapy	Second-line Therapy	Notes and/or Cautions
Hypertension without other compelling indications	Thiazide diuretics, beta-blockers, ACE-inhibitors, ARBs, or long-acting dihydropyridine calcium channel blockers	Combinations of first-line drugs (see Table 5)	Alpha-blockers are not recommended as initial therapy. Beta-blockers are not recommended as initial therapy in those over 60 years of age. Hypokalemia should be avoided by using potassium-sparing agents in those who are prescribed diuretics. ACE inhibitors are not recommended in blacks.
Isolated systolic hypertension without other compelling indications	Thiazide diuretics, ARBs or long-acting dihydropyridine calcium channel blockers	Combinations of first-line drugs	Hypokalemia should be avoided by using potassium-sparing agents in people who are prescribed diuretics.
Diabetes mellitus with nephropathy	ACE inhibitors or ARBs	Addition of one or more of thiazide diuretics, cardioselective beta-blockers, long-acting calcium channel blockers or an ARB/ACE inhibitor combination	N/A
Diabetes mellitus w/o nephropathy	ACE inhibitors, ARBs or thiazide diuretics	Combination of first-line drugs or addition of cardioselective beta-blockers and/or long-acting calcium channel blockers	If the serum creatinine level is > 150 μmol loop diuretic should be used as a replacement for low-dose thiazide diuretics if volume required.
Angina	Beta-blockers (consider adding ACE inhibitors)	Long-acting calcium channel blockers	Avoid short-acting nifedipine
Prior myocardial infarction	Beta-blockers and/or ACE inhibitors	Combinations of additional agents	N/A
Heart failure	ACE inhibitors (thiazide or loop diuretics, beta-blockers, spironolactone as additive therapy)	ARBs or hydralazine/isosorbide dinitrate	Avoid nondihydropyridine calcium channel blockers (diltiazem, verapamil)
Past cerebrovascular accident or TIA	ACE inhibitor/diuretic combinations	N/A	Blood pressure reduction reduces recurring cerebrovascular events
Renal disease	ACE inhibitors (diuretics as additive therapy)	Combinations of additional agents	Avoid ACE inhibitors if bilateral renal art stenosis
Left ventricular hypertrophy	ACE inhibitors, ARBs, dihydropyridine calcium channel blockers, diuretics, (beta-blockers for patients under 55 years)	N/A	Avoid hydralazine and minoxidil
Peripheral arterial disease	Does not affect initial treatment recommendations	Does not affect initial treatment recommendations	Avoid beta-blockers with severe disease
Dyslipidemia	Does not affect initial treatment recommendations	Does not affect initial treatment recommendations	N/A

European Societies of Hypertension and Cardiology Guidelines June 2003[215]

> " Emphasis on identifying the first class of drugs to be used is probably outdated by the need to use two or more drugs in combination in order to achieve goal blood pressure."

Journal of Hypertension, 2003, Vol 21, No. 6.

Fig 1.

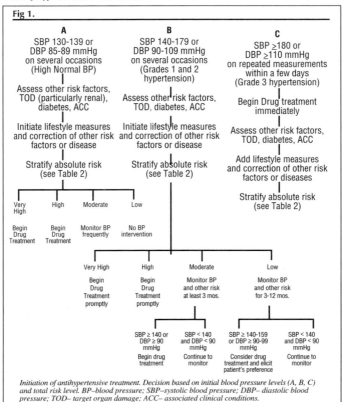

Initiation of antihypertensive treatment. Decision based on initial blood pressure levels (A, B, C) and total risk level. BP–blood pressure; SBP–systolic blood pressure; DBP– diastolic blood pressure; TOD– target organ damage; ACC– associated clinical conditions.

Fig 2.

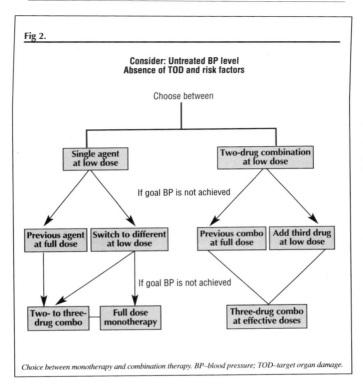

Choice between monotherapy and combination therapy. BP–blood pressure; TOD–target organ damage.

Goals of treatment [215]

• The primary goal of treatment of the patient with high blood pressure is to achieve maximum reduction in the long-term risk of cardiovascular morbidity and mortality. Achieving this goal requires treatment of all reversible risk factors identified, including smoking, obesity, dislipidemia, or diabetes, and the appropriate management of associated clinical conditions, as well as treatment of the raised blood pressure per se.

• On the basis of current evidence from trials, it can be recommended that blood pressure, both systolic and diastolic, be intensively lowered at least below 140/90 mm Hg and to definite lower values, if tolerated, in all hypertensive patients, and below 130/80 mm Hg in diabetics. It is important to keep in mind, however, that systolic values below 140 mm Hg may be difficult to achieve, particularly in the elderly.

Choice of antihypertensive drugs [215]

- The main benefits of antihypertensive therapy are due to lowering of blood pressure per se.

- There is also evidence that specific drug classes may differ in some effect, or in a special groups of patients.

- Drugs are not equal in terms of adverse disturbances, particularly in individual patients.

- The major classes of antihypertensive agents-diuretics, beta-blockers, calcium antagonists, ACE inhibitors, angiotensin receptor antagonists - are suitable for the initiation and maintenance of therapy.

- Emphasis on identifying the first class of drugs to be used is probably outdated by the need to use two or more drugs in combination in order to achieve goal blood pressure.

- Within the array of available evidence, the choice of drugs will be influenced by many factors, including:
  - Previous experience of the patient with antihypertensive agents
  - Cost of drugs
  - Risk profile, presence or absence of target organ damage, clinical cardiovascular or renal disease or diabetes;
  - Patient's preference

International Society of Hypertension in Blacks (ISHIB) Recommendations[216]

Recommendations for African-American patients to initiate monotherapy for newly diagnosed patients with one of these medications:

- Diuretic
- Beta-blocker
- CCB
- ACE-inhibitor
- ARB

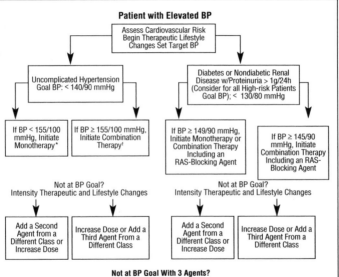

Patient with Elevated BP

Assess Cardiovascular Risk
Begin Therapeutic Lifestyle Changes Set Target BP

Uncomplicated Hypertension
Goal BP: < 140/90 mmHg

Diabetes or Nondiabetic Renal Disease w/Proteinuria > 1g/24h
(Consider for all High-risk Patients Goal BP); < 130/80 mmHg

If BP < 155/100 mmHg, Initiate Monotherapy*

If BP ≥ 155/100 mmHg, Initiate Combination Therapy†

If BP ≥ 149/90 mmHg, Initiate Monotherapy or Combination Therapy Including an RAS-Blocking Agent

If BP ≥ 145/90 mmHg, Initiate Combination Therapy Including an RAS-Blocking Agent

Not at BP Goal?
Intensity Therapeutic and Lifestyle Changes

Not at BP Goal?
Intensity Therapeutic and Lifestyle Changes

Add a Second Agent from a Different Class or Increase Dose

Increase Dose or Add a Third Agent From a Different Class

Add a Second Agent from a Different Class or Increase Dose

Increase Dose or Add a Third Agent From a Different Class

Not at BP Goal With 3 Agents?

- Consider factors that may decrease compliance or efficacy with current regimen
- Consider referral to BP specialist

Clinical alogrithm for achieving target blood pressure (BP) in African American patients with high BP. RAS indicates renin-angiotensin system. Asterik indicates to initiate monotherapy at the recommended starting dose with an agent from any of the following classes: diuretics, B-blockers, calcium channel blockers (CCBs), angiotensin-converting enzyme (ACE) inhibitors, or angiotensin II receptor blockers (ARBs). Dagger indicates to initiate low-dose combination therapy with any of the following combinations: B-blockers, ACE inhibitor/diuretic, ACE inhibitors/CCB, or ARB/diuretic.

Arch Intern Med. Vol. 163, 525-541, March 2003.

Secondary Hypertension

Cause	Signs and Symptoms	Confirmation
Oral contraceptives	Recent onset of hypertension Average 5% increase in BP after 7 years	Cessation of oral contraceptive should be followed by normalization of BP within 6 months
Licorice intoxication	Eating large amounts of licorice Pseudo - hyperaldosteronism	Cessation of licorice intake should cause normalization of BP within 1 month
Primary aldosteronism	Muscle cramps, weakness, polyuria, hypokalemia, metabolic alkalosis	Decreased PRA, increased urinary K^+; increased serum aldosterone, decreased serum K^+, positive saline suppression test, aldosterone /PRA Ratio>25
Pheochromocytoma	Sustained hypertension, intermittent hypertension, headaches, sweating, palpitation, pallor, tachycardia, orthostatic hypotension	24-hr urinary or serum catecholamines, VMA, CT scan, MIBG scan, MRI scan, clonidine suppression test, PET scan, metanephrines
Hyperparathyroidism	Bone pain, constipation, fatigue	Hypercalcemia, hypophosphatemia, increased parathyroid hormone

Secondary Hypertension (continued)

Cause	Signs and Symptoms	Confirmation
Thyroid disease	Hyperthyroidism, hypothyroidism	Free thyroxine index, free triiodothyronine index, thyroid-stimulating hormone
Acromegaly	Physical findings	Growth hormone level
Decongestants	Tachycardia, sudden increased BP	History of OTC medications
Stress/Anxiety Depression	Tachycardia, sweating	Clinical history, anxiolytics and anti-depressants
Obesity	Increase weight/BMI/WC/WHR	Weight loss
Burns	2nd and 3rd degree	Lasts 2 weeks
Sleep apnea	Obesity, snoring, apnea, daytime somnolence	Sleep study, arterial blood gases, PFTs
Cushing's syndrome	Moon face, central obesity, hirsutism, hypokalemia, diabetes, glucose intolerance	Increased urinary 17-hydroxycorticosteroids and 17-ketosteroids and urine and plasma cortisol, loss of diurnal variation of serum cortisol, dexamethasone suppression test
Coarctation of aorta	Headache, lower extremity claudication, leg BP 20 mm Hg lower than arm BP, reduced femoral pulse, abnormal chest x-ray	Arteriography of aorta Chest CT or MRI
Renal disease	Dysuria, nocturia, hematuria, RBC casts, recurrent UTI, edema	Creatinine, BUN, urinalysis, nuclear medicine GFR, ultrasound, renal biopsy

Secondary Hypertension (continued)

Cause	Signs and Symptoms	Confirmation
Renovascular hypertension	Recent-onset, accelerated hypertension, abdominal bruit, DBP ≥110 mm Hg resistant to treatment, atherosclerotic and fibromuscular dysplasia subtypes	Arteriography, renal vein renins, PRA, nuclear medicine GFR and renogram, captopril test (captopril renal scan), renal artery Doppler scan, MRA
Miscellaneous drugs or toxins*	Hypertension or attenuation of antihypertensive drug action	Discontinue medications; serum and urine studies

(NSAIDs, sympathomimetics, cocaine, alcohol, erythropoietin, cyclosporin, tacrolimus, anabolic steroids, cortisone, caffeine, ephedrine, MDMA, methylphenidate, nicotine, phencyclidine, phenylephrine, phenylpropanolamine, ergoatamine, bromocriptine, metoclopramide, TCA, lead, mercury, cadmium, arsenic, digitalis, disulfuram, lithium, herbals, thallium)

Cause	Signs and Symptoms	Confirmation
Neurologic disorders	Brian tumors, head injury, quadraplegia, GBS Baroreceptor dysfunction Autonomic insufficiency	Specific treatment of underlying cause Clonidine Nitroglycerin HS
Peri-operative CV surgery	Transient BP increase	Oberservation
SIADH	Increase volume and weight hypoanemia	Increased intravascular volume Hyponatremia, ↑ Una+, and Uosmols

Indirect Measurement of Blood Pressure [6,7,120]

Equipment
Sphygmomanometer (anaeroid or mercury manometer)

Methodology

1. The patient should be seated for 5 minutes in a quiet, comfortable environment, with the arm free of restrictive clothing or other materials and supported at heart level. The patient should avoid exertion, temperature extremes, eating, caffeine, or smoking for 1 hour before BP measurement.

2. The observer (clinician) should be at eye level of the meniscus of the mercury column or centered in front of the gauge; avoid strained posture.

3. The appropriate cuff size should be selected. The cuff bladder should be 20% wider than the diameter of the extremity. The bladder length should be approximately twice the recommended width.

4. The deflated cuff should be placed at least 2.5 cm above the antecubital space. The cuff should fit smoothly and snugly around the arm, with the bladder centered directly over the brachial artery.

5. Palpate for the brachial pulse. To estimate systolic blood pressure (SBP), rapidly inflate the cuff until the brachial pulse can no longer be felt.

6. Place the bell of the stethoscope over the previously palpated brachial artery. Rapidly inflate the cuff to 30 mm Hg above the point at which the brachial pulse disappears; deflate the cuff at the rate of 2 to 3 mm Hg/sec.

7. Record SBP as the first Korotkoff sound and DBP as the fifth Korotkoff sound.

8. Allow 1 to 2 minutes between BP determinations.

9. BP should then be determined in the upright posture after the patient has been standing for 2 minutes with pulse rate. The arm should be positioned at heart level, with the forearm at the horizontal level of the fourth inter-costal space.

10. On the initial visit, BP readings should be performed in both arms and in the thigh. Subsequent BP determinations should be performed in the arm with the higher reading if there is more than a 10 mm Hg discrepancy in BP reading.

Korotkoff Sounds[7]

Phase I: Marked by the first appearance of faint, clear tapping sounds which gradually increase in intensity. *Phase I should be used as the SBP.*

Phase II: Period during which a murmur or swishing sound is heard.

Phase III: Period during which sounds are crisper and increase in intensity.

Phase IV: Period marked by the distinct, abrupt muffling of sound (soft, blowing quality is heard).

Phase V: The point at which sounds disappear. *Phase V should be used as the DBP* (except on rare occasions, e.g., aortic insufficiency).

Common Mistakes in Blood Pressure Measurement [4,7]

1. Failure to keep the person in the supine position for 5 minutes before measuring the BP.

2. Failure to keep the arm at the level of the heart.

3. If Korotkoff sounds cannot be heard, failure to *completely deflate* the cuff before determining BP and failure to wait 1 to 2 minutes before doing further determinations.

4. Observer error, because of hearing impairment, bias (preferring some digits over others), or unconscious bias toward underreading or overreading BP depending on dividing line of normal.

5. Failure to keep the eyes at the level of the mercury manometer.

6. Deflating cuff too rapidly. The cuff should be deflated at a rate of 2 to 3 mm Hg/sec.

7. Failure to use appropriate cuff size. Use of a regular adult cuff for obese persons leads to a high BP reading. Use a large adult cuff or thigh cuff for obese persons; use a child's cuff for children. The cuff should cover two thirds of the arm above the antecubital space.

8. Failure to position the cuff correctly. The cuff should be placed 2 to 3 cm above the antecubital space.

9. Failure to provide a conducive environment: comfortable room temperature and quiet surroundings free of noises and distracting stimuli.

10. Missing the heartbeat during auscultation in patients with excessive bradycardia.

11. Patient has consumed alcohol, caffeine, smoked recently, or is under stress.

Hypertension-Atherosclerotic Syndrome

Hypertension is not just a disorder of increased intra-arterial pressure. Rather, it is part of a *syndrome* of commonly associated genetic or acquired (or both) metabolic functional and structural abnormalities, including dyslipidemia, insulin resistance (hyperinsulinemia, impaired glucose tolerance, hyperglycemia, diabetes mellitus), central or portal obesity, renal function abnormalities, abnormal vascular and cardiac smooth muscle proliferation, metabolism, hypertrophy, and hyperplasia, abnormal cellular cation transport or membranopathy, endocrine changes, coagulation abnormalities, inflammation and endothelial dysfunction. These abnormalities can lead to acceleration of arterial damage, atherosclerosis, and a greater incidence of atherosclerotic cardiovascular complications. This metabolic and structural syndrome of vascular disease exists in both treated and untreated hypertensives and in children of hypertensive parents.[147] Recognition of this concept should lead to a more rational and logical approach to the treatment of hypertension.[4,147]

Prevalence of Insulin Resistance

- 63% in type 2 diabetes
- 57% in patients with low HDL-C
- 54% in hypertriglyceridemia
- 41% in impaired glucose tolerance
- 37% in hyperuricemia
- 29% in hypertension
- 25% in hypercholesterolemia

Adapted from Bonora E, Kiechel S, Willeit J, et al: Prevalence of insulin resistance in metabolic disorders: The Bruneck Study. Diabetes. 1998;47:1643–1649.

Vascular Changes and CV Risk Factors in Borderline Hypertensives (BP 130/94 mm Hg)

	vs. Normotensives
Vascular resistance	+22%
Vessel structural changes	+11%
Total cholesterol	+8%
HDL cholesterol	−7%
Triglycerides	+42%
Insulin	+43%
Glucose	+4%
Insulin resistance	+29%

From Julius S, Jamerson K, Mejia A, et al. The association of borderline hypertension with target organ changes and higher coronary risk: Tecumseh Blood Pressure study. *JAMA. 1990;264:354-358.*

Normotensive Hypertension and Hypertension Syndromes: [147]

- Hypertension is associated with a constellation of metabolic, biochemical, functional, structural and clinical abnormalities in over 70% of cases.
- These abnormalities precede development of hypertension by years or decades and worsen with progression of hypertension levels.
- Normotensive adults and children with a positive family history of hypertension have a cardiovascular risk profile that is similar to hypertensive patients.
- Early detection, CV risk factor control, lifestyle modification, nonpharmacologic and pharmacologic therapy are mandatory to reduce CV events.

The following metabolic and structural abnormalities have been demonstrated in the "Normotensive Hypertensive" and in the Hypertension Syndrome. [147]

1. Endothelial Dysfunction (ED)
2. Abnormal Ventricular and Arterial Compliance (AC) – Both proximal C-1 and Distal C-2 Arterial compliance
3. Abnormal Glucose/Carbohydrate Metabolism
4. Insulin Resistance (>50%)
5. Endocrine and Neurohormonal Dysfunction (SNS, RAAS, PRA, Aldosterone, ET-1)
6. Renal Function Abnormalities (Na+, uric acid, CrCl, MAU, NAG, B2M)
7. Thrombotic/Coagulation Abnormalities (PAI-1, platelets, fibrinogen, VWF, TxA2)
8. LVH LV Mass Index and diastolic Dysfunction (>50%)
9. Dyslipidemia (80%)
10. Central/Portal Obesity
11. Hyperuricemia (UA)
12. Accelerated Atherogenesis
13. Vascular Inflammation

14. Vascular smooth Muscle Hypertrophy/Dystrophic changes and Abnormality in Remodeling (VSMH)
15. Increased Pulse Wave Velocity (PWV)
16. Increased Adhesion molecules (VCAM, ICAM, E-selectin) and LT
17. Increased Growth Factors (BFGF)
18. Increased ET-1
19. Increased Oxidative Stress (ROS)
20. Abnormal SBP and DBP response to exercise

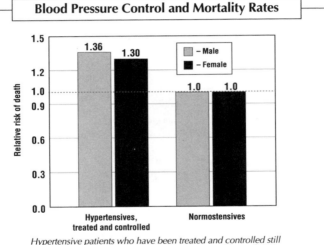

Blood Pressure Control and Mortality Rates

Hypertensive patients who have been treated and controlled still have a higher mortality rate than normotensive subjects of 30%.

Havik RJ et al. Hypertension. 1989; 13 (suppl 1): 1-22—1-32.

Nonpharmacologic Treatment of Hypertension [4,8]

Nonpharmacologic therapy should be an *initial* and *adjunctive* therapy to drug therapy and should be continued during drug therapy to enhance efficacy, reduce dose and number of drugs and limit adverse effects, as well as to promote cardiovascular health. An initial trial of 3 to 6 months should be instituted in patients who have mild elevations in BP without end-organ damage, diabetes mellitus, renal insufficency CHF, CHD, or other compelling indications. In a compliant patient, these measures can be an effective means of BP reduction. (*See JNC-7 Guidelines*).

1. *Weight reduction* (to ideal body weight [IBW]): About 60% of hypertensive patients are 20% over ideal body weight. Weight loss increases cardiac output (CO) and decreases left ventricular filling pressure (LVFP), intravascular volume, reduces insulin, catecholamine levels, systemic vascular resistance (SVR), Na+ retention, sympathetic nervous system activity and renin; and aldosterone improves insulin resistance, reduces cytokines (TNF-alpha) and other inflammatory markers.

2. *Discontinuation of smoking:* Vasoconstriction, sympathetic nervous system activity, norepinephrine (NE), carbon monoxide levels, platelet aggregation and inflammatory markers are reduced.

3. *Discontinuation or limitation of caffeine:* Vasoconstriction, PRA, and NE levels are reduced, and central aortic compliance is improved.

4. *Discontinuation or limitation of alcohol:* More than one or two drinks/day, 8 oz of wine, or 24 oz of beer elevates BP, PRA, aldosterone, and cortisol.

5. *Aerobic exercise and physical training:* 30 to 60 minutes per day to 60% to 80% maximal aerobic capacity for age: heart rate (HR) = (220 − age). Isometric exercises may elevate BP, but progressive resistance training 3 x per week is advised under supervision.

6. *Other behavioral modifications:* Stress management, biofeedback, relaxation, psychotherapy, hypnosis, transcendental meditation.
7. *Discontinuation of concomitant medications that increase BP:*
   a. Oral contraceptives
   b. NSAIDs: Interfere with diuretics, beta-blockers, angiotensin-converting enzyme (ACE) inhibitors, and ARBs
   c. Antihistamines/decongestants and phenylpropanolamine, ephedrine, phenylephrine, pseudoephedrine
   d. Corticosteroids and mineralocorticoids, anabolic steroids
   e. Sympathomimetics and amphetamine-like drugs.
   f. Carbenoxolone or licorice
   g. Tricyclic antidepressants
   h. Monoamine oxidase (MAO) inhibitors
   i. Ergot alkaloids
   j. Diet pills and "energy" pills
   k. Toxins: lead, cadmium, thallium, mercury, arsenic
   l. Erythropoietin
   m. Cyclosporin and tacrolimus
   n. Caffeine
   o. Alcohol
   p. Nicotine
   q. Bromocriptine
   r. Metoclopramide
   s. Digitalis
   t. Disulfuram
   u. Lithium
   v. Herbals
8. *Assurance, patient education, frequent follow-up, and improved patient compliance.*
9. *Nutritional aspects.* [151]

Nutrition, Dietary Supplements and Nutraceuticals in the Prevention and Treatment of Hypertension: [151]*

Introduction:

New and future treatment guidelines for lower target blood pressure (BP) levels in the general hypertensive population as well as in specific populations of hypertensive patients will demand a combination of nonpharmacologic (lifestyle modification) and pharmacologic therapy.[7, 27] Hypertensive patients with diabetes mellitus (DM), renal insufficiency (RI), proteinuria, congestive heart failure (CHF), coronary heart disease (CHD) and those with previous myocardial infarction (MI), cerebrovascular accidents (CVA), or transient ischemic attacks (TIA) often require three to four antihypertensive medications to reach a BP of 140/90 mm Hg or less.[7, 27] Lower recommended target BP goals of 130/80 mm Hg or perhaps 110/70 mm Hg cannot be attained without aggressive use of balanced drug and non-drug treatments. Nutrition, dietary supplements, nutraceuticals, achieving ideal body weight, exercise (aerobic and resistance training), restriction of caffeine and alcohol, and cessation of all tobacco products are crucial ingredients of this combination approach if BP and subsequent target organ damage (TOD) are to be reduced.

Hypertension, Nutrition and Vascular Biology:

Hypertension (HTN) is a consequence of the interaction of our environment and genetics. Macronutrients and micronutrients are crucial in the regulation of BP, subsequent TOD and atherosclerosis (AS). Nutrient-gene interactions, oxidative stress and subsequent gene expression have either positive or negative influences on vascular biology (VB) in humans. Endothelial dysfunction (ED) and vascular smooth muscle (VSM) dysfunction are the initiating and perpetuating factors in essential HTN. The correct combination of macronutrients and micronutrients will significantly influence prevention and treatment of HTN and subsequent vascular complications. Treatment directed at the blood vessel, as well as the BP, should include identification and optimal management of cardiovascular (CV) risk factors and oxidative stress in order to reduce AS and TOD. TOD reduction is dependent on both hypertensive and non-hypertensive mechanisms.

References for this section on nutrition are found on pages 38-40.

Nutritional needs have been imposed on the population during our evolution from a pre-agricultural, hunter-gatherer milieu to a highly technological agricultural industry that is dependent on mechanical processing for our food supply.[18, 48] The paleolithic diet consisted of low sodium, high potassium, high fiber, low fat, lean animal protein, low refined carbohydrate and low cholesterol, an intake composed of fruits, vegetables, berries, nuts, fish, fowl, wild game and other nutrient-dense foods. On the other hand, the modern diet of processed, chemically-altered, fast, fried and frozen food has resulted in an epidemic of nutritionally-related diseases such as HTN, hyperlipidemia, DM, the metabolic syndrome, and obesity.

Nutrition Trials and Hypertension:
Reduction in BP as well as reductions in CV morbidity and mortality have been demonstrated in numerous short-and long-term clinical HTN nutritional trials.[4, 5, 12, 44, 45, 47] Up to 50% of hypertensive patients in the appropriate stage and risk category may be initially treated with lifestyle modifications based on global hypertensive guidelines.[27, 213, 214, 215] However, specific patients with existing CV, cerebrovascular, renal, or other TOD, DM, metabolic syndrome or multiple CV risk factors usually require immediate drug therapy in conjunction with lifestyle modifications.[27] Combined nutrients present in food, especially fruits and vegetables, as well as single and combined nutraceutical and nutrient or dietary supplementation have been demonstrated to reduce BP (Table I).[43]

The combined low sodium Dash II diet[45] reduced blood pressure 11.5/6.8 mm Hg within two weeks, maintained this BP for the duration of the two-month study, and improved quality of life. This level of BP reduction is equivalent to that achieved with pharmacologic monotherapy.

Sodium:

A reduction in sodium intake to 2400 mg per day lowers BP an average of 4-6 mm Hg systolic and 2-3 mm Hg diastolic BP in salt-sensitive hypertensive patients.[3] Reduced sodium intake also reduces renal dysfunction, proteinuria, CHF, CVA, vascular hypertrophy, and left ventricular hypertrophy (LVH). Further reductions of BP can be achieved with progressive restriction from 150 mmol to 100 mmol to 50 mmol of dietary sodium per day in the DASH II diet.[45]

Potassium:

The magnitude of BP reduction with dietary supplementation of 60 to 120 mEq per day of potassium is 4.4 mm Hg systolic and 2.5 mm Hg diastolic BP in hypertensive patients.[3, 49] In addition, potassium may reduce CV events and CVA independent of BP and reduce the risk of cardiac arrhythmias. The recommended dietary intake is a K^+/Na^+ ratio of 5:1.

Magnesium:

Magnesium supplementation in the range of 500 to 1000 mg per day reduces systolic BP 2.7 mm Hg and diastolic BP 3.4 mm Hg.[51] Magnesium lowers systemic vascular resistance (SVR) and reduces arrhythmias. The mechanism is blockade of calcium influx into VSM cells and increased levels of the vasodilating prostaglandin E_1 (PGE_1).

Calcium:

A recent meta-analysis of the effect of calcium supplementation in hypertensive patients demonstrated a reduction in systolic BP of 4.3 mm Hg and diastolic BP of 1.5 mm Hg.[9] Calcium is particularly effective in patients with a high sodium intake and when given in a natural form with potassium and magnesium.[36, 41, 50] Blacks, elderly, diabetic, salt-sensitive, pregnant and postmenopausal women, and low-renin hypertensives have the best response.

Protein:

High intake of non-animal protein (1 g/kg/day) (Intersalt Study, Intermap Study) is associated with a lower BP.[3,19] Hydrolyzed whey protein[29] and sardine muscle extract[28] significantly lower BP in humans through an angiotensin-converting enzyme inhibitor (ACEI) mechanism.

Fats:

Consumption of omega-3 fatty acids (polyunsaturated fatty acids - PUFA) such as EPA (eicosapentaenoic acid) and DHA (docosahexanoic acid) significantly reduce mean BP in humans by 5.8 to 8.1 mm Hg.[8, 32, 37, 42] Combined with omega-9 fatty acids (olive oil) (monounsaturated, oleic acid), low saturated fat, elimination of trans-fatty acids and increased GLA (gamma linolenic acid); these dietary changes may have dramatic effects on BP, VB and AS. The omega-3 to omega-6 fatty acid ratio should be 1:1 to 4:1 with consumption of cold water fish (cod, tuna, mackerel, salmon), or EPA/DHA supplements (3-4 grams per day). The olive oil dose is 40 grams of extra-virgin olive oil per day (4 tablespoons).[20]

Garlic:

The prospective placebo-controlled studies utilizing the correct form (wild garlic is best) and dose of garlic demonstrate only minimal decreases in systolic BP of 5-8 mm Hg or mean BP of 2-3 mm Hg. However, garlic may have numerous other beneficial vascular effects as it is a natural ACEI and calcium channel blocker (CCB).[11]

Seaweed:

Wakame seaweed in doses of 3.3 grams per day significantly lowered BP in hypertensive humans within four weeks due to ACEI activity.[38] The average reduction in BP was 14/5 mm Hg. Long-term use in Japan appears to be safe.

Fiber:

Clinical trials with various types of fiber to reduce BP have been inconsistent.[3, 25] The average BP reduction in prospective studies using 60 grams per day of oatmeal fiber, (3 grams of betaglucan per day, glucomannan, or 7 grams of psyllium per day) is 7.5 mm Hg/5.5 mm Hg.

Vitamin C:

Vitamin C at doses of 250 to 500 mg BID lowers BP, especially in hypertensive patients with initially low plasma ascorbate levels.[16, 21, 39] Vitamin C improves ED, increases nitric oxide levels, is a potent antioxidant, decreases SVR and BP falls an average of 7/4 mm Hg. The greater the initial BP and the lower the plasma ascorbate level, the greater the response. Combinations with other antioxidants and vitamins may have synergistic antihypertensive effects.

Vitamin B-6:

Supplemental vitamin B-6 at 5 mg/kg/day reduced BP 14/10 mm Hg over four weeks.[6] Vitamin B-6 reduces central sympathetic nervous system activity, acts as a central alpha agonist (i.e. Clonidine), a CCB and a diuretic. Pyridoxine also improves insulin sensitivity and carbohydrate metabolism, which improves BP. Daily doses should probably not exceed 200 mg to avoid neuropathy.

Lycopene:

Paran et al[40] evaluated 30 subjects with grade I hypertension given tomato lycopene extract for eight weeks. The BP fell 9/7 mm Hg within eight weeks. Lycopene is found in high concentrations in tomatoes, tomato products, guava, watermelon, papaya, and apricots.

Co-Enzyme Q-10 (Ubiquinone):

Enzymatic assays show a deficiency of Co-Enzyme Q-10 (Co-Q-10) in 39% of essential hypertensive patients versus only a 6% deficiency in controls.[34] Human studies demonstrate significant and consistent reductions in BP averaging 15/10 mm Hg in all reported prospective clinical trials.[13, 14, 15, 31, 33] Doses of 100 to 225 mg per day (1-2 mg/kg/day) to achieve a therapeutic plasma level of over 2-3 micrograms/ml are effective within four to eight weeks in reducing BP. The BP remains steady at this level and returns to baseline at two weeks following discontinuation of Co-Q-10. Co-Q-10 reduces SVR, catecholamine and aldosterone levels, improves insulin sensitivity, and endothelial function and increases nitric oxide levels.[13,14,33] No adverse effects have been noted at these doses with chronic use. Patients have been able to stop or reduce the number of antihypertensive drugs by one to three with chronic ingestion of Co-Enzyme Q-10. A reputable, certified absorbable form, with excellent bioavailability and measurement plasma levels is an important clinical consideration.

L-Arginine:

L-arginine is the natural predominant precursor for vascular nitric oxide. Administration of 10 grams orally per day in food and/or as a supplement significantly reduces BP in human subjects by 6.2/6.8 mm Hg, improves ED and blood flow.[30, 46]

Taurine:

Taurine, a sulfonic beta-amino acid, is significantly reduced in the urine of essential hypertensive patients.[2] Administration of six grams of taurine per day lowers BP 9/4 mm Hg.[22] Taurine induces a sodium-water diuresis, vasodilation, increases atrial natriuretic factor (ANF) and reduces sympathetic nervous system activity and aldosterone levels, improves insulin sensitivity, and reduces homocysteine levels.

Celery:

Celery has antihypertensive properties due to 3-N-butyl phthalide, apigenin, and other substances that act like ACEI or CCB blockers. Four large celery sticks per day or the equivalent in celery juice, oil,or celery seed extract reduces BP in animals and humans.[10, 17, 26, 34, 35]

Combinations:

Combinations of various nutraceutical or dietary supplements, vitamins, and antioxidants may further enhance BP reduction, reduce oxidative stress, and improve vascular function and structure.[24] Optimal doses and combinations are yet to be determined, but future research will provide important data.

Finally, the addition of lifestyle modification with low dose combination antihypertensive drugs provides additive or synergistic BP reduction to achieve these lower BP goals, improves risk factors, metabolic parameters, vascular structure and function and allows for lower doses and number of drugs with reduced side effects to reduce TOD.

Natural Antihypertensive Compounds Categorized by Antihypertensive Class:

As has been discussed previously, many of the natural compounds such as food, nutraceutical and dietary supplements, vitamins, antioxidants or minerals function in a similar fashion to a specific class of antihypertensive drugs. Although the potency of these natural compounds may be less than or equal to the antihypertensive drug and the onset of action slower when used in combination, the antihypertensive effect is magnified. In addition, many of these natural compounds have varied, additive, or synergistic mechanisms of action in lowering BP.

Lifestyle Changes and SBP Meta-analysis of Clinical Diet Trials

Table 1.

Intervention	Reduction in SBP (mmHg)
↑ Mg^{++}	0-1
↑ Ca^{++}	2
↑ K^+	4
↓ ETOH	4
Fish Oil	6
↓ Na^+	6
↓ Weight	8
Exercise	10
DASH diet	12

Nutritional Intervention, Prevention and Treatment of Hypertension Trials and Consensus Reports

1. Health Professionals Follow-up Study: CVA reduction (K^+ intake)
2. Health Professionals Follow-up Study: CHD / MI reduction
3. Multiple Risk Factor Intervention Trial (MRFIT): CHD reduction
4. Lyon diet Heart Study: CHD / MI reduction
5. Trials of Hypertension Prevention (TOHP-I & II): BP prevention
6. Trial of Non-pharmacologic intervention in Elderly (TONE): BP reduction
7. Treatment of Mild Hypertension Study (TOMHS): BP reduction
8. Dietary Approaches to Stop Hypertension (DASH-I): BP reduction
9. Dietary Approaches to Stop Hypertension (DASH-II-Na+): BP reduction
10. Neonatal sodium restriction study: BP prevention x 15 years
11. Mediterranean Diet: BP reduction
12. Inter map: BP reduction (non-animal protein)
13. JNC-7: BP reduction
14. AHA nutritional committee (BP reduction)
15. Cardiovascular Risk Reduction Dietary Intervention Trial (CRRDIT)
16. Intersalt: BP reduction
17. Nurses Health Study (NHS)
18. US Male Health Study (USMHS)
19. National Diet Heart Study (NDHS)
20. Vanguard Study
21. Premier Trial

Natural Antihypertension Compounds Categorized by Antihypertensive Class

Table 2.

Intervention		
Diuretics		
1.Hawthorne Berry	6.Vitamin C (Ascorbic Acid)	10.Protein
2.Vitamin B-6 (Pyridoxine)	7.K+	11.Fiber
3.Taurine	8.Mg++	12.Co-Enzyme Q-10
4.Celery	9.Ca++	13.L-Carnitine
5.GLA		
Beta-Blockers (BB)		
1. Hawthorne Berry		
Central Alpha Agonists (CAA)		
1. Taurine	5.Protein	9. Co-Enzyme Q-10
2. K+	6.Fiber	10. Celery
3. Zinc	7.Vitamin C	11. GLA/DGLA
4. Na+ Restriction	8.Vitamin B-6	12. Garlic
Direct Vasodilators		
1. Omega-3 FA	7. Fiber	12. Co-Enzyme Q-10
2. MUFA (Omega-9 FA)	8. Garlic	13. L-Arginine
3. K+	9. Flavonoids	14. Taurine
4. Mg++	10. Vitamin C	15. Celery
5. Ca++	11. Vitamin E	16. ALA (Alpha lipoic acid)
6. Soy		
Calcium Channel Blockers (CCB)		
1. Alpha Lipoic Acid (ALA)	7. Hawthorne Berry	
2. Vitamin C (Ascorbic Acid)	8. Celery	
3. Vitamin B-6 (Pyridoxine)	9. Omega-3 Fatty Acids (EPA and DHA)	
4. Magnesium (Mg++)	10. Calcium	
5. N-Acetyl Cysteine (NAC)	11. Garlic	
6. Vitamin E		
Angiotensin Converting Enzyme Inhibitors (ACEI)		
1. Garlic	11.Gelatin	
2. Seaweed - various (Wakame, etc.)	12.Sake	
3. Tuna protein/muscle	13.Essential Fatty Acids (Omega-3 FA)	
4. Sardine protein/muscle	14.Chicken Egg Yolks	
5. Hawthorne Berry	15.Zein	
6. Bonito Fish (dried)	16.Dried Salted Fish	
7. Pycnogenol	17.Fish Sauce	
8. Casein	18.Zinc	
9. Hydrolyzed Whey Protein	19.Hydrolyzed Wheat Germ Isolate	
10. Sour Milk		
Angiotensin Receptor Blockers (ARBs)		
1. Potassium (K+)	5. Vitamin B-6 (Pyridoxine)	
2. Fiber	6. Co-Enzyme Q-10	
3. Garlic	7. Celery	
4. Vitamin C	8. Gamma Linolenic Acid (GLA) and DGLA	

Nutrition and Dietary Supplements References

1. Ackermann RT, Mulrow CD, Ramirez G, et al: Garlic shows promise for improving some cardiovascular risk factors. Arch Intern Med 161:813-824, 2001.

2. Ando K, Fujita T: Etiological and physiopathological significance of taurine in hypertension. Nippon Rinsho 50:374-381, 1992.

3. Appel LJ: The role of diet in the prevention and treatment of hypertension. Curr Atheroscler Rep 2:521-528, 2000.

4. Appel LJ, Moore TJ, Obarzanek E, et al. A clinical trial of the effects of dietary patterns on blood pressure. N Engl J Med 336:1117-1124, 1997.

5. Ascherio A, Rimm EB, Hernan MA, et al: Intake of potassium, magnesium, calcium and fiber and risk of stroke among US men. Circulation 98:1198-1204, 1998.

6. Aybak M, Sermet A, Ayyildiz MO, Karakilcik AZ: Effect of oral pyridoxine hydrochloride supplementation on arterial blood pressure in patients with essential hypertension. Arzneimittelforschung 45:1271 -1273, 1995.

7. Bakris GL: A practical approach to achieving recommended blood pressure goals in diabetic patients. Arch Intern Med 161:2661 -2667, 2001.

8. Bao DQ, Mori TA, Burke V, et al: Effects of dietary fish and weight reduction on ambulatory blood pressure in overweight hypertensives. Hypertension 32:710-717, 1998.

9. Bucher HC, Cook RJ, Guyatt GH, et al: Effects of dietary calcium supplementation on blood pressure. A meta-analysis of randomized controlled trials. JAMA 275:1016-1022, 1996.

10. Castleman M: *The Healing Herbs: The Ultimate Guide to the Curative Power of Nature's Medicines.* Emmaus, Pennsylvania:Rodale Press 1991: 105-107.

11. Clouatre D: *European Wild Garlic: The Better Garlic.* San Francisco:Pax Publishing; 1995.

12. De Lorgeril M, Salen P, Martin JL, et al: Mediterranean diet, traditional risk factors and the rate of cardiovascular complications after myocardial infarction: final report of the lyon diet heart study. Circulation 99:779-785, 1999.

13. Digiesi V, Cantini F, Bisi G, et al: Mechanism of action of coenzyme Q10 in essential hypertension. Curr Ther Res 51:668-672,1992.

14. Digiesi V, Cantini F, Brodbeck B : Effect of coenzyme Q10 on essential hypertension. Curr Ther Res 47:841-845, 1990.

15. Digiesi V, Cantini F, Oradei A, et al: Coenzyme Q-10 in essential hypertension. Mol Aspects Med 15:8257-8263, 1994.

16. Duffy SJ, Gokce N, Holbrook M, et al: Treatment of hypertension with ascorbic acid. Lancet 354:2048-2049, 1999.

17. Duke JA: *The Green Pharmacy Herbal Handbook.* Emmaus, Pennsylvania: Rodale Press; 2000: 68-69.

18. Eaton SB, Eaton SB III, Konner MJ: Paleolithic nutrition revisited: a twelve-year retrospective on its nature and implications. Eur J Clin Nutr 51:207-216, 1997.

19. Elliott P, Dennis B, Dyer AR, et al: Relation of dietary protein (total, vegetable, animal) to blood pressure: INTERMAP epidemiologic study. Presented at the 18th Scientific Meeting of the International Society of Hypertension, Chicago, IL, August 20-24, 2000.

20. Ferrara LA, Raimondi S, d'Episcopa I, et al: Olive oil and reduced need for antihypertensive medications. Arch Intern Med 160:837-842, 2000.

21. Fotherby MD, Williams JC, Forster LA, et al: Effect of vitamin C on ambulatory blood pressure and plasma lipids in older persons. J Hypertens 18:411-415, 2000.

22. Fujita T, Ando K, Noda H, et al: Effects of increased adrenomedullary activity and taurine in young patients with borderline hypertension. Circulation 75:525-532, 1987.

23. Gaby AR. The role of co-enzyme Q-10 in clinical medicine: Part II. Cardiovascular disease, hypertension, diabetes mellitus and infertility. Alt Med Rev 1(3): 168-175, 1996.

24. Galley HF, Thornton J, Howdle PD, et al: Combination oral antioxidant supplementation reduces blood pressure. Clin Sci 92:361-365, 1997.

25. He J, Welton PK: Effect of dietary fiber and protein intake on blood pressure. A review of epidemiologic evidence. Clin Exp Hypertens 21:785-796, 1999.

26. Heinerman J. *Heinerman's New Encyclopedia of Fruits and Vegetables.* Paramus, New Jersey:Prentice Hall 1995: 93-95.

27. Joint National Committee on Prevention, Detection, Evaluation, and Treatment of High Blood Pressure: The sixth report of the Joint National Committee on the prevention, detection, evaluation, and treatment of high blood pressure. Arch Intern Med 157:2413-2446, 1997.

28. Kawasaki T, Seki E, Osajima K, et al: Antihypertensive effect of valyl-tyrosine, a short chain peptide derived from sardine muscle hydrolyzate, on mild hypertensive subjects. J Hum Hypertens 14:519-523, 2000.

29. Kawase M, Hashimoto H, Hosoda M, et al: Effect of administration of fermented milk containing whey protein concentrate to rats and healthy men on serum lipids and blood pressure. J Dairy Sci 83:255-263, 2000.

30. Kelly JJ, Williamson P, Martin A, Whitworth JA: Effects of oral L-arginine on plasma nitrate and blood pressure in cortisol-treated humans. J Hypertens 19:263-268, 2001.

31. KendlerBS: Nutritional strategies in cardiovascular disease control: an update on vitamins and conditionally essential nutrients. Prog Cardiovasc Nurs 14:124-129, 1999.

32. Knapp HR, Fitzgerald GA: The antihypertensive effects of fish oil: a controlled study of polyunsaturated fatty acid supplements in essential hypertension. N Engl J Med 320:1037-1043,1989.

33. Langsjoen P, Willis R, Folkers K: Treatment of essential hypertension with coenzyme Q10. Mol Aspects Med 15:8265-8272, 1994.

34. Le OT, Elliott WJ: Dose response relationship of blood pressure and serum cholesterol to 3-N-butyl phthalide, a component of celery oil. Clinical Research 39:750A, 1991. Abstract.

35. Le OT, Elliott WJ: Mechanisms of the hypotensive effect of 3-N-butyl phthalide (BUPH): a component of celery oil. J Am Hypertens 40:326A, 1992. Abstract.

36. McCarronDA: Calcium metabolism in hypertension. Keio J Med 44:105-114, 1995.

37. Morris M, Sacks F, Rosner B: Does fish oil lower blood pressure? A metaanalysis of controlled trials. Circulation 88:523-533, 1993.

38. Nakano T, Hidaka H, Uchida J, et al: Hypotensive effects of wakame. J Jpn Soc Clin Nutr 20:92, 1998.

39. Ness AR, Chee D, Elliot P: Vitamin C and blood pressure - an overview. J Hum Hypertens 11:343-350, 1997.

40. Paran E, Engelhard Y: Effect of tomato's lycopene on blood pressure, serum lipoproteins, plasma homocysteine and oxidative stress markers in grade I hypertensive patients. Am J Hypertens 14:141A, 2001. Abstract P-333.

41. Preuss HG: Diet, genetics and hypertension. J Am Coll Nutr 16:296-305, 1997.

42. Frisco D, Paniccia R, Bandinelli B, et al: Effect of medium-term supplementation with a moderate dose of n-3 polyunsaturated fatty acids on blood pressure in mild hypertensive patients. Thromb Res 91:105-112, 1998.

43. Reaven P, Parthasarathy S, Grasse BJ, et al: Effects of oleate-rich and linoleate-rich diets on the susceptibility of low density lipoprotein to oxidative modification in mildly hypercholesterolemic subjects. J Clin Invest 91:668-676, 1993.

44. Resnick LM, Oparil S, Chait A, et al: Factors affecting blood pressure responses to diet: the Vanguard Study. Am J Hypertens 13:956-965, 2000.

45. Sacks FM, Svetkey LP, Vollmer WM, et al: Effects on blood pressure of reduced dietary sodium and the dietary approaches to stop hypertension (DASH) diet. N Engl J Med 344:3-10,2001.

46. Siani A, Pagano E, Iacone R, et al: Blood pressure and metabolic changes during dietary L-arginine supplementation in humans. Am J Hypertens 13:547-551, 2000.

47. The Treatment of Mild Hypertension Research Group: The Treatment of Mild Hypertension Study: a randomized, placebo-controlled trial of a nutritional hygienic regimen along with various drug monotherapies. Arch Intern Med 151:1413-1423, 1991.

48. Weder AB: Your mother was right: eat your fruits and vegetables. Curr Hypertens Rep 1:11-12,1999.

49. Whelton PK, He J. Potassium in preventing and treating high blood pressure. Semin Nephrol 19:494-499, 1999.

50. Whiting SJ, Wood R, Kim K: Calcium supplementation. J Am Acad Nurse Pract 9:187-192, 1997.

51. Witteman JCM, Grobbee DE, Derk FHM, et al. Reduction of blood pressure with oral magnesium supplementation in women with mild to moderate hypertension. J Clin Nutr 60:129-135, 1994.

The DASH Diets
(DASH-I and DASH-II-Sodium) [4, 45]

Dietary Approaches to Stop Hypertension

The DASH-I diet published in 1997[4] was a landmark nutritional trial in reducing blood pressure in hypertensive patients. The DASH-II sodium diet published in 2001[45] confirmed the value of DASH-I, but proved that moderate to severe sodium restriction further enhanced BP reduction. These nutritional studies are so important in the nonpharmacologic management of hypertension that they will be presented in detail.

The DASH-I diet was a two-month, multicenter, randomized, controlled prospective clinical trial of 379 subjects with borderline or stage I hypertension (SBP < 160 mm Hg and DBP 80-95 mm Hg), no concomitant diseases and on no antihypertensive drugs. The average age was 45 years, two-thirds were minorities (60% black, 6% other races and 34% white). The design of the study and prescribed nutrition for the three treatment groups, which included control subjects, the fruit and vegetable (F + V) group and the combined diet (C) group, are shown. After a three-week control diet in all subjects, randomization was to one of the three treatment groups above for eight weeks. The sodium content remained the same in all three groups at three grams per day. All diets were prepared and were well tolerated with a 93% adherence rate. There was no change in alcohol intake, weight, or sodium excretion during the study. Subjects met weekly with the investigators.

The results of this clinical trial demonstrate significant reductions in BP with a controlled diet including the described modifications of increasing whole grains, nuts, poultry, fish, fruits, vegetables, K+, Mg++, and Ca++, while reducing intake of saturated and trans fatty acids, red meat, sweets, sugars and other refined carbohydrates. The hypertensive subjects on the combined diet had the greatest BP reduction of 11.4/5.5 mm Hg. Minority subjects, especially blacks, had greater reductions in BP compared to white subjects, and hypertensive subjects had greater BP reductions than normotensive subjects. Urinary Mg++ and K+ increased in the "F + V" and "C" groups, while urinary Ca++ decreased in the "F + V" group. The urinary Na+ remained constant in all three groups.

The reduction in BP occurred immediately, reaching near maximum levels at two weeks, but was sustained throughout the eight-week study. In addition, the quality of life improved in subjects on the "F + V" and "C" diets. The combined treatment group had reductions in BP that were equal to that obtained with pharmacologic treatment of mild hypertension. DASH-I emphasizes the importance of combined nutrients as they occur in natural food.

The DASH-II diet took the DASH-I diet one step further, proving that moderate to severe Na+ restriction reduced BP even more in all three study groups. This was a multicenter, randomized, controlled prospective study of 412 subjects on either a control diet or one of three DASH-Na+ diets for 30 days (150 mmol, 100 mmol or 50 mmol Na+ intake). The SBP and DBP reductions were significant with each incremental decrease in Na+ intake. The important conclusions and results of this study are shown. Hypertensive subjects, blacks, and women had the greatest BP reductions.

A comparison of the relative BP reduction in DASH-I and DASH-II in hypertensive subjects is shown. The net BP reduction versus the control patient reduction was greatest in the DASH-II combination, low Na+ (50 mmol) diet (-11.5/6.8 mm Hg). The message from these two studies is clear. Hypertensive patients can achieve significant BP reductions that are equivalent to drug therapy used in mild hypertensive patients by combining a more severe Na+ restriction of 50 mmol/day with the combination DASH-I diet. These benefits are immediate, sustainable, inexpensive, increase nutrient levels, and improve the individual's quality of life.

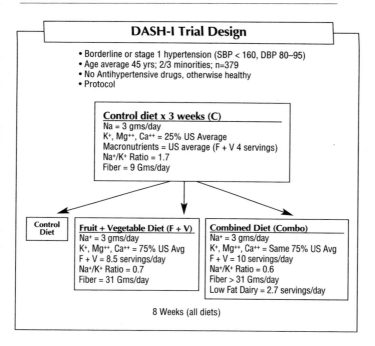

DASH-I Trial Design

- Borderline or stage 1 hypertension (SBP < 160, DBP 80–95)
- Age average 45 yrs; 2/3 minorities; n=379
- No Antihypertensive drugs, otherwise healthy
- Protocol

Control diet x 3 weeks (C)
Na = 3 gms/day
K^+, Mg^{++}, Ca^{++} = 25% US Average
Macronutrients = US average (F + V 4 servings)
Na^+/K^+ Ratio = 1.7
Fiber = 9 Gms/day

Control Diet

Fruit + Vegetable Diet (F + V)
Na^+ = 3 gms/day
K^+, Mg^{++}, Ca^{++} = 75% US Avg
F + V = 8.5 servings/day
Na^+/K^+ Ratio = 0.7
Fiber = 31 Gms/day

Combined Diet (Combo)
Na^+ = 3 gms/day
K^+, Mg^{++}, Ca^{++} = Same 75% US Avg
F + V = 10 servings/day
Na^+/K^+ Ratio = 0.6
Fiber > 31 Gms/day
Low Fat Dairy = 2.7 servings/day

8 Weeks (all diets)

Summary of BP Reductions in DASH-I and DASH-II Na⁺ Diets Hypertensive Patients and Overall

	SBP	DBP
DASH-I Overall Combination Diet vs. Control Diet	-5mmHG	-3mmHg
DASH-I Hypertensive Pts. Combo Diet vs. Control Diet	-10.7 mmHg	-5.2mmHg
DASH-II Overall Comb. Low Na⁺ DASH Diet vs. Control high Na⁺ Diet	-8.9 mmHg*	-4.5mmHg
DASH-II Hypertensive Pts. Comb Low Na⁺ DASH Diet vs. Control high Na⁺ Diet	-11.5 mmHg*	-6.8mmHg*

* = $p < 0.001$

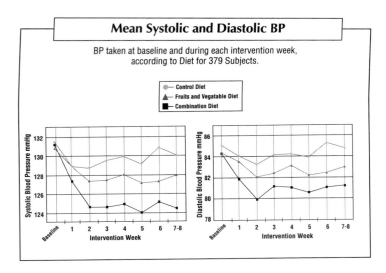

Mean Systolic and Diastolic BP

BP taken at baseline and during each intervention week,
according to Diet for 379 Subjects.

- Control Diet
- Fruits and Vegatable Diet
- Combination Diet

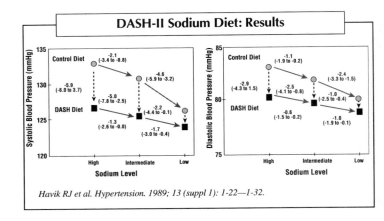

DASH-II Sodium Diet: Results

Havik RJ et al. Hypertension. 1989; 13 (suppl 1): 1-22—1-32.

DASH-II Sodium Conclusions

- Reduction of sodium intake to 50 mmol/day from current recommendations of 100 mmol/day significantly reduces BP.
- DASH combination diet with low sodium intake of 50 mmol/day lowers BP more in combination than either singly.
- Level of dietary sodium had twice BP reducing effect with the control diet than with DASH diet ($p < 0.001$).
- BP reductions occurred in all patients regardless of age, gender, ethnicity, or BP level (normals).
- Hypertensive patients, blacks and women had the greatest BP reductions.
- Low $Na+$ intake attenuated the hypotensive effects of $K+$ and $CA+$.

PREMIER Trial: [211]

A lifestyle study for patients with above-optimal BP who were not taking medication

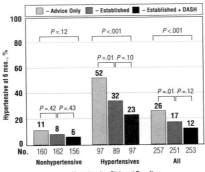

Figure 3. Percentage of Participants with Hypertension at 6 months by Randomized Group Among Nonhypertensive, Hypertensive, and All Participants at Baseline

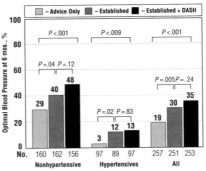

Figure 4. Percentage of Participants with Optimal Blood Pressure at 6 Months by Randomized Group Among Nonhypertensive Participants at Baseline, Hypertensive at Baseline, and All Participants at Baseline

DASH indicates Dietary Approaches to Stop Hypertension

JAMA, April 23/30, 2003—Vol 289, No. 16

Conclusion: Individuals with above-optimal BP, including stage 1 hypertension, can make multiple lifestyle changes that lower BP.

Key point: Patients with suboptimal BP who receive behavioral interventions plus DASH diet have only a 12% chance of developing HTN at 6 mos. and 35% chance of having optimal BP at 6 mos. (3-to-1 odds of beneficial outcome).

Recommendations

Nutrition	Daily Intake
1. DASH I and DASH Il-Na+ diets	
2. Sodium restriction	50-100 mmol
3. Potassium	60-100 mEq
4. Potassium/sodium ratio > 5:1	
5. Magnesium	500-1000 mg
6. Calcium	1000-1500 mg
7. Zinc	25 mg
8. Protein: total intake (30% total calories)	1.0 - 1.5 grams/kg
A. Non-animal sources preferred but lean or wild animal protein in moderation is acceptable	
B. Hydrolyzed whey protein	30 grams
C. Soy protein (fermented is best)	30 grams
D. Hydrolyzed wheat germ isolate	2-4 grams
E. Sardine muscle concentrate extract	3 mg
F. Cold water fish, poultry	3 servings per week
9. Fats: 30% total calories	
A. Omega-3 fatty acids (30%) PUFA (DHA, EPA, cold water fish)	3-4 grams
B. Omega-6 fatty acids (10%) PUFA (flax, GLA, canola oil, nuts)	.75 to 1 gram

    C. Omega-6 fatty acids (30%)
       MUFA (olive oil - extra virgin)   4 tablespoons

    D. Saturated FA
       (lean, wild animal meat) (30%)

    E. P/S ratio
       (polyunsaturated/saturated) fats > 2.0

    F. Omega-3/Omega-6 PUFA, ratio 2:1-4:1

    G. No trans-fatty acids (hydrogenated margarines,
       vegetable oils)

    H. Nuts: almonds, walnuts, hazelnuts, etc.

10. Carbohydrates (40% total calories)

    A. Reduce or eliminate refined sugars and simple
       carbohydrates

    B. Increase complex carbohydrates and whole grain fiber
       (oat, barley, wheat), vegetables, beans, legumes

oatmeal	60 grams
oatbran (dry)	40 grams
beta-glucan	3 grams
psyllium	7 grams

11. Garlic	4 cloves/4 grams
12. Mushrooms (shiitake and maitake)	3 servings per week
13. Guava fruit	500-1000mg
14. Wakame seaweed (dried)	3.0 - 3.5 grams

15. Celery

Celery sticks	4 sticks
Celery juice	8 teaspoons TID
Celery seed extract	1000 mg BID
Celery oil (tincture)	1/2 -1 teaspoon TID

16. Lycopene	10 mg

    Tomatoes and tomato products, guava,
    watermelon, apricots, papaya

Exercise   7 days/week

   • Aerobically at 60-80% MHR
     60 minutes daily
     4200 KJ/week

   • Resistance training   3 days per week

Weight Loss
- To LBW (Lean Body Weight)
- Lose 1-2 pounds/week
- BMI < 25
- Waist circumference
  < 35 inches in female
  < 40 inches in male
- Total body fat
  < 16% in males
  < 22% in females
- Increase lean muscle mass
- Reduce weight hip ratio to below 0.9

Alcohol Restriction < 20 grams/day
Wine < 10 ounces
Beer < 24 ounces
Liquor < 2 ounces (100 proof whiskey)

Caffeine Restriction < 100 mg/day

Tobacco and Smoking   STOP
Avoid drugs and interactions that increase BP

Vitamins, Antioxidants, and Nutraceutical Supplements
	Daily Intake
1. Vitamin C	250 to 500 mg BID
2. Vitamin E (mixed tocopherols/tocotrienols)	400 to 800 IU QD
3. Vitamin B-6	100 mg QD to BID
4. Co-enzyme Q-10	60 mg QD to BID
5. Lipoic acid (with biotin)	100 to 200 mg BID
6. N-acetyl cysteine	1000 mg BID
7. L-arginine (supplement) plus lentils, hazelnuts, walnuts, peanuts	5 grams BID
8. Hawthorne standardized extract	160-900 mg QD
9. L-carnitine	1000 mg BID
10. Taurine	2-3 grams BID

Obesity

1. It is unsafe to lose over 3.3 lbs-week and the preferred weight loss is 1 to 2 lbs-week.
2. Body fat is more important than body weight.
   Males should be < 15% body fat
   Females should be < 22% body fat
3. The number of calories needed per day to keep you at the same weight is your weight in pounds times 10.
   i.e., 160 lbs. = 1600 calories
   1600 calories is your BMR (basal metabolic rate)
4. It takes a 3500 calorie deficit to lose *one pound*.
5. If body mass index (BMI) is over 27, there is a danger of developing *significant health problems*.

   $$BMI = \frac{Weight\ (pounds)}{Height\ in\ inches)^2} \times 703 = kg/m^2$$

6. Four major factors contribute to obesity:
   - Genetics
   - Metabolic factors
   - Diet
   - Physical inactivity
7. Waist circumference over the values below is associated with a high risk of disease, and may be the single best predictor of obesity related CVD and overall morbidity and mortality:
   Men over 40 inches
   Women over 35 inches
8. Neck circumference also correlates with high disease risk.
   Men over 15.6 inches
   Women over 14.4 inches
9. Obesity will increase the risk of morbidity and mortality of the following diseases:
   - Hypertension (high blood pressure)
   - Dyslipidemia and insulin resistance
   - Type II diabetes
   - Coronary heart disease and MI
   - Stroke
   - Gallbladder disease
   - Osteoarthritis
   - Sleep apnea

- Respiratory problems
- Cancer of breast, prostate, colon, and endometrium
- Chronic kidney disease
- Microalbuminuria and proteinuria
10. Ideal body weight calculation: (Depends on body frame)
- Women: 100 lbs. first 5 feet, then 5 lbs. for each additional inch of height
- Men: 106 lbs. first 5 feet, then 6 lbs. for each additional inch of height
- 10% for large frame and delete 10% for small frame

Exercise Activities and Kilocalories Used

Energy Values in Kilocalories per Hour of Selected Activities

	Weight (pounds)					
	95	125	155	185	215	245
Slow walking	86	114	140	168	196	222
Walking, moderate pace	172	228	280	336	392	555
Hiking	285	342	420	504	588	666
Jogging	430	570	700	840	980	1,110
Running	480	770	945	1,134	1,323	1,499
Heavy housework	194	256	315	378	441	500
Sweeping	108	142	175	210	245	278
Scrubbing	237	313	385	462	539	611
Tennis	301	399	490	588	686	777
Golf (carrying clubs)	237	313	385	462	539	611
Golf (in a cart)	151	200	245	294	343	389
Swimming (light laps)	344	456	560	672	784	888
Swimming (hard laps)	430	570	700	840	980	1,110

Exercise: The Prescription

- Aerobic exercise should be combined with resistance training
- Duration: 60 minutes per session/daily
  - Warmup/Condition/Cooldown
  - 300 calories expenditure
- Intensity: Percent of MHR (maximum heart rate)
  for age: MHR = MAC (maximum aerobic capacity)
  Mild:50–60% x (220 – age)
  Moderate:70% x (220 – age)
  Heavy: 80% x (220 – age)
- Methods: walk, run, bicycle, swim, water-jog, treadmill,
  Nordic Ski Track, Health Rider
- Graduated supervised exercise regimen over 6–8 weeks
  of cardiovascular training
- CHD risk reduction plateaus at a level of 4200 KJ week
  (see below):

Relative Risk for Coronary Heart Disease According to Levels of Physical Activity*

| | Energy expended in exercise each week (in KJ) | | | | |
	< 2100	2100-4199	4200-8399	8400-12,599	≥12,600
No. of Men	2002	2354	3481	2145	2534
Relative CHD Risk	1	0.9	0.81	0.8	0.81

1983 through 1997

Relative risk adjusted for age, body mass index, alcohol intake, hypertension, diabetes mellitus, smoking status, and early (<65y) parental death.

Approaches to Selection of Antihypertensive Therapy

1. Stepped-care approach: Limited usefulness.[4,5,9]
2. Demographic approach (race, sex, age).
3. Renin profile analysis: Laragh method (see pg.54) useful for "V" and "R" patients.[11, 12, 218]
4. Subsets of hypertension: Individualized therapy: recommended approach.[4,5,9]
   a. Pathophysiology: Membranopathy, ion transport defects, structural factors, smooth muscle hypertrophy (vascular, cardiac, cerebral, renal), functional factors, vasoconstrictive forces, endothelial dysfunction.
   b. Hemodynamics: SVR, CO, arterial compliance, organ perfusion, BP. Select the appropriate therapy to reverse the circulatory dysregulation..
   c. End-organ damage: Reduce risk factors for *all* end-organ damage.
   d. Concomitant medical diseases and problems: Select antihypertensive medications with favorable or neutral effects.
   e. Demographics: Race, age, gender.
   f. Adverse effects of drugs and quality of life.
   g. Compliance with medication regimen.
   h. Total health care costs: Direct and indirect costs.

Renin Profiling: The Laragh Method[218]

Table 1. Hypertensive patients fall into two basic types

V Hypertension (Volume)	R Hypertension (Renin)
PRA < 0.65 ng/mL/hr	PRA > 0.65 ng/mL/hr
Direct Renin Level < 5μU/mL	Direct Renin Level > 5μU/mL
	Have progressively more renin-angiotensin mediated vasoconstrictor hypertension
Have predominately sodium→volume mediated hypertension	

Table 2. Antihypertensive drugs also fall into two basic types

V Drugs	R Drugs
Reduce sodium→volume factor: spironolactone, diuretics, α-blockers or CCBs	Block plasma renin-angiotensin system: CEIs, ARBs, or β-blockers

Laragh Method

- Individual hypertensive patients differ in underlying pathophysiology and in response to drugs.
- Individual hypertensive patients have V or R forms of hypertension.
- Drugs act against either V or R forms of hypertension; therefore different patients respond to different drugs.
- Targeted monotherapy is the ultimate realizable goal for treating most individual patients.

Hemodynamics in Hypertension

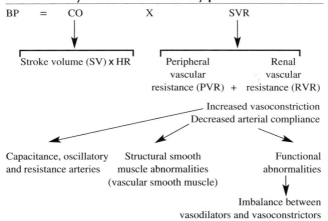

Hemodynamic Progression of Hypertension

1. *Early hypertension:* Increased CO with relative increased SVR (inappropriately increased).
2. *Established hypertension:* Decreased CO and increased SVR.
3. *Late hypertension:* Decreased CO (25%) and markedly increased SVR (25% to 30%).

All patients with essential hypertension have elevated SVR as the primary hemodynamic abnormality. Even in the uncommon case in which the CO may be transiently increased, the SVR is inappropriately elevated. Antihypertensive therapy should reverse the hemodynamic abnormalities.

Hemodynamics: Logical and Preferred Method to Reduce Blood Pressure

1. Reduce SVR.
2. Preserve CO.
3. Improve arterial compliance.
4. Maintain organ perfusion.

Achieve all the above by:

Avoiding compensatory neurohumoral reflexes, such as reflex tachycardia, salt and water overload, and reflex vasoconstrictors (NE, angiotensin II, antidiuretic hormone).

24-hour BP control.

BP control under all circumstances: rest, exercise, stress, mental function, diurnal variation.

Vascular/Arterial Compliance

1. Three vessel wall components contribute to vascular compliance
   a. Elastin: very elastic
   b. Smooth muscle: immediate elasticity
   c. Collagen: very stiff
2. Vascular compliance is composed of three arterial functions
   a. Capacitive: large conduit arteries, store blood in systole
   b. Oscillatory: small branch arteries, contribute to pressure oscillations and to reflected waves.
   c. Resistance: arterioles control blood flow and resistance function.
3. Endothelial dysfunction is first manifested in the elastin components of thin-walled arterioles (oscillatory and resistance). This raises resistance in these thin-walled arterioles prior to any effect on conduit arteries.
4. C_2-oscillatory and resistance arteriolar compliance is reduced markedly in elderly hypertensives and diabetics.

Early hypertensives, normotensive hypertensives and normotensive children of hypertensive parents have reduced C_2. A low C_2-AC predicts an increased risk of future CV events.

5. C_1-capacitance compliance is reduced more in isolated systolic hypertension (ISH) than in essential hypertension.

Hemodynamic Effects of Antihypertensive Drugs [4,5,9,13-30]

1. Reduce SVR, preserve CO, and improve arterial compliance and perfusion.*
   a. Calcium channel blockers (CCB)
   b. ACE inhibitors (ACEI)
   c. Angiotensin II (Ang-II) receptor blockers (ARB)

2. Reduce SVR, preserve CO and perfusion; effects on arterial compliance unknown.*
   a. Central alpha-agonists
   b. Alpha-blockers

3. Reduce SVR, preserve CO and perfusion, but worsen arterial compliance.
   a. Direct vasodilators
   b. Beta-blockers with intrinsic sympathomimetic activity (ISA)
   c. Beta-blockers and alpha-blockers

4. Reduce SVR, CO, and perfusion, and worsen arterial compliance.
   a. Diuretics
   b. Neuronal-inhibiting drugs

5. Increase SVR and reduce CO, perfusion, and arterial compliance.
   a. Beta-blockers without ISA

*The best hemodynamic profile is achieved by calcium channel blockers, ACE inhibitors, Ang-II receptor antagonists. The central alpha-agonists, and alpha-blockers are the next best. Diuretics and beta-blockers have the worst hemodynamic profile.

Hemodynamic Effects of Antihypertensive Drugs

	Diuretics	Beta-Blockers	Calcium Channel Blockers	ACE Inhibitors	Ang-II Receptor Blockers	Central Alpha-Agonists	Alpha-Blockers	Direct Vasodilators	Alpha-Blockers and Beta-Blockers	Beta-Blockers with ISA	Neuronal Inhibitors
SVR	↓/→	←	→/↑	→	→	→	→/←	→	↓/→	↓/→	→
CO	→	→	↑/→	←	←	↑	↑/←	←	↓/→	↓/↑	→
SV	→	→	↑/→	←	←	↑	↑/←	←	↓/→	↓/↑	→
HR	→	→	↑/↓	↑	↑	↓	↑/←	→	↑/←	→/↑	→
RBF	←	←	←	←	←	←	←	→	↓/→	↑	→
RVR	←	→	→	→	→	→	→	←	↓/→	↓/↑	→
GFR	←	→	→	→	→	→	←	→	↓/→	↑	→
Cerebral blood flow	→	←	←	←	←	↑/←	↑/←	←	↑	↑	↑/↓
CABF	→	↑/←	←	→	→	↑/←	↑/↓	→	↑	↑	←
Intravascular volume	→	→	→	←	→	↑/↓	?	←	↑/←	→/↓	→/↑
Arterial compliance	→	→	→	→	→	←	→	←	→	←	↓/↑
Perfusion	↓/→	↓/→	→	→	→	→	→	→	→	←	↓/↑
LVH	↓/→	↑	→/↑	↑	↑	↑	↑	↑	↑/→	→/↓	→
VSM hypertrophy	←		↓/→								
Exercise	→/↓		↑/↑								

↓ Reduced; ↑ increased; → no change; ? unknown.

CABF = coronary artery blood flow, VSM = vascular smooth muscle

58

Hypertension-Related End-Organ Damage [3,31,32]

1. Cerebrovascular
   a. Cerebral infarctions: thrombotic or lacunar infarct
   b. Intracranial hemorrhage: hemorrhagic CVA
   c. Hypertensive encephalopathy
   d. Dementia and cognitive dysfunction (vascular dementia and Alzheimer's disease)
2. Cardiac
   a. CHD
      (1) Angina pectoris
      (2) MI
   b. CHF
      (1) Systolic CHF
      (2) Diastolic CHF (diastolic failure and dysfunction)
   c. LVH
   d. Sudden death
3. Renal
   a. Microalbuminuria and proteinuria
   b. Chronic renal insufficiency
   c. Chronic renal failure (ESRD)
4. Large artery disease
   a. Carotid artery stenosis and obstruction
   b. Lower extremity arterial disease or peripheral vascular disease and claudication
   c. Aortic aneurysm and dissection
5. Progression of hypertension; accelerated and malignant hypertension
6. Retinopathy

Life Expectancy and Blood Pressure (Man, 35 years old) [9,32]

1. | BP (mm Hg) | Life expectancy (years) |
   |---|---|
   | 120/80 | 76 |
   | 130/90 | 67½ |
   | 140/95 | 62½ |
   | 150/100 | 55 |

2. There is a positive correlation between BP level and total mortality.

3. The lower the SBP or DBP in either sex, the lower the mortality; the greater the BP, the higher the mortality.

4. For every 10-mm Hg rise in mean arterial pressure (MAP), there is a 40% rise in cardiovascular risk.

5. The higher the pulse pressure, the greater the morbidity and mortality.

6. SBP is a better predictor of cardiovascular and cerebrovascular morbidity and mortality than DBP in most patients, especially after age 50.

7. Framingham and MRFIT studies indicate reductions in CV morbidity and mortality with BP reductions to perhaps as low as 110/70 mm Hg. Recent meta-analysis supports BP levels of 115/75 mm Hg[197] to optimize target organ damage (TOD) reduction.

Systolic, Diastolic and Pulse Pressure Concepts[152]

- SBP > DBP to predict CVD — qualified
- PP predicts CVD with absolute superiority in some populations
- DBP in elderly if excessively low is associated with ↑CVD

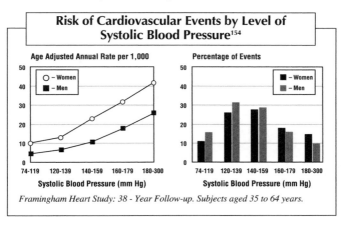

Risk of Cardiovascular Events by Level of Systolic Blood Pressure[154]

Framingham Heart Study: 38 - Year Follow-up. Subjects aged 35 to 64 years.

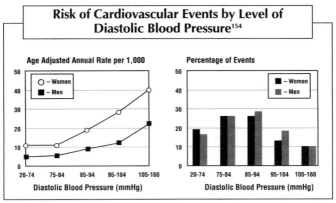

Risk of Cardiovascular Events by Level of Diastolic Blood Pressure[154]

Risk of cardiovascular events by level of diastolic blood pressure - 38 year follow-up. The Framingham Heart Study subjects aged 35 to 64 years.

Arterial Pressure Components by Age[153]

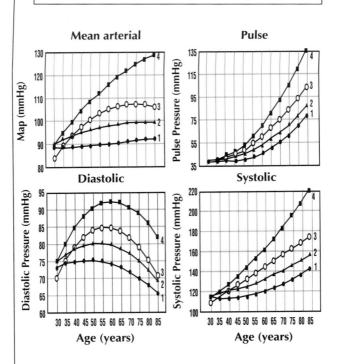

Group averaged individual regression analysis. Curves plotted based on blood pressure-predicted values at 5-year age intervals (age 30-85 years) from least-squares regression equations, developed from individual intercept, slope and quadratic term (curvature), coefficients averaged from individual least-squares mean regressions of each arterial pressure component by age, MAP, mean arterial pressure. Baseline mean systolic blood pressure (SBP) groupings: Group 1, SBP<120 mm Hg; Group 2, SBP 120-139 mm Hg; Group 3 140-159 mm Hg; Group 4, SBP 160+ mm Hg.

Increase in Risk of Cardiovascular Events per SD Increase in Blood Pressure Parameter[154]

30-Year Follow-Up

| | Standardized Increment in Risk | | | |
Types of Hypertension	Men 35-64 yrs.	Women 65-94 yrs.	Men 35-64 yrs.	Women 65-94 yrs.
Systolic	41%*	51%*	43%*	23%*
Mean Arterial	41%*	44%*	42%*	18%*
Pulse Pressure	29%*	42%*	36%*	22%*
Diastolic	35%*	30%*	33%*	9%†

* – p <0.001; † – p =NS.

Framingham Study: According to Age and Sex

Risk of Cardiovascular Events by Type of Hypertension[154]

38-Year Follow-Up

| | Age-Adjusted Risk Ratio* | | | |
| | 35-64 yrs. | | 65-94 yrs. | |
Types of Hypertension	Men	Women	Men	Women
Isolated Diastolic	1.8†	†1.2‖	1.2†	1.6§
Isolated Systolic	2.4§	1.9‡	1.9‡	1.4‡
Combined	2.74%§	2.2%§	2.2%§	1.6%§

* Reference group consists of normotensive persons.

† – p <0.05; ‡ – p <0.01; § – p <0.001; ‖ = NS.

Framingham Study: According to Age and Sex

Risk Associated with Increasing SBP at Fixed Levels of DBP

By Level of Systolic Blood Pressure (SBP) and Diastolic Blood Pressure (DBP)

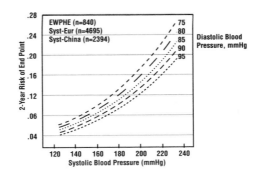

The 2-year probability of a cardiovascular endpoint was adjusted for active treatment, sex, age, previous cardiovascular complications, and smoking by Cox multiple regression with stratification for Trial (European Working Party on High Blood Pressure in the Elderly trial, Systolic Hypertension in Europe Trial, and Systolic Hypertension in China Trial).

Pulse Pressure & Cardiovascular Events

Table 3. Risk of Cardiovascular Events by Pulse Pressure: Framingham Study (30-Year Follow-Up)

| | Age-Adjusted Rate/1,000 | | | |
| | 35-64 yrs. | | 65-94 yrs. | |
Pulse Pressure (mm Hg)	Men	Women	Men	Women
2-39	9	4	2	17
40-49	13	6	16	19
50-59	16	7	32	22
60-69	22	10	39	25
70-182	33	16	58	32

* $p < 0.001$
Reg. = regression; RF = Risk Factor

Am J Cardiol 85:253, 2000

Isolated Systolic Hypertension (ISH)

Systolic Blood Pressure & Vascular Hemodynamics

	Normal Aorta (Young Adults)		Stiff Aorta (Older Adults)
1. Aortic BP	130	Systolic Diastolic	140
2. PWV (m/s)	5.0		10.0
3. Reflected	Early Diastole		Late Systole
4. Pulse Wave Shape			
5. Aortic BP	130 80	Systolic Diastolic	160

Annals Int. Med. 2000; 132 (3): 235.

Clinical Hypertension Trials and Antihypertensive Drug Therapy [32–43]

The pharmacologic treatment of Stage I and II (mild to moderate) hypertension (DBP <110 mm Hg) has reduced only some end-organ damage in the DIURETIC–BETA-BLOCKER trials.

1. BP reduction has reduced consequences of pressure-related arteriolar disease:
   a. Intracranial hemorrhage and cerebral infarction
   b. CHF, systolic CHF*
   c. Progression of hypertension: accelerated and malignant
   d. Retinopathy
   e. Aortic aneurysm and dissection
   f. Hypertensive encephalopathy

2. BP reduction has not achieved expected reduction in the diuretic and beta-blocker trials in:
   a. LVH
   b. Diastolic CHF
   c. Chronic renal insufficiency and failure

3. BP reduction has not reduced consequences of atherosclerotic-related diseases to the predicted extent in diuretic and beta-blocker trials except in ALLHAT which was diuretic (chlorthalidone) based rather than diuretic/BB based therapy (compared to a CCB or ACEI).[150]
   a. CHD
   b. Angina pectoris
   c. MI
   d. Sudden death
   e. Larger artery disease: carotid, lower extremities

Beta-blocker monotherapy does not reduce CHD or MI in the elderly. However, the recent STONE, SYST-EUR, SYST-CHINA, HOT, STOP-2, CHEN-DU, INSIGHT, NORDIL, NIC--EH, CONVINCE, VHAS, PREVENT, ALLHAT, VALUE AND GLANT prospective clinical trials have shown significant reductions in cardiovascular and cerebrovascular morbidity and mortality with the calcium channel blockers, especially with amlodipine in ALLHAT and VALUE. CAPPP, STOP-2, ALLHAT, PROGRESS, HOPE, and ANBP-2 have demonstrated significant reductions in CHD and MI as well as other CV and CVA morbidity and mortality with ACEI. LIFE showed reductions in CVA and CVD morbidity and mortality with an ARB compared to a beta-blocker, and VALUE and MOSES reduced CVD with an ARB. RENAAL, IRMA, IDNT and AASK showed renal protection with ARBs in hypertensive-diabetes.

ALLHAT showed questionable superiority of chlorthalidone to amlodipine and lisinopril in preventing new onset non-fatal CHF in a high risk elderly population. However, unmasking of asymptomatic CHF, study design, demographics, BP differences or other factors may have accounted for this difference (see details on ALLHAT study).

Treatment of Hypertension: Questions Posed*

1. What level of blood pressure requires initiation of treatment and does this level vary depending on demographics, risk factors and concomitant diseases?

2. What is the goal blood pressure to optimally reduce target organ damage and does it vary depending on demographics, risk factors and concomitant diseases?

3. Is there a difference among the various classes of antihypertensive drugs and cardiovascular, cerebrovascular and renal outcomes?

* These questions will be addressed in this section on clinical trials in hypertension and drug treatment.

Clinical Hypertension Trials: Important Clinical Points

1. The risks of CV morbidity and mortality increase with rising BP level.

2. Hypertension becomes more progressive and severe without intervention.
   a. Placebo study patients had more progression of hypertension (>15%)
   b. Drug treatment patients had little or no progression of hypertension (<1%).

3. Higher BP levels induce more vascular damage, arteriosclerosis and atherosclerosis that is synergistic to additional risk factors such as hyperlipidemia, diabetes mellitus or smoking.

4. Elderly hypertensives are those with more CV risk factors or CV or renal disease will show more benefit sooner on any drug treatment at equal BP reduction compared to younger patients and those without concomitant CV or renal disease.

5. Renal outcomes in most of the large prospective clinical hypertension trials have been largely ignored or not reported adequately.

6. The major recent meta-analysis trials (RCTs on hypertension) have been selective in analysis of data and excluded many trials. Conclusions therefore may not only be biased but invalid. [156, 157, 158, 159, 160]

7. All of the diuretic beta-blocker trials done prior to 1985 used high dose diuretic, hydrochlorothiazide (HCTZ) over 50 mg per day; later studies used low doses of 12.5 to 25 mg of HCTZ.

8. Prior to the SHEP study in 1989 the criteria for entry into clinical trials and definition of BP control was based on DBP not SBP. It is now clear that SBP is more important in predicting CV risk in most patients (especially those over 55 years).

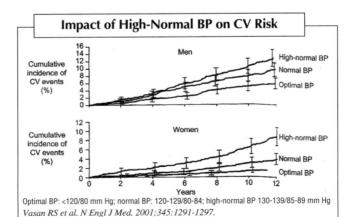

Impact of High-Normal BP on CV Risk

Optimal BP: <120/80 mm Hg; normal BP: 120-129/80-84; high-normal BP 130-139/85-89 mm Hg
Vasan RS et al. N Engl J Med. 2001;345:1291-1297.

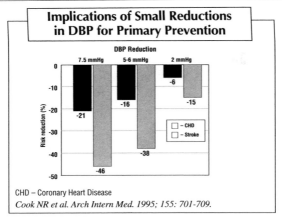

Implications of Small Reductions in DBP for Primary Prevention

CHD – Coronary Heart Disease

Cook NR et al. Arch Intern Med. 1995; 155: 701-709.

Age-specific relevance of usual blood pressure to vascular mortality: a meta-analysis of individual data for one million adults in 61 prospective studies:[197]

Within each decade of age at death, the proportional difference in the risk of vascular death associated with a given absolute difference in usual blood pressure is about the same down to at least 115 mm Hg usual systolic blood pressure (SBP) and 75 mm Hg usual diastolic blood pressure (DBP), below which there is little evidence. At ages 40-69 years, each difference of 20 mm Hg usual SBP (or, approximately equivalently, 10 mm Hg usual DBP) is associated with more than a twofold difference in the stroke death rate, and with twofold differences in the death rates from CHD and other vascular causes. All of these proportional differences in vascular mortality are about half as extreme at ages 80-89 years as at ages 40-49 years, but the annual absolute differences in risk are greater in old age. The age-specific associations are similar for men and women, and for cerebral hemorrhage and cerebral ischemia. For predicting vascular mortality from a single blood pressure measurement, the average of SBP and DBP is slightly more informative than either alone, and pulse pressure is much less informative.

Throughout middle and old age, usual blood pressure is strongly and directly related to vascular (and overall) mortality, without any evidence of a threshold down to at least 115/75 mm Hg.

Completed Trials and Trials in Progress in Hypertension Treatment: [160]

Trial details						Patient Characteristics					Estimated Events	
							ENTRY BLOOD PRESSURE LEVELS					
ACRONYM	**TITLE**	**PATIENTS, n**	**PLANNED FOLLOW-UP, Y**	**RANDOMIZED TREATMENTS (FACTORIAL ASSIGNMENTS)**	**COMPLETION DATE**	**ENTRY CRITERIA**	**AGE, Y**	**DBP**	**SBP**		**CHD**	**Stroke**
AASK	African-American Study of Kidney Disease and Hypertension	1200	5	ACE, Beta, DCA (more, less)	2001	HBP+RD	18-70	=95	any		144	72
ABCD	Appropriate Blood Pressure Control in Diabetes Trial	950	5	ACE, DCA	1998	DM	=40 =70	any	No ISH		119	59
ACTION	A Coronary Disease Trial Investigating Outcome with Nifedipine GITS	6000	5	DCA,plac	2003	CAD	>34	none	none		918	333
ADVANCE	Action in Diabetes and Vascular Disease	11,140	4.5	Perindopril + Indapamide vs. Placebo	2006	DM	>30	none	none		—	—
ALLHAT	Antihypertensive Therapy and Lipid-Lowering Heart Attack Prevention Trial	40,000	6	ACE, alph, DCA, diur (chol, open)	2002	HBP+ CVD risk	>55	>89 <110	>139 <180		2580	2790
ANBP2	Australian National Blood Pressure Study 2	6000	5	ACE, diur	2002	HBP	65-84	>89	>159		300	150
ASCOT	Anglo-Scandinavian Cardiac Outcomes Trial	18,000	5	DCA±ACE, Beta±diur (chol, plac)	2003	HBP+ CVD risk	>39-79	>89	>139		1150	400

Trial details

ACRONYM	TITLE	PATIENTS, n	PLANNED FOLLOW-UP, Y	RANDOMIZED TREATMENTS (FACTORIAL ASSIGNMENTS)	COMPLETION DATE	ENTRY CRITERIA	AGE, Y	ENTRY BLOOD PRESSURE LEVELS DBP	ENTRY BLOOD PRESSURE LEVELS SBP	Estimated Events CHD	Estimated Events Stroke
BENEDICT	Bergamo Nephrology Diabetes Complication Trial	2400	3	ACE, NCA, plac	2001	Dm	>39	>80	>139	200	100
CAPPP	Captopril Prevention Project	10,800	5	ACE, Beta/diur	1998	HBP	23-66	>99	any	324	162
CHEN-DU	Nifedipine Trial										
CLEVER	Chinese Lacidipine Event Reduction Trial	10,000	3	DCA, plac	2002	HBP+ CVD risk	50-79	95-115	160-210	200	400
CSG	Collaborative Study Group of Irbesartan										
CONVINCE	Controlled onset Verapamil Investigation for Cardiovascular Endpoints	15,000	5	NCA, Beta/diur	2001	HBP+ CVD risk	>54	>89 <110	>139 <190	1250	750
DIAB-HYCAR	Diabetes hypertension Cardiovascular Morbidity-Mortality and Ramipril	4000	3	ACE, plac	1999	DM+prot	>50	any	any	300	150
ELSA	European Lacidipine Study of Atherosclerosis	2251	4	DCA,Beta	2000	HBP	45-75	>94 <116	<149 <211	89	44
EUROPA*	European Trial on Reduction of Cardiac Events with Perindopril	10,500	3	Ace, plac	2004	CAD	>18	any	any	964	350
FACET	Fosinopril and Amlodipine Cardiac Events Trial	380	3.5	CCB,ACE	1998	NIDDM+HBP	—	>90	>140	—	—

Completed Trials and Trials in Progress in Hypertension Treatment: [160]

ACRONYM	TITLE	PATIENTS, n	PLANNED FOLLOW-UP, Y	RANDOMIZED TREATMENTS (FACTORIAL ASSIGNMENTS)	COMPLETION DATE	ENTRY CRITERIA	AGE, Y	DBP	SBP	CHD	Stroke
GLANT	Study Group on 1 Long-term Antihypertensive Therapy	1936		ACE,CCB		HBP	60+	90-114	>160	2	5
HDS	Hypertension in Diabetes Study	1148	8.2	ACE, Beta, open (ins, sul, diet)	1998	HBP+DM	25-75	>84	>149	244	122
HOPE	Heart Outcomes Prevention Evaluation Study	9541	4.7	ACE, plac(vit E,plac)	2000	CVD risk	54	any	any	1200	550
HOT	Hypertension Optimal Treatment Trial	19196	3.5	More, Less(asp, plac)	1997	HBP	50-80	>99 <116	any	552	276
HYVET	Hypertension in the VeryElderly Trial	2100	5	ACE,diur, plac	2001	HBP	>89	>89 <110	>159 <220	683	341
IDNT	Irbesartan Diabetes Nephropathy Trial	1650	3	AIIA, DCA, plac	2000	DM+prot	30-70	>84	>134	124	62
INSIGHT	Int'l Nifedipine GITS Study Intervention as a Goal for Hypertension Therapy	6592	3	DCA, diur	1999	HBP+ CVD risk	55-80	>94	>149	246	123
INVEST	International Verapamil/ Trandolapril Study	27000	2	NCA, Beta	2001	HBP+ CAD	>49	none	none	581	268
LIFE	Losartan Intervention for Endpoint Reduction in Hypertension	9194	4	AIIA, Beta	2001	HBP+LVH	55-80	95-115	160-200	693	347
MIDAS	Multicenter Isradipine Diuretic Atherosclerosis Study	883		dCA, diur	1996	HBP	50-64	>96 <101	>149 <165	—	—
MOSES	Morbidity and Mortality After Stroke: Eprosartan vs. Nitrendipine in Secondary Prevention	1400	2.5	CCB, ARB	2004	Stroke during last 24 mos.	any	any	any	—	—

ACRONYM	TITLE	PATIENTS, *n*	PLANNED FOLLOW-UP, Y	RANDOMIZED TREATMENTS (FACTORIAL ASSIGNMENTS)	COMPLETION DATE	ENTRY CRITERIA	Patient Characteristics AGE, Y	ENTRY BLOOD PRESSURE LEVELS DBP	SBP	Estimated Events CHD	Stroke
NICS – EH	National Intervention Cooperative Study in Elderly Hypertensives	1000	5	DCA, diur	1997	HBP	>59	<115	>159 <220	30	1
NORDIL	Nordic Diltiazem Study	11,000	5	NCA, Beta/diur	2002	HBP	50-69	>99	any	360	180
OPERA	Omapatrilat in Persons with Enhanced Risk of Atherosclerotic Events	12,600		Omapatrilat vs. Placebo							
PART2	Prevention of Atherosclerosis with Ramipril	617	4	ACE, plac	1998	Athero	18-75	any	any	40	14
PATE	Practitioners Trial on the efficacy of Antihypertensive Treatment in the Elderly hypertension	1748	3	ACE,CCB	2000	HBP	>60	>84	>150	45	37
PEACE	Prevention of Events with Angiotensin Converting Enzyme Inhibition	8000	5	ACE, plac		CAD	>50	any	any	1224	444
PHYLLIS	Plaque Hypertension Lipid Lowering Italian Study	450	3	ACE, plac (chol, plac)	2000	CIT	45-70	95-115	>150 <211	7	4
PRESERVE	Prospective Randomized Enalapril Study Evaluation Regression of Ventricular Enlargement	303	none	CCB,ACE	2001	> 50+ LV Mass	> 50	> 90	>150	—	—

Completed Trials and Trials in Progress in Hypertension Treatment: [160]

Trial details						Patient Characteristics					Estimated Events	
								ENTRY BLOOD PRESSURE LEVELS				
ACRONYM	TITLE	PATIENTS, n	PLANNED FOLLOW-UP, Y	RANDOMIZED TREATMENTS (FACTORIAL ASSIGNMENTS)	COMPLETION DATE	ENTRY CRITERIA	AGE, Y	DBP	SBP		CHD	Stroke
PREVENT	Prospective Randomised Evaluation of Vascular Effects of Norvasc	825	5	DCA, plac	1997	ang CHD	30-80	any	any		20	6
PROGRESS	Perindopril Protection Against Recurrent Stroke Study	6000	5	ACE, plac	2000	Stroke or TIA	any	any	any		600	300
PROTECT	Perindopril Regression of Vascular Thickening European Community Trial											
QUIET	Quinapril Ischemia Event Trial	1750	3	ACE, plac	1996	ang CHD	18-75	any	any		500	350
RENAAL	Randomized Evaluation of NIDDM with the AII Antagonist Losartan	1500	4	ANA, plac	2002	DM	31-70	<110	<200		100	50
SCAT	Simvastatin/Enalapril Coronary Atherosclerosis Trial	460	5	ACE, plac (chol, plac)	1998	CAD	any	any	any		42	15
SCOPE	Study of Cognition and Prognosis in Elderly Patients with Hypertension	4000	2.5	AIIA, plac	2003	HBP	70-89	90-99	160-179		60	30
SHELL	Systolic Hypertension in the Elderly Lacidipine Long-Term Study	4800	3.5	DCA, diur	1999	HBP	>59	<95	>160		101	50

Trial details

ACRONYM	TITLE	PATIENTS, n	PLANNED FOLLOW-UP, Y	RANDOMIZED TREATMENTS (FACTORIAL ASSIGNMENTS)	COMPLETION DATE	ENTRY CRITERIA	AGE, Y	ENTRY BLOOD PRESSURE LEVELS DBP	ENTRY BLOOD PRESSURE LEVELS SBP	Estimated Events CHD	Estimated Events Stroke
STONE	Shanghai Trial of Nifedipine in the Elderly	1632	2.5	CCB, plac	1995	HBP	60-79	any	any	—	—
STOP-2	Swedish Trial in Old Patients with Hypertension	6628	4	ACE, Beta/diur, dCA	1998	HBP	70-84	>104	>179	318	167
SYST-EUR	SYST-EUR Multicentre Trial	4695	1.6	dCA, plac	1997	ISH	>59	<95	160-119	500	250
SYST-CHINA	SYST-CHINA Systolic Hypertension in China	2400	2.8	CCB, pla		ISH	>60				
VALUE*	Diovan Antihypertensive Long-term Use Evaluation	14,400	6	AIIA, dCA	2004	HBP+ CVD risk	>49	<115	<210	1450	869
VHAS	Verapamil in Hypertension Atherosclerosis Study	1414	2	nCA, diur	1996	HBP	40-65	>94	>159	40	20

* Collaboration pending

ACE—angiotensin-converting enzyme inhibitor, AHA—angiotensin II antagonist; alph—alpha blocker, ang CHD—angiographic coronary heart disease; asp—aspirin; athero—atherosclerosis; beta—beta-blocker, CAD—coronary artery disease; CCB—calcium channel blocker CHD—coronary heart disease; chol—cholesterol lowering; CIT—carotid intimal thickness; CVD—cardiovascular disease; DBP—diastolic blood pressure; dCA—dihydropyridine calcium antagonist; diur—diuretic; DM—diabetes mellitus; HBP—high blood pressure; ins—insulin; ISH—isolated systolic hypertension; less—less intensive blood pressure lowering; LVH—left ventricular hypertrophy; more—more intensive blood pressure lowering; na—not available; nCA—non-dihydropyridine calcium antagonist; open—open control; plac—placebo; pla—placebo; prot—proteinuria; RD—renal disease; SBP—systolic blood pressure; sul—sulphonamide; TIA—transient ischemic attack; vit E—vitamin E.

Twenty-Three Controlled, Randomized Clinical Trials with Diuretics and Beta-Blockers in Mild to Moderate Hypertension and Coronary Heart Disease, 1979–1992

Trial (Date)	Blind	Initial No. of Patients	DBP (mm Hg)	Treatment	Mean Duration (years)	CHD Incidence
1 HDFP (1979)[33]	No	10,940	90–114	Referred care vs. stepped care	5	Decreased
2. VA Cooperative II (1970)[34]	Double	380	90–114	Placebo vs. diuretics + reserpine + hydralazine	3.8	No difference
3. Oslo (1980)[37]	No	785	90–109	None vs. diuretics + methyldopa + propranolol	10	Increased
4 Australian (1980)[38]	Double	3427	95–110	Placebo vs. diuretics + methyldopa + propranolol + pindolol	4.1	No difference
5. MRC (1984)[39]	Single	17,354	90–109	Placebo vs. bendrofluazide or propranolol	5	No difference
6. MRFIT (1982)[40]	Open	8012	90–114	Thiazide diuretics	7	No difference
7. EWPHE (1985)[41]	Double	840	90–120	Placebo vs. thiazide diuretics + triamterene + methyldopa	4.8	No difference
8. MPPCD (1985)[42]	No	1203	95–110	No drug vs. pindolol + propranolol, diuretics, hydralazine	5	Increased
9. USPHS (1977)[45]	Double	389	90–115	Placebo vs. diuretics reserpine	7–10	No difference
10. VA-NHLBI (1978)[46]	Double	1012	85–105	Placebo vs. chlorthalidone + reserpine	1–5	No difference
11. IPPPSH (1972)[47]	Double	6357	100–125	No treatment vs. oxprenolol	3–5	No difference

Trial (Date)	Blind	Initial No. of Patients	DBP (mm Hg)	Treatment	Mean Duration (years)	CHD Incidence
12. HEP (1986)[48]	No	884	105–120	No treatment vs. atenolol + thiazide diuretics	8	No difference
13. HAPPHY (1987)[49]	No	6500	100–130	Diuretics vs. atenolol or metoprolol	4	No difference
14. MAPHY (1988)[50]	No	3234	100–130	Metoprolol vs. thiazide diuretics	5	Less in metoprolol vs. thiazides
15. SHEP (1991)[51]	Double	4736	SBP>160 DBP<90	Placebo vs. thiazide diuretics + beta-blockers	5	Decrease in nonfatal MI only
16. STOP (1991)[52]	Double	1627	105–120	Moduretic, atenolol, metoprolol, or pindolol	5	No difference
17. VA COOP I (1967)[167]	Double	143	SBP>186 DBP>121	Placebo vs. diuretics, reseryne hydralazine	1.5	Reduced (Severe HBP study*)
18. CARTER (1970)[181]	Double	97	SBP>160 DBP>110	Diuretics vs. Placebo	4.0	CHD not reported Reduced CVA only
19. BARRACLOUGH (1973)[182]	Double	116	109	Diuretics vs. Placebo	2.0	Reduced (NS)
20. HYPERTENSION-STROKE COOP (1974)[183]	Double	452	SBP>167 DBP>100	Diuretics vs. Placebo	2.3	Reduced CVA, No CHD Data
21. Kuramoto (1981)[184]	Double	91	SBP>168 DBP>86	Diuretics vs. Placebo	4.0	Reduced
22. SHEP-P (1989)[185]	Double	551	SBP>172 DBP>75	Diuretics (low dose)	2.8	Reduced CVA, No CHD Data
23. MRC-II (1992)[186]	Double	4396	SBP>185 DBP>91	Diuretics (low dose) + BB OSP	5.8	Reduced in Diuretic group but *not* BB group

HDFP–Hypertension Detection and Follow-up Program; MRC–Medical Research Council Trial; MRFIT–Multifactorial Risk Factor Intervention Trial; EWPHE–European Working Party on Hypertension in the Elderly; MPPCD–Multifactorial Primary Prevention of Cardiovascular Diseases; USPHS–U.S. Public Health Service Trial; VA-NHLBI–Veterans Administration–National Heart, Lung, and Blood Institute; IPPPSH–International Prospective Primary Prevention Study in Hypertension; HEP–Hypertension in the Elderly; HAPPHY–Heart Attack Primary Prevention in Hypertension; MAPHY–Metoprolol Atherosclerosis Prevention in Hypertension Trial; SHEP–Systolic Hypertension In the Elderly Program; SHEP P–Pilot; STOP–Swedish Trial In Old Patients with Hypertension.

Meta-Analysis of 18 Randomized, Placebo-Controlled Diuretic-Beta-Blocker Clinical Trials in Hypertension[157, 202 203 204 206]

Total of over 47,000 Hypertensive Patients

Outcome Drug Regimen	Dose	No.of Trials	Events, Active Treatment/Control	RR(95% CI)	RR (95% CI)
Stroke					
Diuretics	High	9	88/232	0.49 (0.39-0.62)	
Diuretics	Low	4	191/347	0.66 (0.55-0.78)	
β-Blocker		4	147/335	0.71 (0.59-0.86)	
HDFP	High	1	102/158	0.64 (0.50-0.82)	
Coronary Heart Disease					
Diuretics	High	11	211/331	0.99 (0.83-1.18)	
Diuretics	Low	4	215/363	0.72 (0.61-0.85)	
β-Blocker		4	243/459	0.93 (0.80-1.09)	
HDFP	High	1	171/189	0.90 (0.73-1.10)	

Scale: 0.4 — 0.7 — 1.0 (Treatment Better / Treatment Worse)

Diuretic High = High Dose > 50mg HCTZ
Diuretic Low = Low Dose < 50mg HCTZ (12.5-25 mg HCTZ)

Note:

1. Beta-blocker and diuretics both significantly reduced *stroke* but diuretics were more effective, at either high or low dose compared to beta-blocker (34 to 54% vs. 29%).

2. Diuretics at high doses did not reduce CHD. Diuretics at low dose reduced CHD by 28%, beta-blocker did not reduce CHD.

3. This meta-analysis is selective and does not include all 23 reported studies on the previous pages. It includes only 18 of 23 studies. It excludes studies numbers 6, 8, 11, 13, 14. Three studies did <u>not</u> report the CHD events (18,20,22).

4. Older patients benefited more and sooner than younger patients with equal BP reductions.

Diuretic and Beta-Blocker Clinical Trials in Mild to Moderate Hypertension and Coronary Heart Disease: *Summary*

CHD Mortality Increase

Oslo	1980
MPPCD	1985

Sudden Death Increased (Abnormal electrocardiogram [ECG])

MRFIT	1982
HDFP	1979

CHD Mortality Decreased

HDFP	1979	
SHEP	1991	(SBP > 160)
MRC #2	1992	(diuretic group only, not beta-blocker group)
MAPHY	1988	(beta-blocker better than diuretic; no placebo)

No Difference in CHD Mortality Between Control vs. Treatment or Aggressive vs. Less Aggressive Treatment

VA Cooperative	1970
Barraclough	1973
USPHS	1977
VA-NHLBI	1978
Australian	1980
MRC	1984
MRFIT	1982
EWPHE	1985
IPPPSH	1972
HEP	1986
HAPPHY	1987
STOP	1991

Summary of Clinical Trials with Diuretics

1. Diuretics (non loop diuretics) are equally effective in reducing blood pressure compared to most other anti-hypertensive drug classes.

2. Low dose and not high dose diuretics are preferred (i.e. HCTZ or chlorthalidone at 6.25 to 25mg per day, or indapamide at .625 to 2.5 mg per day. However, indapamide may be preferred.

3. CVA is reduced about 38-51% which is similar to other antihypertensive drug classes.

4. CHD and MI are reduced by about 28% with low dose diuretics in some studies but high dose diuretics (with the exception of indapamide) do not reduce CHD or MI. There is a suboptimal reduction in CHD in most clinical trials with the recent exception of ALLHAT. There may also be increased risk for sudden death due to cardiac arrhythmias in predisposed patients with CHD, electrolyte disorders, or those on digitalis.

5. Renal insufficiency, reduction in GFR, ESRD and proteinuria are not improved with diuretic monotherapy and may be nephrotoxic with chronic use. These nephrotoxic effects do not apply to indapamide.

6. CHF is reduced about 52%.

7. New-onset DM and hyperglycemia are more common with diuretics (except indapamide) than other anti-hypertensive drug classes.

8. Promote atherogenesis compared to other agents as evidenced by increases in carotid IMT and coronary artery calcification by EBT. These atherogenic effects do not apply to indapamide which is anti-atherogenic.

9. Metabolic and biochemical abnormalites are common and include hypokalemia, hypomagnesemia, hyperglycemia, hyperuricemia and gout, hyperhomocysteinemia, hyperlipidemia, increased PAI-1, metabolic alkalosis, hypercalcemia, hyponatremia, and insulin resistance.

10. Increased risk of renal cell cancer and colonic cancer.
11. No improvement in structure or function of arterioles with chronic therapy; endothelial dysfunction and abnormalities of arterial compliance remain despite normalization of blood pressure.
12. High adverse effect profile and low compliance rate.

Summary of Clinical Trials with Beta-Blockers

1. Blood pressure reduction is inferior to other agents in the black and elderly population.
2. CVA is reduced but less compared to diuretics, CCB, ACEI and ARBs. The reduction in CVA is about 29%.
3. CHD and MI are not significantly reduced with beta-blocker monotherapy (7% NS).
4. CHF is reduced and prevented.
5. Patients post-MI should receive non-ISA beta-blockers.
6. Renal protection and reduction in proteinuria may be inferior to ACEI, ARB and CCB, but perhaps better than thiazide and thiazide-like diuretics.
7. The adverse effects are high and the compliance rates are low.
8. Metabolic abnormalities such as dyslipidemia. hyperglycemia and insulin resistance are common.
9. Drug-induced new onset type-2 DM and glucose intolerance occurs most frequently with diuretics (HCTZ and chlorthalidone) and beta-blockers, due to insulin resistance.

Meta-Analysis of Randomized Controlled Clinical Hypertension Trials with Anti-Hypertensive Drug Therapy

Several recent meta-analysis studies have been published that review the clinical cardiovascular and cerebrovascular outcomes in the treatment of hypertension using various classes of new antihypertensive drugs[156, 158, 159, 197, 202-206] and compare to results in diuretic/beta-blocker trials.

Meta-analysis may provide clinical results that are suggestive of CV outcomes and specific influences by anti-hypertensive drug class but by no means are these results definitive. Numerous flaws exist in such analysis:

1. Study selection bias and incomplete review of published clinical trials.

2. Statistical analysis of varied study designs, sample size different demographics, inclusion and exclusion criteria, defined primary and secondary outcomes, initial and post treatment BP levels. Concomitant CV risk factors, specific drugs used as well as doses and administration frequency, confounders of all types such as concomitant non-antihypertensive therapy, varied definitions of outcomes and subject adherence to assigned treatment.

3. Lack of critical analysis of the validity of the reported results of such trials with blanket assumption of accuracy and then subsequent inclusion in the meta-analysis renders conclusions circumstantial.

1. The summary of these meta-analyses suggest the following reductions in clinical CV outcomes compared to placebo:

    A. CHF reduced 52%

    B. CVA reduced 38%-42%

    C. MI/CHD reduced 16%-20%

This assumes a SBP reduction of 10-12 mm Hg and DBP reduction of 5-6 mm Hg.

2. Regarding specific drug classes, there appears to be no significant difference in CHF, CVA, CHD or MI outcomes. Despite trends in favor of one drug class over another, none of these reached statistical significance. Total mortality was equal among drug classes as well.

These meta-analyses will be reviewed in detail in following pages.

Meta-Analysis by Pahor, Pasty, Alderman et al:[159]

• This review included nine trials of 27,743 subjects.

• The trial selection was biased and incomplete. It included trials that were of small sample size and inappropriate for such a meta-analysis.

- The results and conclusions are invalid and open to major criticism.
- The incidence of CVA and total mortality was equal among drug classes.
- The suggestion that MI, CHF and CV events were higher with CCBs is *not valid* due to biased study selection, inclusion of short-acting CCB trials, small samples studies with inability to define outcome that are statistically significant and inclusion of inappropriate studies. Subsequent larger prospective clinical trials as well as better and more accurate meta-analysis *totally refute this meta-analysis.*
- See reference for details. This is, at best, a mediocre meta-analysis with inappropriate biased inferential conclusions.

Meta-Analysis by Blood Pressure Lowering Treatment Trialists Collaboration:[158]

This overview included a total of 74,696 patients (15 trials)

1. 4 placebo-controlled ACEI trials with 12,124 patients.
   CVA reduced 30%
   CHD reduced 20%
   CV events reduced 21%
2. 2 placebo-controlled CCB trials with 5,520 patients.
   CVA reduced 39%
   CV events reduced 28%
3. More intensive BP reduction in 3 trials with 20,408 patients reduced events more than less intensive treatment.
   CVA reduced 20% more
   CHD reduced 19% more
   Major CV events reduced 15% more
4. 8 trials comparing different drug classes with 37,872 patients showed no significant differences among any CV outcomes.
5. Mean age of 62 years and 53% male subjects in the 15 included trials.

Table 1: Trials included in the first round of analyses;[158]

Acronym	Main treatments compared	Type of data provided	Number of patients	Disease history	Mean age (years)	Proportion of male patients (%)
TRIALS COMPARING ACTIVE TREATMENT AND PLACEBO						
HOPE[26]	Ramipril vs. placebo	Tabular	9297	CHD,CVD, orDM+CVDRF	66	73
PART[227]	Ramipril vs. placebo	IPD	617	CHD or CVD	61	82
QUIET[79]	Quinapril vs. placebo	Tabular	1750	CHD	58	82
SCAT[40]	Enalapril vs. placebo	Tabular	460	CHD	61	89
PREVENT[38]	Amlodipine vs. placebo	IPD	825	CHD	57	80
SYST-EUR[41]	Nitrendipine vs. placebo	IPD	4695	HBP	70	33
TRIALS COMPARING MORE INTENSIVE AND LESS INTENSIVE BLOOD-PRESSURE-LOWERING STRATEGIES						
ABCD[28]	Target DBP S75 mm Hg re <90 mm Hg	Tabular	470	HBP+DM	58	67
HOT[42]	Target DBP <80 mm Hg vs. <85 or <90 mm Hg*	Tabular	18790	HBP	62	53
UKPDS-HDS[34, 35]	Target DBP <85 mm Hg vs. <105 mm Hg	IPD	1148	HBP+DM	56	55
TRIALS COMPARING REGIMENS BASED ON DIFFERENT DRUG CLASSES						
CAPPP[209]	Captopril vs. Beta-blocker (not specified) or diuretic (not specified)	Tabular	10985	HBP	53	53
STOP-[233]	Enalapril or Lisinopril vs. Felodipine or Isradipine vs. Atenolol or Metoprolol or Pindolol or Hydrochlorothiazide+Amiloride	Tabular	6614	HBP	76	33
UKPDS-HDS[34, 35]	Captopril vs. Atenolol	IPD	758	HBP+DM	56	54
INSIGHT[30]	Nifedipine GITS vs. Hydrochlorothiazide+Amiloride	Tabular	6321	HBP+CVD RF	65	46
NICS-EH[31]	Nicardipine vs. Trichlormethiazide	IPD	429	HBP	70	33
NORDIL[32]	Diltiazem vs. beta-blocker (not specified) or diuretic (not specified)	Tabular	10881	HBP	60	49
VHAS[43, 44]	Verapamil vs. Chlorthalidone	Tabular	1414	HBP	54	49
ABCD-hypertensive[29]	Enalapril vs. Nisoldipine	Tabular	470	HBP+DM	58	67

CHD=coronary heart disease, CVD=other cardiovascular disease, CVD RF=other CVD risk factor, DSP=diastolic blood pressure, GITS=gastrointestinal transport system, IPD=individual participant data, DM=diabetes mellitus, HBP=high blood pressure. *Felodipine was the first-line drug used in all randomised groups in HOT.

Table 2: Blood-pressure differences, proportion remaining on randomised treatments, and proportion achieving blood-pressure goals: [158]

Acronym	SBP/DBP at entry (mm Hg)	Blood-pressure differences (treatment–control)* between randomized groups during follow-up (mm Hg)		Proportion remaining on randomized treatment or achieving blood-pressure goal (%)		Duration of follow-up(years)
		SBP	DBP	Study Treatment	Control*	
TRIALS COMPARING ACTIVE TREATMENT AND PLACEBO						
HOPE	139/79	-3	-1	71	73	5
PART2	133/79	-6	-4	72	75	4
QUIET	123/74	NA	NA	72	75	2
SCAT	130/78	-4	-3	NA	NA	5
PREVENT	129/79	-5	-4	69	78	3
SYST-EUR	174/86	-10	-5	72	66	2
TRIALS COMPARING MORE INTENSIVE AND LESS INTENSIVE BLOOD-PRESSURE-LOWERING STRATEGIES						
ABCD-hypertensive†	155/98	-6	-8	49	89	5
HOT‡	169/105	-3	-3	55	80	4
UKPDS-HDS§	160/94	-10	-5	56	91	8
TRIALS COMPARING REGIMENS BASED ON DIFFERENT DRUG CLASSES*						
CAPPPH	161/99	+3	+1	67	86	6
STOP-2¶	194/98	<3	<1	64	62	5
UKPDS-HDS	160/94	+1	+2	78	65	8
INSIGHT	173/99	<1	<1	60	67	4
NICS-EH	172/94	0	+2	92	94	4
NORDIL	173/106	+3	<1	77	93	5
VHAS	169/102	<1	<1	78	77	2
ABCD-hypertensive†	155/98	<1	<1	45	40	5

SBP=systolic blood pressure, DBP=diastolic blood pressure, NA=not available. *In all studies except ABCD, group randomised to _-blocker and/or diuretic therapy designated control. †Group randomised to calcium antagonist designated control, group randomised to ACE inhibitor designated treatment. Mean BP levels achieved: 132/78 mm Hg in more intensive vs. 138/86 mm Hg in less intensive group. ‡Most intensive BP lowering regimen (target DBP < 80 mm Hg) designated treatment, less Intensive regimens designated control. Mean BP levels achieved: 140/81 mm Hg in more intensive vs 143/84 mm Hg in less intensive group. §Mean BP levels achieved: 144/82 mm Hg in more Intensive vs. 154/87 mm Hg In less intensive group. _Blood pressure difference (2/2 mm Hg) present between randomised groups at study entry. ¶Group randomised to _-blockers/diuretics designated control, group randomised to ACE inhibitors or calcium antagonists designated treatment (in this table only). Elsewhere, groups randomised to ACE inhibitor or calcium antagonists are considered as separate study treatments.

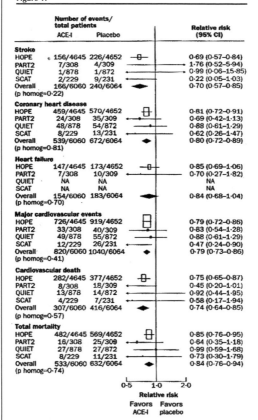

Comparisons of ACE-Inhibitor-based Therapy with Placebo

Figure 1.

	Number of events/ total patients		Relative risk (95% CI)
	ACE-I	Placebo	
Stroke			
HOPE	156/4645	226/4652	0·69 (0·57–0·84)
PART2	7/308	4/309	1·76 (0·52–5·94)
QUIET	1/878	1/872	0·99 (0·06–15·85)
SCAT	2/229	9/231	0·22 (0·05–1·03)
Overall (p homog=0·22)	166/6060	240/6064	0·70 (0·57–0·85)
Coronary heart disease			
HOPE	459/4645	570/4652	0·81 (0·72–0·91)
PART2	24/308	35/309	0·69 (0·42–1·13)
QUIET	48/878	54/872	0·88 (0·61–1·29)
SCAT	8/229	13/231	0·62 (0·26–1·47)
Overall (p homog=0·81)	539/6060	672/6064	0·80 (0·72–0·89)
Heart failure			
HOPE	147/4645	173/4652	0·85 (0·69–1·06)
PART2	7/308	10/309	0·70 (0·27–1·82)
QUIET	NA	NA	NA
SCAT	NA	NA	NA
Overall (p homog=0·70)	154/6060	183/6064	0·84 (0·68–1·04)
Major cardiovascular events			
HOPE	726/4645	919/4652	0·79 (0·72–0·86)
PART2	33/308	40/309	0·83 (0·54–1·28)
QUIET	49/878	55/872	0·88 (0·61–1·29)
SCAT	12/229	26/231	0·47 (0·24–0·90)
Overall (p homog=0·41)	820/6060	1040/6064	0·79 (0·73–0·86)
Cardiovascular death			
HOPE	282/4645	377/4652	0·75 (0·65–0·87)
PART2	8/308	18/309	0·45 (0·20–1·01)
QUIET	13/878	14/872	0·92 (0·44–1·95)
SCAT	4/229	7/231	0·58 (0·17–1·94)
Overall (p homog=0·57)	307/6060	416/6064	0·74 (0·64–0·85)
Total mortality			
HOPE	482/4645	569/4652	0·85 (0·76–0·95)
PART2	16/308	25/309	0·64 (0·35–1·18)
QUIET	27/878	27/872	0·99 (0·59–1·68)
SCAT	8/229	11/231	0·73 (0·30–1·79)
Overall (p homog=0·74)	533/6060	632/6064	0·84 (0·76–0·94)

0·5　　1·0　　2·0

Relative risk

Favors ACE-I　　Favors placebo

Boxes and horizontal lines represent risk and 95% CI for each trial. Size of boxes is proportional to inverse of variance of that trial result. Diamond represents the 95% CI for pooled estimates of effect and are centered on pooled relative risk. ACE-I=Ace inhibitor, p homog=p value from x^2 test for homogeneity, NA=data not available.

Comparisons of Calcium-antagonist-based Therapy with Placebo

Figure 2.

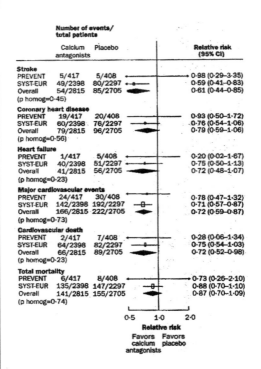

Boxes and horizontal lines represent risk and 95% CI for each trial. Size of boxes is proportional to inverse of variance of that trial result. Diamond represents the 95% CI for pooled estimates of effect and are centered on pooled relative risk. ACE-I=Ace inhibitor, p homog=p value from x^2 test for homogeneity, NA=data not available.

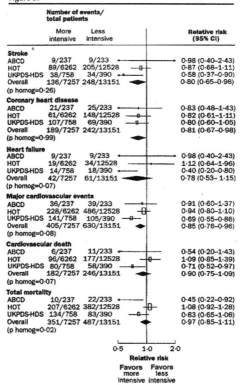

Comparisons of More Intensive Blood Pressure Lowering Strategies with Less Intensive Strategies

Figure 3.

| | Number of events/ total patients | | Relative risk |
	More intensive	Less intensive	(95% CI)
Stroke			
ABCD	9/237	9/233	0·98 (0·40–2·43)
HOT	89/6262	205/12528	0·87 (0·68–1·11)
UKPDS-HDS	38/758	34/390	0·58 (0·37–0·90)
Overall	136/7257	248/13151	0·80 (0·65–0·98)
(p homog=0·26)			
Coronary heart disease			
ABCD	21/237	25/233	0·83 (0·48–1·43)
HOT	61/6262	148/12528	0·82 (0·61–1·11)
UKPDS-HDS	107/758	69/390	0·80 (0·60–1·05)
Overall	189/7257	242/13151	0·81 (0·67–0·98)
(p homog=0·99)			
Heart failure			
ABCD	9/237	9/233	0·98 (0·40–2·43)
HOT	19/6262	34/12528	1·12 (0·64–1·96)
UKPDS-HDS	14/758	18/390	0·40 (0·20–0·80)
Overall	42/7257	61/13151	0·78 (0·53–1·15)
(p homog=0·07)			
Major cardiovascular events			
ABCD	36/237	39/233	0·91 (0·60–1·37)
HOT	228/6262	486/12528	0·94 (0·80–1·10)
UKPDS-HDS	141/758	105/390	0·69 (0·55–0·86)
Overall	405/7257	630/13151	0·85 (0·76–0·96)
(p homog=0·08)			
Cardiovascular death			
ABCD	6/237	11/233	0·54 (0·20–1·43)
HOT	96/6262	177/12528	1·09 (0·85–1·39)
UKPDS-HDS	80/758	58/390	0·71 (0·52–0·97)
Overall	182/7257	246/13151	0·90 (0·75–1·09)
(p homog=0·07)			
Total mortality			
ABCD	10/237	22/233	0·45 (0·22–0·92)
HOT	207/6262	382/12528	1·08 (0·92–1·28)
UKPDS-HDS	134/758	83/390	0·83 (0·65–1·06)
Overall	351/7257	487/13151	0·97 (0·85–1·11)
(p homog=0·02)			

0·5   1·0   2·0
Relative risk
Favors   Favors
more   less
intensive   intensive

p homog=p value from x^2 test for homogeneity, NA=data not available.

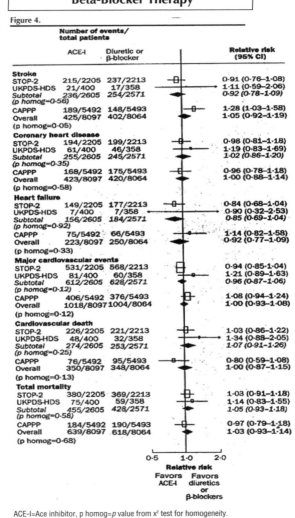

Comparisons of Ace-Inhibitor Based Therapy with Diuretic-based or Beta-Blocker Therapy

Figure 4.

ACE-I=Ace inhibitor, p homog=*p* value from x^2 test for homogeneity.

Comparisons of Calcium-antagonist-based Therapy with Diuretic-based or Beta-Blocker-based Therapy

Figure 5.

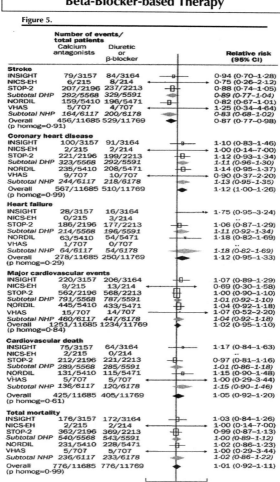

	Number of events/ total patients		Relative risk (95% CI)
	Calcium antagonists	Diuretic or β-blocker	
Stroke			
INSIGHT	79/3157	84/3164	0·94 (0·70–1·28)
NICS-EH	6/215	8/214	0·75 (0·26–2·12)
STOP-2	207/2196	237/2213	0·88 (0·74–1·05)
Subtotal DHP	*292/5568*	*329/5591*	*0·89 (0·77–1·04)*
NORDIL	159/5410	196/5471	0·82 (0·67–1·01)
VHAS	5/707	4/707	1·25 (0·34–4·64)
Subtotal NHP	*164/6117*	*200/6178*	*0·83 (0·68–1·02)*
Overall (p homog=0·91)	456/11685	529/11769	0·87 (0·77–0·98)
Coronary heart disease			
INSIGHT	100/3157	91/3164	1·10 (0·83–1·46)
NICS-EH	2/215	2/214	1·00 (0·14–7·00)
STOP-2	221/2196	199/2213	1·12 (0·93–1·34)
Subtotal DHP	*323/5568*	*292/5591*	*1·11 (0·96–1·30)*
NORDIL	235/5410	208/5471	1·14 (0·95–1·37)
VHAS	9/707	10/707	0·90 (0·37–2·20)
Subtotal NHP	*244/6117*	*218/6178*	*1·13 (0·95–1·35)*
Overall (p homog=0·99)	567/11685	510/11769	1·12 (1·00–1·26)
Heart failure			
INSIGHT	28/3157	16/3164	1·75 (0·95–3·24)
NICS-EH	0/215	3/214	··
STOP-2	186/2196	177/2213	1·06 (0·87–1·29)
Subtotal DHP	*214/5568*	*196/5591*	*1·11 (0·92–1·34)*
NORDIL	63/5410	54/5471	1·18 (0·82–1·69)
VHAS	1/707	0/707	··
Subtotal NHP	*64/6117*	*54/6178*	*1·18 (0·82–1·69)*
Overall (p homog=0·29)	278/11685	250/11769	1·12 (0·95–1·33)
Major cardiovascular events			
INSIGHT	220/3157	206/3164	1·07 (0·89–1·29)
NICS-EH	9/215	13/214	0·69 (0·30–1·58)
STOP-2	562/2196	568/2213	1·00 (0·90–1·10)
Subtotal DHP	*791/5568*	*787/5591*	*1·01 (0·92–1·10)*
NORDIL	445/5410	433/5471	1·04 (0·92–1·18)
VHAS	15/707	14/707	1·07 (0·52–2·20)
Subtotal NHP	*460/6117*	*447/6178*	*1·04 (0·92–1·18)*
Overall (p homog=0·84)	1251/11685	1234/11769	1·02 (0·95–1·10)
Cardiovascular death			
INSIGHT	75/3157	64/3164	1·17 (0·84–1·63)
NICS-EH	2/215	0/214	··
STOP-2	212/2196	221/2213	0·97 (0·81–1·16)
Subtotal DHP	*289/5568*	*285/5591*	*1·01 (0·86–1·18)*
NORDIL	131/5410	115/5471	1·15 (0·90–1·48)
VHAS	5/707	5/707	1·00 (0·29–3·44)
Subtotal NHP	*136/6117*	*120/6178*	*1·15 (0·90–1·46)*
Overall (p homog=0·61)	425/11685	405/11769	1·05 (0·92–1·20)
Total mortality			
INSIGHT	176/3157	172/3164	1·03 (0·84–1·26)
NICS-EH	2/215	2/214	1·00 (0·14–7·00)
STOP-2	362/2196	369/2213	0·99 (0·87–1·13)
Subtotal DHP	*540/5568*	*543/5591*	*1·00 (0·89–1·12)*
NORDIL	231/5410	228/5471	1·02 (0·86–1·23)
VHAS	5/707	5/707	1·00 (0·29–3·44)
Subtotal NHP	*236/6117*	*233/6178*	*1·02 (0·86–1·22)*
Overall (p homog=0·99)	776/11685	776/11769	1·01 (0·92–1·11)

0·5   1·0   2·0

DHP=dihydropyridine, NHP=non-dihydropyridine, p homog=*p* value from x^2 test for homogeneity.

Comparisons of ACE-Inhibitor-based Therapy with Calcium-antagonist-based Therapy

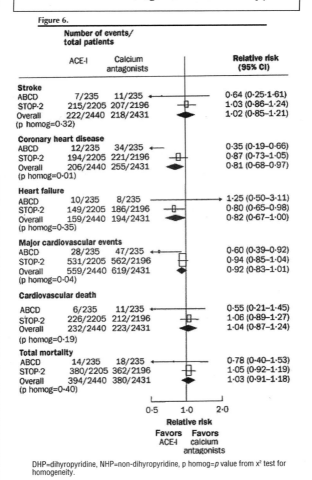

Figure 6.

DHP=dihyropyridine, NHP=non-dihyropyridine, p homog=p value from x² test for homogeneity.

Staessen, Wang and Thijs Meta-Analysis. Summary of Clinical Trials in Hypertension and Clinical Outcomes: [156]

A reduction in SBP of 10-12 mm Hg and a reduction in DBP of 5-6 mm Hg results in the following reductions in cardiovascular end-points based on meta-analysis studies of 27 trials on over 136,124 patients: [156]

CHF	reduced	52%
CVA	reduced	38%-42%
CHD and MI	reduced	16%-21%

The conclusion was that results of the outcome trials for antihypertensive drugs can be explained by BP differences between randomized groups. All antihypertensive drugs had similar long-term efficacy and safety.

It was suggested that calcium channel blockers provided more reduction in CVA (13.5% 95% CI 1.3-24.2, p=0.03) and less reduction in the risk of myocardial infarction (19.2%, 3.5-37.3, p=0.01). The CVA reduction trend was confirmed in ALLHAT (NS) and in a recent meta-analysis, but the MI risk was not confirmed in ALLHAT (CCB (amlodipine) = chlorthalidone).
Specific BP reduction related to outcomes:

- SBP reduction of 10 mm Hg and DBP reduction 4 mm Hg
    - CVA decreased 30%
    - MI decreased 23%

- DBP reduction (if DBP was predominant) of 5-6 mm Hg
    - CVA decreased 38%
    - MI decreased 16%

Table 1: Characteristics of trials in hypertension comparing different active treatments:[156]

Characteristics	UKPDS[16,27]*	STOP[26]	CAPPP[4]	NORDIL[9]	INSIGHT[8]	ALLHAT[10]	MIDAS[3]	NICS[5]	VHAS[88]†
Masking type	Open	Open	Open	Open	Double	Double	Double	Double	Open
Number of patients	1148	6614	10985	10881	6321	24335	883	414	1414
Treatment									
Reference	Atenolol <180/105	HCTZ/A or β-blockers	Diuretic or β-blockers	Thiazide or β-blockers	HCTZ/A	Chlorthalidone	HCTZ	Trichlorme-Thiazide	Chlorthalidone
Experimental	<Captopril <150/85	ACEIs DHPs	Captopril	Diltiazem (SR)	Nifedipine (GITS)	Doxazosin	Isradipine	Nicardipine (SR)	Verapamil (SR)
Age (mean [SD], years)	56(8)	76(..)	53(8)	60(7)	65(7)	67(8)	59(9)	70(7)	53(7)
Mean systolic/diastolic blood pressure (mm Hg)									
At entry	160/94	194/98	161/99	173/106	167/96	145/83‖	150/97	172/94	169/102
Difference during follow-up§	-1/-1	-0.3/+0.5	-3/-1	-3.1/-0.2	-0/-0	-2/+1	-3.5/-0	-0.7/-1.2	-1.0/+0.4
Proportion of patients (%)									
Women	45	67	47	51	54	47	22	67	51
Cardiovascular complications	..	~20	4	~8	~20	45	~4	~28	5
Diabetes mellitus	100	11	5	7	21	36	..	..	4‖
Follow-up (years)									
Median	8.4	5.0	6.1	4.5	3.5	3.3	3.0	4.3	2.0
Mean	..	..	..	..	..	..	..	..	..

ACEIs=angiotensin-converting enzyme inhibitors; DHPs=dihydropyridine calcium-channel blockers (felodipine or isradipine); GITS=gastro-intestinal therapeutic system; HCTZ=hydrochlorothiazide; HCTZ/A=hydrochlorothiazide plus amiloride; SR=sustained release. Acronyms of trials are explained in the appendix. *UKPDS compared captopril with atenolol and tested two levels of control of systolic/diastolic blood pressure. †In VHAS, study drug was given in the initial 6 months and thereafter in an open way. ‡90% of ALLHAT patients had blood pressure control on old drug treatment. §Negative values indicate tighter blood pressure measured at entry while on antihypertensive treatment. ‖Patients on antidiabetic drug treatment.

Table 2: Pooled estimates of advantage of new versus old antihypertensive drugs with respect to cause-specific mortality[156]

	Zelen's p-value*	Pooled estimates of advantage of new versus old drugs expressed In percent†		
		Estimate (SD)	95% CIs	p
Cause of death‡				
Stroke				
CCBs	0.95	-5.3 (17.9)	-31.4 to 30.7	0.79
ACEIs	0.89	-5.6 (18.6)	-32.5 to 31.8	0.79
CCBs and ACEIs	0.99	-5.4 (14.0)	-26.8 to 22.5	0.70
Myocardial Infarction				
CCBs	0.13	22.6 (16.6)	-9.2 to 65.8	0.19
ACEIs	0.32	-6.3 (15.1)	-28.9 to 23.4	0.68
CCBs and ACEIs	0.10	7.9(12.1)	-13.6 to 35.0	0.53
Sudden death				
CCBs	0.46	-8.8 (18.4)	-34.5 to 26.8	0.64
ACEIs	0.07	3.8 (19.3)	-26.5 to 46.7	0.89
CCBs and ACEIs	0.12	-5.3 (15.1)	-28.0 to 25.1	0.74
Myocardial Infarction plus sudden death				
CCBs	0.92	7.9 (12.2)	-13.8 to 35.2	0.53
ACEIs	0-07	-2.5(11.6)	-21.4 to 20.9	0.85
CCBs and ACEIs	0.20	2.5(9.3)	-13.8 to 22.1	0.81

ACEIs=angiotensin-converting enzyme inhibitors; CCBs=calcium-channel blockers.
*The hypothesis of heterogeneity across the reviewed trials was rejected for all fatal outcomes. †Negative values indicate better outcome on the new drugs. ‡The reviewed trials are those listed in table 1 with the exception of ALLHAT, because cardiovascular mortality was unavailable from the published report. Cause-specific cardiovascular mortality was also not reported for MIDAS,3 NICS,5 and VHAS,63.

Effects of Antihypertensive Treatment on Cardiovascular Mortality and All Cardiovascular Events in Trials Comparing Old with New Drugs

Figure 5.

Trials	Number of events old/new	Odds ratios and 95% CIs	Difference (SD)
Cardiovascular mortality			
MIDAS/NICS/VHAS	7/10		
UKPDS	32/48		
STOP2	221/438		
STOP2/CCBs	221/212		
STOP2/ACEIs	221/226		
CAPPP	95/76		
NORDIL	115/131		
INSIGHT	52/60		
All CCBs	395/413		5.8% (7.7) 2P = 0.46
Heterogeneity P = 0.58			
All ACEIs	348/350		−0.5% (8.4) 2P = 0.98
Heterogeneity P = 0.13			
CCBs and ACEIs	522/763		3.6% (6.2) 2P = 0.57
Heterogeneity P = 0.31			
Cardiovascular events			
MIDAS/NICS/VHAS	37/39		
UKPDS	78/107		
STOP2	637/1222		
STOP2/CCBs	637/636		
STOP2/ACEIs	637/586		
CAPPP	401/438		
NORDIL	453/466		
INSIGHT	397/383		
ALLHAT	2245/1592		
All CCBs	1524/1524		0.9% (4.1) 2P = 0.90
Heterogeneity P = 0.90			
All ACEIs	1116/1131		0.8% (4.9) 2P = 0.89
Heterogeneity P = 0.03			
CCBs and ACEIs	2003/2655		1.8% (3.4) 2P = 0.60
Heterogeneity P = 0.38			
All trials	4248/4247		11.2% (2.5) 2P < 0.0001
Heterogeneity P = 0.001			

0   1   2   3

New drugs   New drugs
better   worse

Solid squared=treatment-to-control odds ratios in trials and have a size proportional to number of events. 95% CI for individual trials are denoted by lines and those for pooled odds ratios by diamonds.

Effects of Antihypertensive Treatment on Fatal and Non-Fatal Stroke and Myocardial Infarction in Trials Comparing Old with New Drugs

Figure 2.

Trials	Number of events old/new	Odds ratios and 95% CIs	Difference (SD)
Fatal and non-fatal stroke			
MIDAS/NICS/VHAS	15/19		
UKPDS	17/21		
STOP2	237/422		
STOP2/CCBs	237/207		
STOP2/ACEIs	237/215		
CAPPP	148/189		
NORDIL	196/159		
INSIGHT	74/67		
ALLHAT	351/244		
All CCBs Heterogeneity p=0·82	522/452		−13·5% (7·0) 2p=0·03
All ACEIs Heterogeneity p=0·05	402/425		5·8% (7·6) 2p=0·45
CCBs and ACEIs Heterogeneity p=0·05	687/877		−3·9% (5·6) 2p=0·47
All trials Heterogeneity p=0·02	1038/1121		1·7% (4·7) 2p=0·72
Fatal and non-fatal myocardial infarction			
MIDAS/NICS/VHAS	16/16		
UKPDS	46/61		
STOP2	154/318		
STOP2/CCBs	154/179		
STOP2/ACEIs	154/139		
CAPPP	161/162		
NORDIL	157/183		
INSIGHT	61/77		
ALLHAT	608/365		
All CCBs Heterogeneity p=0·95	388/455		19·2% (7·5) 2p=0·01
All ACEIs Heterogeneity p=0·45	361/362		−1·3% (8·1) 2p=0·90
CCBs and ACEIs Heterogeneity p=0·80	595/817		10·1% (5·8) 2p=0·09
All trials Heterogeneity p=0·79	1203/1182		6·4% (4·4) 2p=0·16

0   1   2   3
New drugs better   New drugs worse

Effects of Antihypertensive Treatment on Fatal and Non-Fatal Congestive Heart Failure in Trials Comparing Old with New Drugs

Figure 3.

Trials	Number of events old/new	Odds ratios and 95% CIs	Difference (SD)
MIDAS/NICS/VHAS	3/4		
UKPDS	9/12		
STOP2	177/335		
STOP2/CCBs	177/186		
STOP2/ACEIs	177/149		
CAPPP	66/75		
NORDIL	53/63		
INSIGHT	12/26		
ALLHAT	420/491		
All CCBs Heterogeneity p=0·25	245/279		15·8% (9·7) 2p=0·11
All ACEIs Heterogeneity p=0·27	252/236		−6·9% (10·0) 2p=0·47
CCBs and ACEIs Heterogeneity p=0·25	320/515		7·1% (7·8) 2p=0·37
All trials Heterogeneity p<0·0001	740/1006		52·4% (5·3) 2p<0·0001

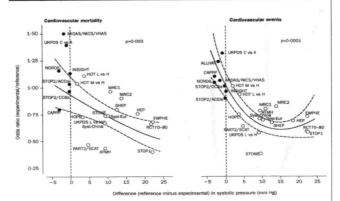

Relation Between Odds Ratios for Cardiovascular Mortality and All Cardiovascular Events, and Corresponding Differences in Systolic Blood Pressure[156]

Figure 4.

Odds ratios were calculated for experimental versus reference treatment. Blood pressure differences were calculated by subtracting achieved levels in experimental groups from those in reference groups. Negative differences indicate tighter blood pressure control on reference treatment. Regression lines were plotted with 95% CI and were weighted for the inverse of individual odds ratios. Closed symbols denote trials that compared new with old drugs. Acronyms and references of trials are in the appendix.

Relation Between Odds Ratios for Fatal and Non-Fatal Myocardial Infarction, and Corresponding Differences in Systolic Blood Pressure[156]

Figure 5.

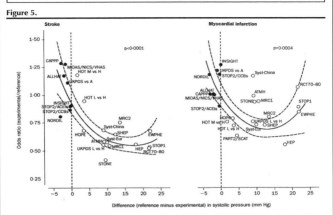

Difference (reference minus experimental) in systolic pressure (mm Hg)

Fatal and non-fatal myocardial infarction includes sudden death. Odds ratios were calculated for experimental versus reference treatment. Blood pressure differences were calculated by subtracting achieved levels in experimental groups from those in reference groups. Negative differences indicate tighter blood pressure control on reference treatment. Regression lines were plotted with 95% CI and were weighted for the inverse of individual odds ratios. Closed symbols denote trials that compared new with old drugs.

Table 3: Variance explained by initial blood pressure and blood pressure difference[156]

	Variance explained and corresponding probability					
	Overall Model		**Initial Blood Pressure**		**Blood Pressure Difference**	
	R^2	p	R^2	p	R^2	p
Outcome						
Cardiovascular Mortality						
Systolic	0.47	0.002	0.11	0.05	0.36	0.0004
Diastolic	0.42	0.005	0.10	0.08	0.32	0.001
Cardiovascular Events						
Systolic	0.66	<0.0001	0.006	0.56	0.65	<0.0001
Diastolic	0.51	0.002	~0	0.99	0.51	0.001
Stroke						
Systolic	0.71	<0.0001	0.004	0.48	0.71	<0.0001
Diastolic	0.66	0.0001	0.007	0.55	0.65	<0.0001
Stroke						
Systolic	0.55	0.001	0.02	0.37	0.53	0.0005
Diastolic	0.54	0.001	0.09	0.06	0.45	0.002

Every metaregression model included blood pressure at entry and blood pressure difference between study groups as independent variables and was weighted by the inverse of the variance odds ratios.

Table 4: Observed odds ratios and odds ratios predicted by differences In systolic blood pressure In metaregression: [156]

	Observed odds ratio* (95% CIs)	Predicted mean odds ratio (95% CIs)†	Difference (% [95% CIs]) ‡	P§
ALLHAT[10]				
Cardiovascular events	1.24 (1.15-1.33)	1.14 (0.98-1.32)	-8.4 (-27.0 to 7.4)	0.32
Stroke	1.18 (0.99-1.39)	1.06 (0.92-1.22)	-11.3 (-38.1 to 10.3)	.33
Myocardial infarction	1.01 (0.88-1.16)	1.13 (0.98-1.31)	10.7 (-8.2 to 26.2)	0.25
CAPPP[4]				
Cardiovascular mortality	0.80 (0.58-1.09)	0.99 (0.81-1.22)	19.8 (-16.1 to 44.6)	0.24
Cardiovascular events	1.10 (0.95-1.27)	1.23 (1.03-1.46)	10.3 (-11.5 to 27.9)	0.33
Stroke	1.29 (1.03-1.61)	1.14 (0.96-1.34)	-13.4 (-49.0 to 13.8)	0.37
Myocardial infarction	1.01 (0.80-1.26)	1.21(1.02-1.44)	17.0 (-9.8 to 37.2)	0.19
HOPE[7]				
Cardiovascular mortality	0.73 (0.62-0.86)	0.86 (0.74-0.99)	14.4 (-5.7 to 30.6)	0.15
Cardiovascular events	0.76 (0.67-0.85)	0.82 (0.75-0.91)	8.4 (-6.2 to 21.0)	0.24
Stroke	0.68 (0.52-0.86)	0.77 (0.69-0.85)	11.1 (-12.3 to 29.6)	0.32
Myocardial infarction	0.79 (0.69-0.90)	0.85 (0.77-0.93)	7.2 (-8.6 to 20.6)	0.35
NORDIL[9]				
Cardiovascular mortality	1.16 (0.89-1.50)	1.00 (0.81-1.22)	-16.1 (-60.8 to 16.2)	0.37
Cardiovascular events	1.04 (0.91-1.20)	1.24 (1.04-1.47)	15.5 (-4.8 to 31.9)	0.13
Stroke	0.81 (0.65-1.01)	1.14 (0.97-1.35)	28.8 (6.8 to 45.5)	0.01
Myocardial infarction	1.19 (0.95-1.48)	1.22 (1.02-1.46)	3.0 (-28.1 to 26.5)	0.83
PART2/SCAT[12, 15]				
Cardiovascular mortality	0.47 (0.21-0.98)	0.83 (0.73-0.95)	43.3 (-19.8 to 73.2)	0.14
Cardiovascular events	0.64 (0.44-0.94)	0.78 (0.70-0.86)	17.3 (-22.8 to 44.3)	0.35
Myocardial infarction	0.63 (0.38-1.05)	0.80 (0.73-0.88)	21.2 (-31.1 to 52.7)	0.36

* – Odds ratio reported in the published articles. † – Mean odds ratio (95% CI) predicted by metaregression lines (figures 4 and 5). ‡ – Difference between predicted minus observed odds ratio (95% CI) expressed in percent of predicted odds ratio. § – Significance of difference between observed and predicted odds ratios.

Health Outcomes Meta-Analysis[219]

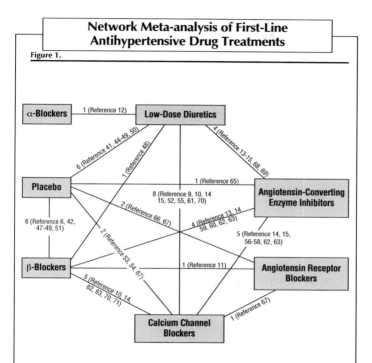

Network Meta-analysis of First-Line Antihypertensive Drug Treatments

Figure 1.

Each first-line drug treatment is a node in the network. The links between the nodes are trials or pairs of trial arms. The numbers along the link lines indicate the number of trials or pairs of trial arms for that link in the network. Reference numbers indicate the trials contributing to each link. A trial such as the Antihypertensive and Lipid-Lowering Treatment to Prevent Heart Attack Trial[12, 15] (ALLHAT) with multiple arms appears along several links (diuretic-angiotensin-converting enzyme (ACE) inhibitors, diuretics-calcium channel blockers (CCBs), ACE inhibitors-CCBs, and diuretics-α-blockers). High-dose diuretics trials were excluded.

JAMA, May 21, 2003–vol 289, No. 19.

Note: All references for this figure are found on page 103.

Network Meta-Analysis of First-Line Treatment Strategies in Randomized Controlled Clinical Trials in Hypertension

Figure 2.

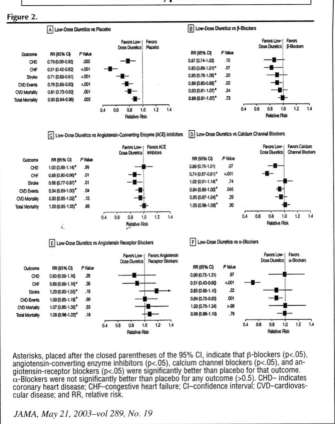

Asterisks, placed after the closed parentheses of the 95% CI, indicate that β-blockers (p<.05), angiotensin-converting enzyme inhibitors (p<.05), calcium channel blockers (p<.05), and angiotensin-receptor blockers (p<.05) were significantly better than placebo for that outcome. α-Blockers were not significantly better than placebo for any outcome (>0.5). CHD– indicates coronary heart disease; CHF–congestive heart failure; CI–confidence interval; CVD–cardiovascular disease; and RR, relative risk.

JAMA, May 21, 2003–vol 289, No. 19

Conclusion: Low-dose diuretics are the most effective first-line treatment for preventing the occurrence of cardiovascular disease morbidity and mortality. **Author's Critique:** This meta-analysis did not examine the incidence of treatment related to non-cardiovascular side effects such as new onset DM or renal disease.

1. Joint National Committee on Prevention, Detection, Evaluation and Treatment of High Blood Pressure. The Sixth Report of the Joint National Committee on Prevention, Detection, Evaluation, and Treatment of High Blood Pressure. Arch Intern Med. 1997:157:2413-2446.

2. Joint National Committee on Detection, Evaluation, and Treatment of High Blood Pressure. The Fifth Report of the Joint National Committee on Detection, Evaluation, and Treatment of High Blood Pressure (JNC V). Arch Intern Med. 1993:153:154-183.

3. Psaty BM, Smith NS, Siscovick DS, et al. Health out comes associated with antihypertensive therapies used as first-line agents: a systematic review and meta-analysis. JAMA. 1997:277:739-745.

4. Veterans Administration Cooperative Study Group on Antihypertensive Agents. Effects of treatment on morbidity in hypertension: results in patients with diastolic blood pressures averaging 115 through 129 mm Hg. JAMA. 1967:202:116-122.

5. Veterans Administration Cooperative Study Group on Antihypertensive Agents II. Effects of treatment: results in patients with diastolic blood pressure aver-aging 90 through 114 mm Hg. JAMA. 1970;213: 1143-1152.

6. Medical Research Council Working Party. MRC trial of treatment of mild hypertension: principal results. BMJ. 1985:291:97-104.

7. Hypertension Detection and Follow-up Program Co-operative Group. The effect of treatment on mild hy-pertension: results of the Hypertension Detection and Follow-up Program. N Engl J Med. 1982:307:976-980.

8. Hypertension Detection and Follow-up Program Co-operative Group. Five-year findings of the Hypertension Detection and Follow-up Program, III: reduction in stroke incidence among persons with high blood pressure. JAMA. 1982:247:633-638.

9. Brown MJ, Palmer CR, Castaigne A, et al. Morbidity and mortality in patients randomized to double-blind treatment with a long-acting calcium channel blocker or diuretic in the international nifedipine GITS study: Intervention as a Goal in Hypertension Treatment (INSIGHT). Lancet. 2000:356:366-372.

10. Hansson L, Hedner T, Lund-Johansen P, etal. Randomised trial of effects of calcium antagonists compared with diuretics and beta-blockers on cardiovascular morbidity and mortality in hypertension: the Nordic Diltiazem (NORDIt) study. Lancet. 2000;356: 359-365.

11. Dahlof B, Devereux RB, Kjeldsen SE, et al. Cardiovascular morbidity and mortality in the Losartan Intervention For Endpoint reduction in hypertension study (LIFE): a randomised trial against atenolol. Lancet. 2002; 359:995-1003.

12. ALLHAT Officers and Coordinator for the ALLHAT Collaborative Research Group. Major cardiovascular events in hypertensive patients randomized to doxazosin vs. chlorthalidone: the Antihypertensive and Lipid-lowering Treatment to Prevent Heart Attack Trial (ALLHAT). JAMA. 2000:283:1967-1975.

13. Hansson L, Lindholm LH, Niskanen L, et al. Effect of angiotensin-converting-enzyme inhibition compared with conventional therapy on cardiovascular morbidity and mortality in hypertension: the Captopril Prevention Project (CAPPP) randomized trial. Lancet. 1999; 353:611-616.

14. Hansson L, Lindholm LH, Ekbom T, et al. Randomized trial of old and new antihypertensive drugs in elderly patients: cardiovascular mortality and morbidity the Swedish Trial in Old Patients with Hypertension-2 study. Lancet. 1999;354:1751-1756.

15. ALLHAT Officers and Coordinators for the ALLHAT Collaborative Research Group. Major outcomes in high-risk hypertensive patients randomized to angiotensin converting enzyme inhibitor or calcium-channel blocker vs diuretic: the Antihypertensive and Lipid Lowering Treatment to Prevent Heart Attack Trial (ALLHAT). JAMA. 2002:288:2981-2997.

16. Pahor M, Psaty BM, Alderman MH, et al. Health outcomes associated with calcium antagonists compared with other first line antihypertensive therapies: a meta-analysis of randomised controlled trials. Lancet. 2000:356:1949-1954.

17. Blood Pressure Lowering Treatment Trialists' Collaboration. Effects of ACE inhibitors, calcium antagonists, and other blood pressure lowering drugs: results of prospectively designed overviews of randomised trials. Lancet. 2000:356:1955-1964.

18. MacMahon S, Neal B. Differences between blood pressure lowering drugs. Lancet. 2000;356:352-353.

19. Lumley T. Network meta-analysis for indirect treatment comparisons. StatMed. 2002;21:2313-2324.

20. MacMahon SW, Cutler JA, Furberg CD, Payne GH. The effects of drug treatment for hypertension on morbidity and mortality from cardiovascular disease: a review of randomized controlled trials. Prog Cardiovasc Dis. 1986;29(suppl 1):99-118.

21. Collins R, Peto R, MacMahon S, et al. Blood pressure, stroke, and coronary heart disease, part 2: short-term reductions in blood pressure: overview of randomised drug trials in their epidemiologic context. Lancet. 1990:335:827-838.

22. Mulrow CD, Cornell JA, Herrera CR, Kadri A, Farnett L, Aguilar C. Hypertension in the elderly: implications and generaliability of randomized trials. JAMA. 1994;272:1932-1938.

23. Hebert PR, Moser M, Mayer J, Glynn RJ, Hennekens CH. Recent evidence on drug therapy of mild to moderate hypertension and decreased risk of coronary heart disease. Arch Intern Med. 1993:153:578-581.

24. Cutler JA, Psaty BM, MacMahon S, Furberg CD. Public health issues in hypertension control: what has been learned from clinical trials. In: Laragh JH, Brenner BM, eds. Hypertension: Pathophysiology, Diagnosis and Management 2nd ed. New York, NY: Raven Press. 1995:253-279.

25. Carter AB. Hypotensive therapy in stroke survivors. Lancet. 1970:1:485-489.

26. Hegeland A. Treatment of mild hypertension: a five-year controlled drug trial: the Oslo Study. Am J Med. 1980:69:725-732.

27. Liu L, Wang JG, Gong L, et al. Comparison of active treatment and placebo in older Chinese patients with isolated systolic hypertension. J Hypertens. 1998; 16:1823-1829.

28. Multiple Risk Factor Intervention Trial Research Group. Multiple Risk Factor Intervention Trial: risk factor changes and mortality results. JAMA. 1982:248: 1465-1477.

29. Miettinen TA, Huttunen JK, Naukkarinen V, et al. Multifactorial primary prevention of cardiovascular diseases in middle-aged men: risk factor changes, incidence and mortality. JAMA. 1985:254:2097-2102.

30. Wolff FW, Lineman RD. Effects of treatment in hypertension: results of a controlled study. J Chronic Dis. 1966:19:227-240.

31. Sprackling ME, Mitchell JRA, Short AH, Watt G. Blood pressure reduction in the elderly: a randomised controlled trial of methyldopa. BMJ. 1981:283:1151-1153.

32. The IPPPSH Collaborative Group. Cardiovascular risk and risk factors in a randomized trial of treatment based on the beta-blocker oxprenolol: the International Prospective Primary Prevention Study in Hypertension (IPPPSH). J Hypertens. 1985:3:379-392.

33. SCOPE Trial Investigators. Primary results of SCOPE. Presented at: International Society of Hypertension. June 27, 2002; Prague, Czech Republic.

34. Hansson L, Lithell H, Skoog I, et al. study on cognition and prognosis in the elderly (SCOPE). Blood Press. 1999;8:177-183.

35. Barraclough M, Joy MD, MacGregor GA, et al. Control of moderately raised blood pressure: report of a co-operative randomized controlled trial. BMJ. 1973;3: 434-436.

36. Hypertension-Stroke Cooperative Study Group. Effect of antihypertensive treatment on stroke recurrence. JAMA. 1974;229:409-418.

37. Smith WM. Treatment of mild hypertension: results of a ten-year intervention trial. Circ Res. 1977; 40(5 suppl 1):l98-1105.

38. Perry Jr HM, Goldman Al, Lavin MA, et al. Evaluation of drug treatment in mild hypertension: VA-NHLBI feasibility study. Ann N YAcadSci. 1978:304: 267-288.

39. The Australian therapeutic trial in mild hypertension: report by the Management Committee. Lancet. 1980:1:1261-1267.

40. Kuramoto K, Matsushita S, Kuwajima I, Murakami M. Prospective study on the treatment of mild hypertension in the aged. Jpn Heart J. 1981;22:75-85.

41. Amery A, Birkenhager W, Brixko P, et al. Mortality and morbidity from the European working party on high blood pressure in the elderly trial. Lancet. 1985; 1:1349-1354.

42. Coope J, Warrender TS. Randomised trial of treatment of hypertension in elderly patients in primary care. BMJ. 1986:293:1145-1151.

43. Wilhelmsen I, Berglund G, Elmfeldt D, et al. Beta-blockers versus diuretics in hypertensive men: main results from the HAPPHY trial. J Hypertens. 1987;5:561-572.

44. Perry MH Jr, Smith WM, McDonald RH, et al. Morbidity and Mortality in the Systolic Hypertension in the Elderly Program (SHEP) pilot study. Stroke. 1989;20:4-13.

45. SHEP Cooperative Research Group. Prevention of stroke by antihypertensive drug treatment in older persons with isolated systolic hypertension: final results of the Systolic Hypertension in the Elderly Program (SHEP). JAMA. 1991;265:3255-3264.

46. Kostis JB, Davis BR, Cutler J, et al. Prevention of heart failure by antihypertensive drug treatment in older persons with isolated systolic hypertension. JAMA. 1997; 278:212-216.

47. Dahlof B, Lindholm LH, Hansson L, Schersten B, Ekbom T, Wester PO. Morbidity and mortality in the Swedish Trial in Old Patients with Hypertension (STOP-Hypertension). Lancet. 1991;338:1281-1285.

48. Medical Research Council Working Party. Medical Research Council trial of treatment of hypertension in older adults: principal results. BMJ. 1992;304: 405-412.

49. The Dutch TIA Trial Study Group. Trial of secondary prevention with atenolol after transient ischemic at-tack or nondisabling ischemic stroke. Stroke. 1993;24: 543-548.

50. PATS Collaborating Group. Post-Stroke Antihypertensive Treatment Study: a preliminary report. Chin Med J. (Engl). 1995;108:710-717.

51. Eriksson S, Olofsson BO, Wester PO. Atenolol in secondary prevention after stroke. Cerebrovasc Dis. 1995;5:21-25.

52. Borhani NO, Mercuri M, Borhani PA, et al. Final outcome results of the Multicenter Isradipine Diuretic Atherosclerosis Study (MIDAS): a randomized controlled trial. JAMA. 1996;276:785-791.

53. Staessen JA, Fagard R, Thijs L, et al, for the Systolic Hypertension in Europe Trial Investigators. Randomized double-blind comparison of placebo and active treatment for older patients with isolated systolic hypertension. Lancet. 1997;350:757-764.

54. Staessen JA. Thijs L, Birkenhager WH, Bulpitt CJ, Fagard R. Update on the Systolic Hypertension in Europe (SYST-EUR) Trial. Hypertension. 1999:33:1476-1477.

55. Rosei EA, Dal Palu C, Leonetti G, et al, for the VHAS Investigators. Clinical results of the Verapamil in Hypertension and Atherosclerosis Study (VHAS). J Hypertens. 1997; 15:1337-1344.

56. Estacio RO, Jeffers BW, Hiatt MR, Biggerstaff SL, Gifford N, Schrier RW. The effect of nisoldipine as compared with enalapril on cardiovascular outcomes in patients with non-insulin-dependent diabetes and hypertension. N Engl J Med. 1998;338:645-652.

57. Schrier RW, Estacio RO. Additional follow-up from the ABCD trial in patients with type 2 diabetes and hypertension. N Engl J Med. 2000;343:1969.

58. Tatti P, Pahor M, Byington RP, et al. Outcome results of the Fosinopril versus Amlodipine Cardiovascular Events Trial (FACET) in patients with hypertension and non-insulin dependent diabetes mellitus. Diabetes Care. 1998;21:597-603.

59. UK Prospective Diabetes Study Group. Tight blood pressure control and risk of macrovascular and micro-vascular complications in type 2 diabetes: UKPDS 38. BMJ, 1998;317:703-713.

60. UK Prospective Diabetes Study Group. Efficacy of atenolol and captopril in reducing risk of macrovascular and microvascular complications in type 2 diabetes: UKPDS 39. BMJ 1998:317:713-720.

61. National Intervention Cooperative Study in Elderly Hypertensives Study Group. Randomized double-blind comparison of a calcium antagonist and a diuretic in elderly hypertensives. Hypertension. 1999;34: 1129-1133.

62. Agodoa LY, Appel L, Bakris GL, et al. Effect of ramipril vs amlodipine on renal outcomes in hypertensive nephrosclerosis. JAMA. 2001;285:2719-2728.

63. Wright JT Jr, Bakris G, Green T, et al. Effect of blood pressure lowering and antihypertensive drug class on progression of hypertensive kidney disease: results from the AASK trial. JAMA. 2002:288:2421-2431.

64. Wright J, for the AASK Study Group Investigators. The African-American Study of Kidney Disease and Hypertension. Presented at: American Society of Hypertension; May 18, 2002; New York, NY.

65. PROGRESS Collaborative Group. Randomised trial of perindopril-based blood pressure-lowering regimen among 6105 individuals with previous stroke or transient ischaemic attack. Lancet. 2001:358:1033-1041.

66. Parving HH, Lehnert H, Brochner-Mortensen J, et al, for the Irbesartan in Patients with Type 2 Diabetes and Microalbuminuria Study. The effect of irbesartan on the development of diabetic nephropathy in patients with type 2 diabetes. N Engl J Med 2001 ;345: 870-878.

67. Lewis EJ, Hunsicker LG, Clarke WR, et al. Reno-protective effect of angiotensin-receptor antagonist irbesartan in patients with nephropathy due to type 2 diabetes. N Engl J Med 2001 ;345:851 -860.

68. The ANBP2 Investigators. Primary results of the Australian National Blood Pressure 2 Trial. Presented at: International Society of Hypertension; June 23-27,2002; Prague, Czech Republic.

69. Wing LMH, Reid CM, Ryan P, et al, for the Second Australian National Blood Pressure Study Group. A comparison of outcomes with angiotensin-converting enzyme inhibitors and diuretics for hypertension in the elderly. N Engl J Med 2003:348:583-592.

70. Black HR, Grimm J RH, Hansson L, et al. Con-trolled Onset Verapamil Investigation of Cardiovascular Endpoints: CONVICE primary results. Presented at: American Society of Hypertension; May 18,2002; New York, NY.

71. Zanchetti Z, Bond G, Hennig M, et al. Calcium antagonist lacidipine slows down progression of asymptomatic caroitd atherosclerosis: principal results of the European Lacidipine Study on Atherosclerosis (ELSA): a randomized, double-blind, long-term trial. Circulation. 2002:106:2422-2427.

72. Sewester CS, Dombek CE, Olin BR, Scott JA, Hebel SK, Novak KK, eds. Drug Facts and Comparisons. St Louis, Mo: Wolters Kluwer Co; 1996.

73. Berlin JA, Laird NM, Sacks HS, Chalmers TC. A comparison of statistical methods for combining event rates from clinical trials. Stat Med. 1989:8:141-151.

74. Bucher HC, Guyatt GH, Griffith LE, Walter SD. The results of direct and indirect treatment comparisons in meta-analysis of randomized controlled trials. J Clin Epi-demiol. 1997;50:683-691.

75. Ekbom T, Dahlof B, Hansson L, Lindholm SH, Schersten B, Wester PO. Antihypertensive efficacy and side effects of three beta-blockers and a diuretic in elderly hypertensives: a report from the STOP-Hypertension study. J Hypertens. 1992;10:1525-1530.

76. Alderman MH, Furberg CD, Kostis JB, et al. Hypertension guidelines: criteria that might make them more clinically useful. Am J Hypertens. 2002;15:917-923.

77. Yusuf S, Wittes J, Friedman L. Overview of results of randomized clinical trials in heart disease, I: treatments following myocardial infarction. JAMA. 1988; 260:2088-2093.

78. Soriano JB, Hoes AW, Meems L, Grobbee DE. Increased survival with beta-blockers: importance of ancillary properties. Prog Cardiovasc Dis. 1997;39: 445-456.

79. Heidenreich PA, McDonald KM, Hastie T, et al. Meta-analysis of trials comparing β-blockers, calcium antagonists, and nitrates for stable angina. JAMA. 1999; 281:1927-1936.

80. Heidenreich PA, Lee TT, Massie BM. Effect of beta-blockers on mortality in patients with heart failure: a meta-analysis of randomized clinical trials. J Am Coll Cardiol. 1997;30:27-34.

81. Lechat P, Packer M, Chalon S, Cucherat M, Arab T, Boissel JP. Clinical effects of beta-adrenergic blockade in chronic heart failure: a meta-analysis of double-blind, placebo-controlled, randomized trials. Circulation. 1998:98:1184-1191.

82. Task Force on the Management of Stable Angina Pectoris. Management of stable angina pectoris: recommendations of the Task Force of the European Society of Cardiology. Eur Heart J. 1997:18: 394-413.

83. Gibbons RJ, Chatterjee K, Daley J, et al. ACC/ AHA/ACP-ASIM guidelines for the management of patients with chronic stable angina: executive summary and recommendations. Circulation. 1999;99:2829-2848.

84. Ryan TJ, Antman EM, Brooks NH, et al. 1999 Update: ACC/AHA guidelines for the management of patients with acute myocardial infarction: executive summary and recommendations. Circulation. 1999;100: 1016-1030.

85. Braunwald E, Antman EM, Beasley JW, et al. ACC/ AHA guidelines for the management of patients with unstable angina and non-ST-segment elevation myocardial infarction: executive summary and recommendations. Circulation. 2000:102:1193-1209.

86. Williams SV, Fihn SD, Gibbons RJ. Guidelines for the management of patients with chronic stable angina: diagnosis and risk stratification. Ann Intern Med. 2001;135:530-547.

87. The Heart Outcomes Prevention Evaluation Study Investigators. Effects of an angiotensin-converting-enzyme inhibitor, ramipril, on cardiovascular events in high-risk patients. N Engl J Med 2000:342:145-153.

88. Flather MD, Yusuf S, Kober L, et al, for the ACE-Inhibitor Myocardial Infarction Collaborative Group. Long-term ACE-inhibitor therapy in patients with heart failure or left-ventricular dysfunction: a systematic overview of data from individual patients. Lancet. 2000; 355:1575-1581.

89. Garg R, Yusuf S, for the Collaborative Group on ACE Inhibitor Trials. Overview of randomized trials of angiotensin-converting enzyme inhibitors on mortality and morbidity in patients with heart failure. JAMA. 1995:273:1450-1456.

90. Pahor M, Psaty BM, Alderman MH, Applegate WB, Williamson JD, Furberg CD. Therapeutic benefits of ACE inhibitors and other antihypertensive drugs in patients with type 2 diabetes. Diabetes Care. 2000:23:888-892.

91. Cupples LA, D'Agostino RB. Some risk factors related to the annual incidence of cardiovascular disease and death using pooled repeated biennial measurements: Framingham Heart Study, 30-year follow-up. In: Kannel WB, Wolf PA, Garrison RJ, eds. The Framingham Study: an Epidemiological Investigation of Cardiovascular Disease. Bethesda, Md: National Institutes of Health; 1987. NIH No. 87-2703.

92. Song F, Altman DG, Glenny AM, Deeks JJ. Validity of indirect comparisons for estimated efficacy of competing interventions: empirical evidence from published meta-analyses. BMJ. 2003326:472.

93. BlackwelderWC. "Proving the null hypothesis" in clinical trials. Control Clin Trials. 1982:3:34 5-353.

94. Blackwelder WC, Chang MA. Sample size graphs for "proving the null hypothesis." Control Clin Trials. 1984:5:97-105.

95. Neaton JD, Grimm Jr RH, Prineas RJ, et al, for the Treatment of Mild Hypertension Research Group. Treatment of Mild Hypertension Study (TOMHS): final results. JAMA. 1993:270:713-724.

Combination Meta-Analysis of 354 Randomized Trials[220]

Design: Meta-analysis of 354 randomized double-blind placebo controlled trials of thiazides, beta-blockers, angiotensin-converting enzymes (ACE) inhibitors, angiotensin II receptor antagonists, and calcium channel blockers in fixed dose.

Conclusions: Combination low dose drug treatment increases efficacy and reduces adverse effects. From the average blood pressure in people who have strokes (150/90 mm Hg), three drugs at half standard dose are estimated to lower blood pressure by 20 mm Hg systolic and 11 mm Hg diastolic thereby reducing the risk of stroke by 63% and ischemic heart disease events by 46% at age 60-69.

Key Points:
- The efficacies of five categories of drugs are similar at standard doses and only 20% lower at half standard doses; adverse effects are much less common at half standard dose than at standard dose.
- The drugs are effective from all pretreatment levels of blood pressure.
- Reductions in blood pressure with drugs in combinations are additive; adverse effects are less than additive.
- Using three blood pressure lowering drugs in low dose combination would reduce stroke by two thirds and heart disease by half.

Prospective Clinical Trials in Hypertension Comparing Calcium Channel Blockers to Other Antihypertensive Therapy: Total of 29 Trials[160]

1. Placebo Controlled Published Trials (6 Trials)
   a. IDNT: Irbesartan Diabetes Nephrology Trial
   b. PREVENT: Prospective Randomized Evaluation of Vascular Effects of Norvasc Trial
   c. STONE: Shanghai Trial of Nifedipine in the Elderly
   d. SYSTEUR: Systolic Hypertension in Europe Trial
   e. CHEN DU: Nifedipine Trial in China
   f. SYST CHINA: Systolic Hypertension in China Trial

2. Placebo Controlled Trials in Progress (unpublished) (3 Trials)
   a. CLEVER: China's Lacidipine Event Reduction Trial
   b. BENEDICT: Bergamo Nephrology Diabetes Complication Trial
   c. ACTION: A Coronary Disease Trial Investigating Outcome with Nifedipine GITS

3. Comparison of Different Antihypertensive Drug Classes: Published Trials (15 Trials)
   a. AASK: African American Study of Kidney Disease and Hypertension
   b. ABCD: Appropriate Blood Pressure Control in Diabetes Trial
   c. ALLHAT: Antihypertensive Therapy and Lipid Lowering Heart Attack Prevention Trial
   d. CONVINCE: Controlled Onset Verapamil Investigation of Cardiovascular Endpoints
   e. INSIGHT: International Nifedipine GITS Study: Intervention as a Goal in Hypertension Trial

      f. NICS-EH: National Intervention Cooperative Study in Elderly Hypertensives

      g. NORDIL: Nordic Diltiazem Study

      h. STOP-2: Swedish Therapy in Old Patients with Hypertension

      i. VHAS: Verapamil in Hypertension and Atherosclerosis Study

      j. MIDAS: Multicenter Isradipine Diuretic Atherosclerosis Study

      k. HOT: Hypertension Optimal Treatment Trial

      l. PATE: Practioners Trial on the Efficacy of Antihypertensive Treatment in the Elderly

      m. GLANT: Study Group on Long-term Antihypertensive Therapy

      n. FACET: Fosinopril and Amlodipine Cardiac Events Trial

      o. PRESERVE: Prospective Randomized Enalapril Regression Study

4. Comparison of Different Antihypertensive Drug Classes: Unpublished Trials in Progress (5 Trials)

      *a. ELSA: European Lacidipine Study of Atherosclerosis

      b. INVEST: International Verapamil Trandolapril Study

      *c. SHELL: Systolic Hypertension in the Elderly Lacidipine Long-Term Study

      d. ASCOT: Anglo-Scandinavian Cardiac Outcomes Trial

      f. VALUE: Valsartan Antihypertensive Long-Term Use Evaluation

*Note: Recently Published

Clinical Hypertension Trials with Calcium Channel Blockers

1. STONE: Shanghai Trial of Nifedipine in the Elderly
2. SYST-EUR: Systolic Hypertension in Europe Trial
3. CHEN-DU: Nifedipine Trial
4. SYST-CHINA: Systolic Hypertension in China Trial
5. HOT: Hypertension Optimal Treatment Trial
6. NICS-EH: National Intervention Cooperative Study in Elderly Hypertensives
7. INSIGHT: International Nifedipine GITS Study: Intervention as a Goal in Hypertension Trial
8. NORDIL: Nordic Diltiazem Study
9. CONVNCE: Controlled Onset Verapamil Investigation of Cardiovascular Endpoints
10. PREVENT: Prospective Randomized Evaluation of Vascular Effects of Norvasc Trial
11. VHAS: Verapamil in Hypertension and Atherosclerosis Study
12. PATE: Practioners Trial on the Efficacy of Antihypertensive Treatment in the Elderly (Japan)
13. ALLHAT: Antihypertensive Therapy and Lipid Lowering Heart Attack Prevention Trial
14. STOP-2: Swedish Therapy in Old Patients with Hypertension
15. IDNT: Irbesartan Diabetes Nephrology Trial
16. AASK: African American Study of Kidney Disease and Hypertension
17. ABCD: Appropriate Blood Pressure Control in Diabetes Trial
18. ELSA: European Lacidipine Study of Atherosclerosis
19. INVEST: International Verapamil Trandolapril Study
20. SHELL: Systolic Hypertension in the Elderly Lacidipine Long-Term Study
21. MIDAS: Multicenter Isradipine Diuretic Atherosclerosis Study

1. **STONE** (*Journal of Hypertension* 1996;14:1237–1245)
   - Single blind
   - 1632 men and women (Chinese)
   - Age 60–79
   - 3-year study with 30-month mean followup
   - Nifedipine tablets 10 mg (not GITS)
   - Placebo control
   - Add on treatment: Captopril or HCTZ

Number and Significance of High-Incidence Endpoints

Original Treatment Assignment

	Number of Events		Significance (p)
	Placebo	Nifedipine	
All events	77	32	0.0001
CV events	59	24	0.0001
Strokes	36	16	0.0030
Severe arrhythmia	13	2	0.0007
Non-CV events	18	8	0.0366
All deaths	26	15	0.0614
CV deaths	14	11	0.4870

2. SYST–EUR (Lancet 1997; 350:757–764)
- Study Dates: 1990–1996, 198 centers
- 4695 patients > 60 years (average age 70)
- Two-thirds female
- BP: SBP 160–219 mm Hg
    DBP < 95 mm Hg
- Drugs
  Nitrendipine 10–40 mg qd
    (two-thirds on monotherapy)
  Enalapril 5–20 mg qd
  HCTZ 12.5–25 mg qd

SYST-EUR Results

	Placebo	Treatment
SBP (mm Hg)	13	23
DBP (mm Hg)	2	7

	Placebo (1000 pt. yrs)	Treatment (1000 pt. yrs)	% Reduction (p)
Total CVA	13.7	7.9	42% (.003)
Non-fatal CVA	10.1	5.7	44% (.007)
Cardiac total events	20.5	15.1	26% (0.03)
Non-fatal cardiac events	12.6	8.5	33% (0.03)
CV total	33.9	23.3	31% (.001)
CV mortality	13.5	9.8	27% (0.07)
CHF events	8.7	6.2	29% (0.12)
MI	8.0	5.5	30% (0.12)
MI deaths	2.6	1.2	56% (0.08)

Conclusions of SYST-EUR Study

1. Treatment of elderly patients with isolated systolic hypertension with nitrendipine reduces the rate of cardiovascular and cerebrovascular complications.
2. Treatment of 1000 patients for 5 years prevents 29 CVA or 53 major cardiovascular endpoints.

3. There was no increase in bleeding or cancer with nitrendipine compared with placebo.

4. Diabetic hypertensives had dramatic reductions in total mortality CV events, CVA, and coronary events on a CCB that was superior to diuretics and BB in SHEP (see pg. 57).

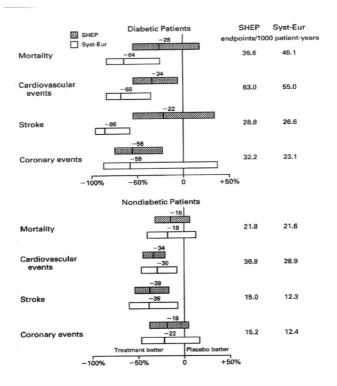

Outcomes in the Systolic Hypertension in the Elderly Program (SHEP) Trial. For these comparisons, the endpoints were standardized according to the definitions used in the SHEP trial. The two right-hand columns show the number of events per 1000 patient-years in the placebo groups in the two trials. The bars indicate the 95% confidence intervals. The numbers above the bars indicate the benefit of the active treatment as compared with placebo. (From Tuomilehto J, Rastenyte D, Birkenhäger W, et al: Effects of calcium-channel blockade in older patients with diabetes and systolic hypertension. N Engl J Med 1999; 340:677–684, with permission).

3. CHEN-DU Nifedipine Trial
- 683 hypertensive patients
- Cardiovascular events at 6 years reduced from 14.0% to 5.2% (p = 0.05) in treated group

4. Systolic Hypertension in China Trial[128]
- 2400 patients over 60 with ISH
- Nitrendipine vs. placebo
  Some received captopril or HCTZ
- Goal SBP < 150 mm Hg or 20 mm Hg decrease
- Median follow-up 2 years 10 months

SYST-CHINA Results

• All cause mortality	↓ 79%
• Cardiovascular mortality	↓ 32%
• Total fatal and non-fatal cardiovascular events	↓ 37%
• Congestive heart failure	↓ 58%
• Cerebrovascular accidents	↓ 58%
• Myocardial infarction	No difference
• Fatal cancer	No difference

5. Hypertension Optimal Treatment (HOT) Trial #1
- 18,700 patients, 26 countries, age 50–80
- DBP 100–115 mm Hg
- Randomized to 3 treatment groups
  DBP ≤ 90 mm Hg → 85.2% achieved
  DBP ≤ 85 mm Hg → 83.2% achieved
  DBP ≤ 80 mm Hg → 81.1% achieved
- Felodipine   78%
  ACEI   41%
  Beta-blockers   28%
  Diuretics   22%
- ASA vs. placebo

HOT Trial #2 Results
- Lowest incidence of major CV events at DBP 82.6 mm Hg
- Optimal SBP at 138.5 mm Hg
- CV risk reduced by 30% and is lower than that observed in prospective trials using diuretics or beta-blockers ($p < .05$)
- Quality of Life (QOL) improved in all groups, but most in DBP < 80 mm Hg
- ASA reduced CV events by 15%, MI by 36%, but no change in CVA. Non-fatal bleeds greater, but no difference in fatal bleeds
- No increased risk of CV even down to DBP of 70 mm Hg
- CV risk reduction was even more significant in diabetic hypertensives ($p < .005$)

6. **National Intervention Cooperative Study in Elderly Hypertensives (NICS-EH)**
   CCB vs. Diuretic
   - 414 patients, age > 60, started 1989
   - SBP 160-220 mm Hg
   - DBP < 115 mm Hg
   - Treatment: Nicardipine SR 20 mg bid vs. Trichlormethiazide 2 mg qd
   - 5 year follow-up in Japan
     CCB: 172/94 mm Hg → 147/81 mm Hg
     Diuretic: 173/93 mm Hg → 147/79 mm Hg
   - Results:
     Cardiovascular endpoints:
     CCB: 10.3%, Diuretic: 8.6%, P-value: NS
     Cardiovascular morbidity
     CCB: 27.8%, Diuretic: 26.8%, P-value: NS
     Rates per 1000 persons per year

Modified from National Intervention Cooperative Study in Elderly Hypertensives Study Group: Randomized double-blind comparison of a calcium antagonist and a diuretic in elderly hypertensives. Hypertension 1999;34:1129-1133.

Insight: [168]

1. Double-blind, prospective, randomized, 703 centers, 8 countries
2. Men and women 55-80 years of age with hypertension plus one additional risk factor
3. Nifedipine GITS vs. HCTZ/ amiloride + atenolol/ enalapril
4. Endpoints: fatal or non-fatal stroke, MI, or CHF
5. 4.5 year follow up. ITT analysis
6. 6321 patients
7. BP > 150/95 mm Hg or SBP > 160 mm hg (mean 173%)
8. Results:

Adverse effects

	Nifedipine (n=3157)		Co-amilozide (n=3164)		p
	n (%)	Number of patients withdrawn	n (%)	Number of patients withdrawn	
Adverse events					
All adverse events	1546 (49%)	539	1327 (42%)	304	<0.0001
Serious adverse events	796 (25%)	198	880 (28%)	245	0.02
Symptomatic adverse events					
Peripheral edema	896 (28%)	267	137 (4-3%)	14	<0.0001
Syncope	47 (1.5%)	9	89 (2.8%)	6	0.0004
Headache	384 (12%)	63	292 (9.2%)	32	0.0002
Palpitation	81 (2.5%)	4	86 (2.7%)	8	0.71
Peripheral vascular disorder	95 (3-0%)	3	168 (5.3%)	13	<0.0001
Impotence	50 (1.6%)	5	60 (1.9%)	6	0.34
Rushing	135 (4.3%)	40	74 (2.3%)	18	<0.001
Diabetes	96(3.0%)	1	137 (4.3%)	8	0.01
Dizziness	254 (8.0%)	21	318 (10.0%)	17	0.006
Gout	41 (1.3%)	0	67 (2.1%)	1	0-01
Accidental injury	41 (1.2%)	4	69 (2.2%)	4	0.007
Depression	124 (3.9%)	6	182 (5.7%)	13	0.0009
Metabolic adverse events					
Hypokalemia	61 (1.9%)	0	195 (6.2%)	8	<0.0001
Hyponatremia	8	0	61 (1.9%)	12	<0.0001
Hyperlipidemia	127 (4.0%)	0	202 (6.3%)	0	<0.0001
Hyperglycemia	178 (5.6%)	0	244 (7.7%)	4	0.001
Hyperuricemia	40 (1.3%)	3	201 (6.4%)	1	<0.001
Impaired renal function	58 (1.8%)	3	144 (4.6%)	18	<0.0001

Cardiovascular Endpoints

	Nifedipine	Co-amilozide	Odds ratio (95% CI)	P-value
Primary outcomes				
Composite	200 (6.3%)	182 (5.8%)	1.11(0.90-1.36)	0.34*
Myocardial infarction				
Non-fatal	61 (1.9)	56 (1.8)	1.09(0.76-1.58)	0.52
Fatal	16 (0.5)	5 (0.2)	3.22 (1.18-8.80)	0.017
Sudden death	17 (0.5)	23 (0.7)	0.74 (0.39-1.39)	0.43
Stroke				
Non-fatal	55 (1.7)	63 (2.0)	0.87 (0.61-1.26)	0.52
Fatal	12 (0.3)	11 (0.3)	1.09 (0.48-2.48)	0.84
Heart failure				
Non-fatal	24 (0.8)	11 (0.3)	2.20 (1.07-4.49)	0.028
Fatal	2 (0.1)	1 (<0.1)	2.01(0.18-2213)	0.63
Other cardiovascular death	13 (0.4)	12 (0.4)	1.09 (0.50-2.38)	0-85
Secondary outcomes				
Composite†	383(12.1)	397 (12.5)	0.96 (0.83-1.12)	0.62
Deaths				
All (first event)*	153 (4.8)	152 (4.8)	1.01 (0.80-1.27)	0.95
Noncardiovascular	71 (2.2)	66 (2.1)	1.08 (0.77-1.52)	0.67
Unknown cause	22 (0.7)	34 (1.1)	0.65 (0.38-1.11)	0.14
Cardiovascular	60 (1.9)	52 (1.6)	1.16(0.80-1.69)	0.4
Non-fatal	230 (7.3)	245 (7.7)	0.94 (0.78-1.13)	0.50
cardiovascular events				
Primary events	140 (4.4)	130 (4.1)	1.08 (0.85-1.38)	0.53
Angina (worsening or new)	57 (1.8)	77 (0.4)	0.74 (0.52-1.04)	0.10
Transient ischemic attacks	25 (0.8)	25 (0.8)	1.00(0.57-1.75)	1.0
Renal failure	8 (0.3)	13 (0.4)	0.62 (0.26-1.49)	0.38

* Myocardial infarction, stroke, heart failure, and cardiovascular death. †Primary * outcomes plus non-cardiovascular deaths, renal failure, angina, and transient 23 additional in nifedipine group and 20 in co-amilozide group occurred after a previous endpoint.

9. Conclusions

  a. More metabolic disorder on co-amilozide than Nifedipine including hypokalemia, hyponatremia, hyperuricemia, hyperglycemia and renal impairment.

  b. Fewer serious adverse effects with Nifedipine than co-amilozide.

  c. Equal BP reduction by 22/17 mm Hg to 138/82 mm Hg.

  d. More new onset DM with co–amilozide (p=0.02).

  e. Nifedipine and co-amilozide were equally effective in preventing overall cardiovascular and cerebrovascular morbidity and mortality.

  f. Wide CI and numbers of patients do not allow for definitive statistical analysis of some of the 10 and 20 endpoints with presumed significant p values such as fatal MI and non-fatal CHF.

  g. More decline in GFR with co-amilozide ($\downarrow$GFR by

2.3 ml/min/yr more than nifedipine (p=.001).

h. Incidence of impaired renal function with co-amilozide group was 4.6% vs. 1.8% in the nifedipine group (p=.001).

i. Nifedipine slowed cardiac calcification by EBT better than co-amilozide. At year 3 progression of coronary calcification was 77.85% with co-amilozide and only 40% with nifedipine.

NORDIL:[169]

1. Open-Blinded endpoint (probe) design
2. Men and women 50-69 (mean age 60) years of age with primary hypertension
3. Treatment: Diltiazem retard vs. diuretic and/or beta-blocker
4. Endpoints: Fatal and non-fatal MI, stroke or sudden death
5. Follow-up: 5 years (mean, 4.5 yr) ITT analysis
6. Sample size: 10,881 in 1032 in centers in Norway and Sweden
7. Blood pressure: DBP > 100 mm Hg mean study BP was diuretic = 151.7/88.7 mm Hg and diltiazem = 154.9/88.6 m
8. Results: (see charts on next page)

Relative Risk and Occurrence of Endpoints

	Number of patients with events		Event rate per 1000 patient-years		Relative risk (95% CI)*	p
	Diltiazem group	Diuretics and β-blocker group	Diltiazem group	Diuretics and β-blocker group		
Primary endpoint	403	400	16.6	16.2	1.00 (0.87-1.15)	0.97
All stroke	159	196	6.4	7.9	0.80 (0.65-0.99)	0.04
Fatal stroke	21	22	0.8	0.9	0.96 (0.52-1.74)	0.89
All stroke plus TIA	200	236	8.1	9.5	0.84 (0.70-1.01)	0.07
All myocardial infarction	183	157	7.4	6.3	1.16 (0.94-1.44)	0.17
Fatal myocardial infarction	28	25	1.1	1.0	1.10 (0.64-1.88)	0.74
Cardiovascular death	131	115	5.2	4.5	1.11 (0.87-1.43)	0.41
Total mortality	231	228	9.2	9.0	1.00 (0.83-1.20)	0.99
All cardiac events	487	470	20.2	19.2	1.04 (0.91-1.18)	0.57
Diabetes mellitus	216	251	9.4	10.8	0.87 (0.73-1.04)	0.14
Atrial fibrillation	105	128	4.2	5.1	0.82 (0.64-1.07)	0.14
CHF	63	53	2.5	2.1	1.16 (0.81-1.67)	0.42

TIA=transient ischemic attack; CHF=congestive heart failure. *Cox's regression model adjusted for age, sex, systolic pressure, and baseline status of diabetes mellitus and smoking.

Relative Risk and Occurrence of Endpoints with Diabetes Mellitus at Baseline

	Number of patients with events		Event rate per 1000 patient-years		Relative risk (95% CI)*	p
	Diltiazem group	Diuretics and β-blocker	Diltiazem group	Diuretics and β-blocker		
Primary endpoint	44	44	29.8	27.7	1.01 (0.66-1.53)	0.98
All stroke	20	20	13.3	12.3	0.97 (0.52-1.81)	0.92
Fatal stroke	1	3	0.6	1.8	0.29 (0.03-2.86)	0.29
All stroke plus TIA	20	23	13.3	14.2	0.85 (0.46-1.55)	0.6
All myocardial infarction	17	18	11.2	11.1	0.99 (0.51-1.94)	0.99
Fatal myocardial infarction	5	2	3.2	1.2	2.45 (0.47-12.8)	0.29
Cardiovascular death	15	13	9.7	7.8	1.16 (0.55-2.44)	0.71
Total mortality	28	26	18.1	15.6	1.07 (0.63-1.84)	0.80
All cardiac events	54	52	37.2	33.3	1.04 (0.71-1.53)	0.82
Atrial fibrillation	9	14	5.9	8.5	0.63 (0.27-1.46)	0.28
CHF	13	7	8.5	4.2	1.46 (0.57-3.72)	0.43

TIA=transient ischemic attack; CHF=congestive heart failure. *Cox's regression model adjusted for age, sex, systolic pressure, and smoking.

9. Conclusions
   a. Blood pressure reduction
      SBP: diuretic ↓23.3 mm Hg vs. diltiazem ↓20.3 mm Hg (p<0.001)
      DBP: diuretic = diltiazem (18.7 mm Hg)
   b. Fatal and non-fatal stroke more common in diuretic than diltiazem group despite lower BP (p=.04), a 20% reduction with diltiazem (corrected 32% for difference in SBP).
   c. Fatal and non-fatal MI were equal between groups (p=0.1) but the wide confidence intervals and lack of power make this conclusion more difficult to interpret.
   d. Significantly more adverse effects with diuretics related to fatigue, dyspnea and impotence (p<0.001) and with diltiazem related to headaches.
   e. Cardiovascular endpoints in DM were equal between the two treatment groups.

CONVINCE:[170, 210]

1. Double blind
2. Men and women 55 years or older with hypertension and one additional risk factor
3. Treatment: coer-verapamil vs. HCTZ or atenolol
4. Endpoints: first occurrence of non-fatal stroke, non-fatal MI or any CV-disease related death
5. Follow up: 6 years terminated early at 3 years.
6. 16,602 patients in 661 sites world-wide
7. Mean initial BP 157/87 mm Hg was reduced equally among the two groups.
8. All cause and CV mortality were equal between treatment groups but due to premature termination of the study only 729 events were reached (2200 events were projected for significance).

Results were consistant with meta-analysis done by ISH. (presented at ASH 2002 NY, NY).

Convince Trial[210]
Primary and Secondary Events by Treatment Assignment

	No. (%) of Participants with events			
	COER Verapamil	Atenolol or Hydrochlorothiazide	Hazard Ratio (95% Confidence Interval)	P Value
Primary (composite) outcome*	364 (4.5)	365 (4.4)	1.02 (0.88-1.18)	.77
Fatal or non-fatal myocardial infarction	133 (1.6)	166 (2.0)	0.82 (0.65-1 .03)	.09
Fatal or non-fatal stroke	133 (1.6)	118 (1.4)	1.15 (0.90-1.48)	.26
Cardiovascular disease-related death	152 (1 .9)	143 (1.7)	1.09 (0.87-1 .37)	.47
Primary event or cardiovascular hospitalization	793 (9.7)	775 (9.3)	1.05 (0.95-1.16)	.31
Angina pectoris	202 (2.5)	190 (2.3)	1.09 (0.89-1.33)	.39
Cardiac revascularization/cardiac transplant	163 (2.0)	166 (2.0)	1.01 (0.82-1.26)	.91
Heart failure	126(1.5)	100 (1.2)	1 .30 (1 .00-1 .69)	.05
Transient ischemic attack and/or carotid endarterectomy	89 (1.1)	105 (1.3)	0.87 (0.66-1.15)	.33
Accelerated/malignant hypertension	22 (0.3)	18(0.2)	1 .26 (0.67-2.34)	.47
Renal failure (acute/chronic)	27 (0.3)	34 (0.4)	0.81 (0.49-1.35)	.43
Death	337 (4.1)	319 (3.8)	1.08 (0.93-1.26)	.32
New cancer (excluding nonmelanoma skin cancer)	310 (3.8)	299 (3.6)	1.06 (0.91-1.24)	.46
Death	95 (1 .2)	93 (1.1)	1 .04 (0.79-1 .39)	.76
Death or hospitalization due to bleeding	118 (1.4)	79 (1.0)	1.54 (1.15-2.04)	.003
Deaths from bleeding	6 (0.1)	6 (0.1)	1.02 (0.33-3.17)	.97
Death or hospitalization due to serious adverse event	1381 (16.9)	1363 (16.4)	1.04 (0.97-1.12)	.29
Hospitalization for serious adverse event	1150 (14.1)	1143 (13.8)	1.03 (0.95-1.12)	.44

Abbreviation: COER, controlled-onset extended-release. *First occurrence of stroke, myocardial infarction, or cardiovascular disease-related death. † Does not include intracerebral bleeding, which was counted as a primary endpoint (stroke).

Incidence of Primary Outcome Measure Over Time

Figure 3.

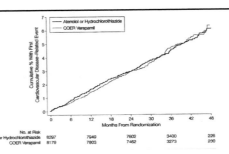

COER indicates controlled-onset extended-release. The COER verapamil group experienced 364 cardiovascular disease-related events and the atenolol or hydrochlorothiazide group experienced 365 (hazard ration, 1.02; 95% confidence interval, 0.88-1.18).

PREVENT:[171]

- 3 years, 825 patients with CHD
- Amlodipine vs. placebo
- No difference in CHD lesion by QCA
- Significantly reduced carotid atherosclerosis
    1. B-mode ultrasound (p <0.009)
    2. CWT decreases .0024 mm/year (amlodipine)
    3. CWT increased .0121 mm/year (placebo)
- 31% reduction in composite cardiovascular morbidity and mortality
    1. Non-fatal vascular events (CHF, unstable angina) 35% (p=0.02)
    2. Revascularization (CABG, PTCA) reduced by 46% (p=0.001)
- Amlodipine is effective in promoting regression of CWT which parallels a lower CV morbidity and mortality.

VHAS:[172]

- 498 hypertensive patients, 4 years
- Verapamil SR 240 mm Hg vs. chlorthalidone 25 mm Hg
- Mean thickness of carotid artery by B-mode ultrasound
  Verapamil – 0.082 mm/year/mm
  Chlorthalidone – 0.037 mm/year/ mm (p<.02)
- Total fatal and non-fatal CV events
  Verapamil – 19
  Chlorthalidone – 35 (p<.01)
- More metabolic abnormalities with chlorthalidone (glucose, K+, uric acid)
- BP reduction equal between groups
- Verapamil was more effective than the diuretic chlorthalidone in promoting regression of thicker carotid lesions which paralleled a lower CV event rate with verapamil.

PATE:[173]

1. Patients age 60 years and older with essential hypertension (mean BP 150/83 mm Hg)
2. Treatment: ACEI (delapril) vs. CCB (manidipine)
3. 3-year study in 699 patients
4. Results:
   a. Total mortality was equal
   b. Total CV morbidity and mortality was equal
   c. Possible "J curve" with SBP below 120 mm Hg related to cardiac events but not CVA
   d. BP reductions equal
   e. No difference in metabolic changes
   f. No difference in cancer morbidity and mortality

Incidence of Fatal and Non-fatal Cardiovascular Events[173]

	ACE-I (n = 699)			Calcium- Antagonist (n = 1049)		
	Event	Fatal	Ratio*	Event	Fatal	Ratio*
Cardiovascular events Fatal and non-fatal	34	7	22.5 X²test	50 P = .78 (event) P = .92 (fatal)	10	19.7
Cerebrovascular events	14	3	9.3 X²test	23 P = .79 (event) P = .68 (fatal)	6	9.1
Cerebral hemorrhage	3	2	2.0	4	4	1.6
Cerebral infarction	9	1	6.0	16	2	6.3
Transient ischemic attack (TIA)	2	1.3	3			1.2
Cardiac events	20	4	13.3 X²test	25 P = .54 (event) P = .35 (fatal)	3	9.9
Angina pectoris	12	8.0	16	1		6.3
Myocardial infarction	3	2	2.0	6	1	2.4
Heart failure	3	2	2.0	1	1	0.4
Severe arrhythmia	2		1.3	2		0.8
Other cardiovascular events Aortic aneurysm				2	1	0.8

* Number of events/1000 patient-years. ACE-I, angiotensin converting enzyme inhibitor.

Survival Analysis

	ACE-I	Calcium Antagonist	Risk Reduction*	CI	Statistics†
Total deaths	11 (1.6%)	18(1.7)	0.785	±0.019	0.9030
Cardiovascular event	7 (1.0%)	10 (1.0%)	0.788	±0.019	0.7127
Cerebrovascular event	3 (04%)	6 (0.6%)	0.787	±0.019	0.8317
Cardiac event	4 (06%)	3 (0.3%)	0.791	±0.019	0.2636
Other Cardiovascular event‡	0 (0.0%)	1 (0.1%)	0.788	±0.019	0.4278
Cancer	4 (0.6%)	8 (0.8%)	0.7886	±0.019	0.8033

* Reduced risk of endpoint on ACE-I compared with calcium antagonist with age adjustment.
† Log-rank test (survival analysis) with age adjustment.
‡ Other cardiovascular event, aortic aneurysm
CI–95% confidence interval; other abbreviations as in Table 2.

Incidence of Primary Outcome Measure Over Time

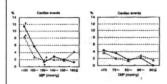

Incidence of cardiac events as a function of SBP and DBP reached by the treatment.
—●— : ACE-I group, - -△- - : Ca-antagonist group, * : p< .01; SBP 130~139 mm Hg v SBP < 120 mm Hg in both ACE-I group and Ca-antagonist group.

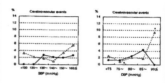

Incidence of cardiac events as a function of SBP and DBP reached by the treatment.
—●— : ACE-I group, - -△- - : Ca-antagonist group, * : p< .01; DBP≥ 90 mm Hg v DBP < 75~79 mm Hg in both ACE-I group and Ca-antagonist group.

Incidence of Cancer Morbidity and Mortality

	ACE-I (n = 699)			Calcium-Antagonist (n = 1049)		
Total	Event	Fatal	Ratio*	Event	Fatal	Ratio*
Cancer Cases	20	4	13.3	23	8	9.1
			X^2test	p = .538 (event)		
				p = .64 (fatal		

* Number of events/1000 patient-years. Abbreviations as in Table 2.

ALLHAT: [150]

On December 17, 2002, the National Heart, Lung and Blood Institute (NHLBI) released the Antihypertensive Lipid Lowering Heart Attack Trial (ALLHAT) study. This is the largest prospective clinical hypertension study to date with 42,418 patients randomized for 4 to 8 years (mean follow-up 4.9 years) in 623 clinical sites. This was a double-blind, randomized, multi-center clinical trial with a primary endpoint of fatal coronary heart disease (CHD) or non-fatal myocardial infarction (MI), and secondary endpoints of all cause mortality, stroke, combined CHD (non-fatal MI, CHD, death, coronary artery bypass graft [CABG], and hospitalization for angina), combined cardiovascular disease (CVD) (combined CHD, stroke, lower extremity revascularization, treated angina, fatal, hospitalized or treated congestive heart failure [CHF], hospitalized or outpatient peripheral arterial disease [PAD]), and finally other events such as renal outcomes (reciprocal serum creatinine, end-stage renal disease [ESRD], estimated glomerular filtration rate [GFR]) and cancer. Metabolic parameters such as cholesterol, potassium, glucose and new onset diabetes mellitus were also measured.

It is our belief that the results of this study have been largely misinterpreted and misquoted by the media. In fact, in the news release to the media, even the NHLBI had a misleading title with commissions and omissions that read as follows...."NHLBI finds Traditional Diuretics Better Than Newer Medications for Treating Hypertension." Patients and physicians are once again confused about the data and what to do in the treatment of hypertension. The Hypertension Institute was one of the study sites for ALLHAT, and the following is our interpretation of this hypertensive trial.

It is important to note that this study was performed in high risk patients with vascular disease or CHD risk factors in an older age group over 55 years of age (average age was 67 years) and a large percentage of women (47%), African Americans (35%), and type 2 diabetic patients (36%). The drugs compared were Chlorthalidone, Amlodipine, Lisinopril and Doxazosin (dropped early in the trial). The drugs were given once a day in the AM as follows:

Chlorthalidone 12.5 to 25 mg, Amlodipine 2.5 to 10 mg, and Lisinopril 10 to 40 mg. Add-on therapy (tier 2 drugs) could be Reserpine, Clonidine, Atenolol and finally Hydralazine as a tier 3 drug. The BP criteria for entry was untreated systolic or diastolic hypertension defined as greater than or equal to 140/90mm Hg, but less than or equal to 180/110mm Hg at two visits or treated by hypertension defined as less than or equal to 160/100mm Hg on 1 to 2 antihypertensive drugs at visit one, or less than or equal to 180/110 mm Hg at visit 2 when medication may have been withdrawn partially. The mean BP at entry was 146/84mm Hg. There were crossovers among the treatment groups of 7 to 9% at year five and about 40% of the patients in each group were on tier 2 medications with an average of at least 2 antihypertensive medications per patient.

What are the Primary Results?

1. Blood pressure:

   SBP: Amlodipine group was 1 mm Hg higher than the Chlorthalidone group (p < 0.05). Lisinopril group was 2 mm Hg higher than the Chlorthalidone group (p < 0.05). However the SBP was 4 mm Hg higher in the black population treated with Lisinopril than with Chlorthalidone (p < 0.01).

   DBP: Amlodipine group was 1mm Hg lower than the Chlorthalidone group (significant), and the Lisinopril group was the same as Chlorthalidone group.

   Therefore, **Amlodipine** was equally effective as **Chlorthalidone** in reducing mean arterial blood pressure. As is evident, although these small differences reached statistical significance because of the larger group sizes, the absolute differences are quite small. If one compares Chlorthalidone directly with Amlodipine, since each had <1 mm Hg difference compared to the other with systolic and diastolic respectively, there was no real difference. It should also be pointed out that significantly more patients enrolled in the Chlorthalidone arm than the other two (15,255 Chlorthalidone versus 9,048 for Amlodipine and 9,054 for Lisinopril) by design of the investigators. It was a "Heart Attack Trial" (HAT).

2. Primary endpoint of non-fatal MI and CHD death

Amlodipine = Chlorthalidone = Lisinopril. THERE WAS
NO SIGNIFICANT DIFFERENCE AMONG THE THREE
DRUGS (p =.65 for A/C and p =.81 for L/C.) C = 11.5%;
A = 11.3%; L = 11.4% (all 6 year rates).

The lack of any difference in the **primary endpoint** in this
study is a key and significant finding that was not clearly
emphasized in the press (remember this is a high risk, elderly,
hypertensive population). It also points out that the small BP
group differences had no clinical significance.

3. Secondary endpoints:

   a. **Stroke:** There was a trend towards Amlodipine being better
than Chlorthalidone with a 7% reduction in the Amlodipine group but this reduction was nonsignificant (p=.28).
Chlorthalidone was better than Lisinopril by 15% overall
(6.3% vs 5.6%; RR 1.15; 95% CI 1.02 - 1.30) (p < 0.02).
This was 40% less in the black population only, but there
was NO DIFFERENCE IN NON-BLACK POPULA-
TION... i.e. Lisinopril was as effective as Chlorthalidone
(NS) in the non-black population.

   b. **CHF:** Chlorthalidone was better than Amlodipine by 38%
(10.2% vs. 7.7%; RR 1.38; 95% CI 1.25 - 1.52 [6 years])
(p < 0.001) in preventing new onset non-fatal CHF.
Chlorthalidone was better than Lisinopril by 20% (8.7%
vs 7.7%; RR 1.19; 95% CI 1.07 - 1.31) (p < 0.001) in
preventing new onset of non-fatal CHF.

   c. **All cause mortality:**
The three treatment groups were identical for mortality.
For A/C p = .20 and for L/C p = .90.

   d. **Combined CVD** (combined CHD, stroke, lower extremity
revascularization, treated angina, fatal, hospitalized or
treated CHF, hospitalized or outpatient PAD); Amlodipine
equals Chlorthalidone

Lisinopril had a 10% higher rate compared to Chlorthalidone
(33.3% vs. 30.9%; RR 1.10; 95% CI 1.05 -1.16) (p< 0.001).

e. **Biochemical Results:**

Chlorthalidone caused significantly more hypokalemia despite supplementation (.3 to .4 mmol/L), which has been linked to sudden death, hyperglycemia, (3-5 mg%) hypercholesterolemia (1-2 mg%) and new onset diabetes mellitus (1.8 to 3.5%) than Amlodipine or Lisinopril ($p < 0.05$).

Chlorthalidone also induced significantly more reduction in GFR (7-8 ml/min decrease) over 4.9 years and increased serum creatinine more than either Amlodipine or Lisinopril ($p < 0.05$). This demonstrates a potentially greater risk for CRI and ESRD and future need for renal replacement therapy such as dialysis or transplant in the Chlorthalidone treated patients. The expected decrease in GFR over 4.9 years is about 3 to 5 ml/min. Thus, Chlorthalidone approximately doubled the expected decline in GFR.

There was no increased risk of cancer or GI bleeding in the Amlodipine or Lisinopril group.

Conclusions:

1. There is no difference in the **primary endpoint** of the study, fatal CHD, or non-fatal MI among the three treatment drug groups.

2. **All cause mortality** was identical among the three treatment groups.

3. Chlorthalidone was superior to Amlodipine and Lisinopril in the prevention of new onset, non-fatal CHF. With Lisinopril, this superiority was much more apparent in the black population.

4. Chlorthalidone was superior to Lisinopril in stroke prevention in blacks but not in non-blacks. Chlorthalidone was NOT better than Amlodipine in any subgroup of patients in stroke prevention.

5. Chlorthalidone induced more biochemical abnormalities such as hypokalemia, hyperglycemia and hypercholesterolemia than Amlodipine and Lisinopril.

6. Chlorthalidone produced significantly more new onset diabetes mellitus than Lisinopril and Amlodipine.

7. Chlorthalidone produced a significantly greater decline in GFR than Amlodipine and Lisinopril (7-8 ml/min). Expected rate is 3 to 5 ml/min. Thus, Chlorthalidone approximately doubled the decline in GFR during the study period.

8. Amlodipine trended toward superiority compared to Chlorthalidone in stroke prevention but it did not reach statistical significance.

9. Blood pressure control was better with Chlorthalidone than Lisinopril, but this control varied among the drugs, racial groups and between SBP and DBP. Chlorthalidone reduced SBP more than Amlodipine and Lisinopril, but Amlodipine reduced DBP more than Chlorthalidone. Thus, Amlodipine was equally effective as Chlorthalidone in lowering mean arterial pressure.

10. In order to get blood pressure from 146/86 to 134/75 required an average of 2 drugs.

Interpretation and Implications for Treatment of Hypertension

Most of the secondary outcome results in ALLHAT are driven by the reductions in CHF and the reductions in stroke in the black population. Some, but not all of the differences can be explained by the differences in blood pressure control as opposed to the specific drug class. For example, there was a 4 mm Hg difference in SBP in black patients in the Lisinopril vs. the Chlorthalidone groups. Based on meta-analysis studies this difference could account for up to a 16% difference in stroke incidence. In the CHF patients, a 4 mm Hg difference in SBP could account for up to a 21% difference in CHF and 6% reduction in CHD and MI. Therefore, if one corrects for the SBP difference of 4 mm Hg in the Lisinopril group, then the stroke and CHF reduction with Chlorthalidone are not as impressive (i.e. 24% and 0%) respectively. In fact, Lisinopril may have been better than Chlorthalidone related to CHD and MI risk by 6%. In addition, both Chlorthalidone and Amlodipine are long-acting antihypertensive agents that control BP beyond 24 hours, whereas Lisino-pril loses its antihypertensive effect at about 16 hours. Would longer acting ACEIs or those with tissue selectivity have done better as was seen in HOPE and PROGRESS? In both of these trials, a long acting tissue-selective ACEI was administered resulting in significant reductions in cardiovascular and cere-brovascular morbidity and mortality. In the HOPE trial, the small reduction in BP did not account for the dramatic reduc-tions in CV events, suggesting that the ACEI had non-hypoten-sive effects that were beneficial to the vascular system. The finial BP results could have been affected by the timing of the BP measurements. Also, the inaccuracy, observer bias or "rounding off effect," as well as the infrequency of cuff BP must be considered in ALLHAT.

The CHF differences may be explained by several theories:

1. Chlorthalidone is superior to other drugs.

2. Withdrawal of diuretics or other drugs at initiation of the study during randomization may have unmasked asympto-matic CHF and resulted in a greater frequency in the non-Chlorthalidone treated patients.

3. The improvement in other CVD endpoints may have shifted the CVD to CHF due to longer survival.

4. The definitions or clinical evaluation and diagnosis for CHF may not be accurate or consistent among the various clinical sites.

5. This is an elderly, high risk population with possible unrec-ognized CHF and, thus, a different population subset than younger, lower risk hypertensives, or it may simply reflect the better follow-up and evaluation in study patients.

6. The Chlorthalidone treated patients may have masked mild or silent CHF symptoms prospectively that would have bi-ased clinical evaluation.

7. It should be remembered that in controlled clinical trials of patients with CHF, over 10,000 patients have been treated with ACEI vs. placebo and the ACEI (or ARBs), improvement in CHF was better. This result is difficult to explain in contrast to ALLHAT.

What should physicians do now to treat Hypertension?

This study addresses only Chlorthalidone, not other diuretics, and suggests that new onset non-fatal CHF is reduced more than with the other two drugs studied. It also suggests that strokes in blacks (but not non-blacks) are reduced more than with Lisinopril, but not when compared to Amlodipine. However, with the caveats and BP differences above, is Chlorthalidone really better for CHF and strokes? How can these results be explained in view of the LIFE trial where an ARB was superior to a beta-blocker and in the HOPE and PROGRESS trials that used ACEIs?

What are the long-term implications for the kidney and decline in GFR with Chlorthalidone? How can ALLHAT be explained in view of the data with RENAAL, IDNT, IRMA, AASK, INSIGHT, HOPE and other studies? ESRD and dialysis are very expensive. Are there differences in specific drugs related to target organ protection?

What are the implications, long term, i.e. more than the 4-8 years of this study and the new onset diabetes and probable insulin resistance in the Chlorthalidone group related to CVD and ESRD? Type II diabetes mellitus is the most common cause of kidney failure in the U.S., but is not usually seen until more than a decade after onset. This increased risk of diabetes has enormous economic, morbidity and mortality issues that are not addressed in ALLHAT.

Based on the ALLHAT Trial, it is not recommended that Chlorthalidone or diuretics should be used as first-line initial treatment of hypertension.

What are the long-term implications for the biochemical abnormalities with Chlorthalidone?

Practically, most hypertensive patients will be on 3 to 4 hypertensive agents to reach new goal BP levels. These agents will need to be Chlorthalidone (or other low dose diuretic), Amlodipine, or other CCB, ACEI, or ARB, or possibly other medications. Control of BP and combination drugs must be paramount in the therapeutic regimen. Studies have suggested that in certain populations, the CCB, ACEI and ARB may actually be the preferred agents.

One must weigh the results of ALLHAT with other studies (HOT, LIFE, HOPE, PROGRESS, SYST-EUR, INSIGHT, MRFIT, NORDIL, MRC, OSLO, RENAAL, IDNT, IRMA, AASK and others). ALLHAT results do not support the results in all of these other clinical trials.

One must also evaluate the patient demographics, underlying CVD and renal diseases and risk factors to select the most appropriate initial drug or drug combinations. Side effects and contraindications to Chlorthalidone are important as well (sulfa allergy, pregnancy, metabolic and renal problems, etc.).

ALLHAT will create guidance, some clarifications but also confusion and criticism as the data is analyzed more carefully and the later subset studies are published. In the mean time, it is not clear just how much new data has really been generated from ALLHAT, and just how much it will change the practice of treating hypertension in practical terms. This story is unfolding and is far from over. All data is good if only to increase our questions and awareness of the complexity of treating hypertension. More studies are on the way with better and different designs and different population demographics that may challenge ALLHAT's ambiguous conclusions. It is known that elderly patients and those with concomitant CV risk factors, CV or renal disease respond sooner and with more benefit at equal BP reductions compared to younger patients and those without concomitant CV or renal disease. After all, ALLHAT was really a study of high risk, elderly hypertensives (average age = 67 years) and correlations to a younger population with different CV risks may not be accurate or appropriate.

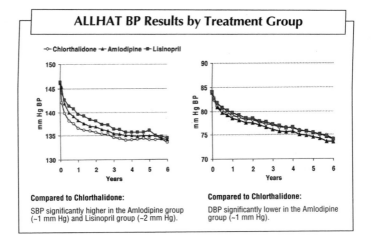

ALLHAT BP Results by Treatment Group

-○- Chlorthalidone -▲- Amlodipine -■- Lisinopril

Compared to Chlorthalidone:

SBP significantly higher in the Amlodipine group (~1 mm Hg) and Lisinopril group (~2 mm Hg).

Compared to Chlorthalidone:

DBP significantly lower in the Amlodipine group (~1 mm Hg).

ALLHAT Biochemical Results

	Chlorthalidone	Amlodipine	Lisinopril
Serum cholesterol – mg/dL			
Baseline	216.1 (43.8)	216.5 (44.1)	215.6 (42.4)
4 Years	197.2 (42.1)	195.6 (41.0)*	195.0 (40.6)*
Serum potassium – mmol/L			
Baseline	4.3 (0.7)	4.3 (0.7)	4.4 (0.7)*
4 Years	4.1 (0.7)	4.4 (0.7)*	4.5 (0.7)*
Estimated GFR† – mL/min/1.73m²			
Baseline	77.6 (19.7)	78.0 (19.7)	77.7 (19.9)*
4 Years	70.0 (19.7)	75.1 (20.7)*	70.7 (20.1)*

* p< .05 compared to Chlorthalidone

† Ann Itern Med. 1999; 130: 461-470

ALLHAT Biochemical Results
Fasting Glucose – mg/dL

	Chlorthalidone	Amlodipine	Lisinopril
Total			
Baseline	123.5 (58.3)	123.1 (57.0)	122.9 (56.1)
4 Years	126.3 (55.6)	123.7 (52.0)	121.5 (51.3)*
Among Baseline nondiabetics with baseline <126 mg/dL			
Baseline	93.1 (11.7)	93.0 (11.4)	93.3 (11.8)
4 Years	104.4 (28.5)	103.1 (27.7)	100.5 (19.5)*
Diabetes Incidence (follow-up fasting glucose ≥ 126 mg/dL)			
4 Years	11.6%	9.8%*	8.1%*

* p< .05 compared to Chlorthalidone

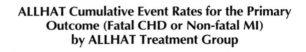

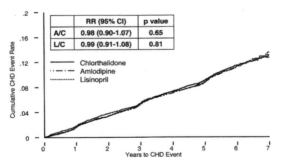

ALLHAT Cumulative Event Rates for the Primary Outcome (Fatal CHD or Non-fatal MI) by ALLHAT Treatment Group

	RR (95% CI)	p value
A/C	0.98 (0.90-1.07)	0.65
L/C	0.99 (0.91-1.08)	0.81

Chlorthalidone
Amlodipine
Lisinopril

Number at Risk:

Chlorthalidone	15,255	14,477	13,820	13,102	11,362	6,340	2,956	209
Amlodipine	9,048	8,576	8,218	7,843	6,824	3,870	1,878	215

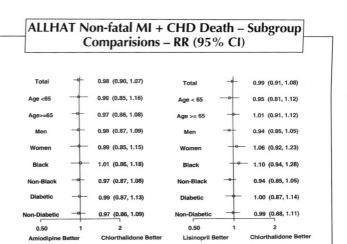

ALLHAT Non-fatal MI + CHD Death – Subgroup Comparisions – RR (95% CI)

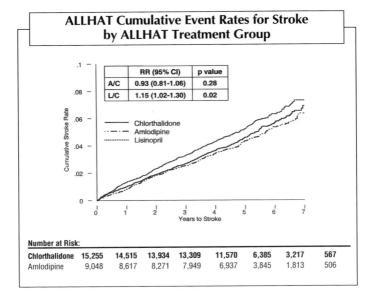

ALLHAT Cumulative Event Rates for Stroke by ALLHAT Treatment Group

	RR (95% CI)	p value
A/C	0.93 (0.81-1.06)	0.28
L/C	1.15 (1.02-1.30)	0.02

Number at Risk:

| Chlorthalidone | 15,255 | 14,515 | 13,934 | 13,309 | 11,570 | 6,385 | 3,217 | 567 |
| Amlodipine | 9,048 | 8,617 | 8,271 | 7,949 | 6,937 | 3,845 | 1,813 | 506 |

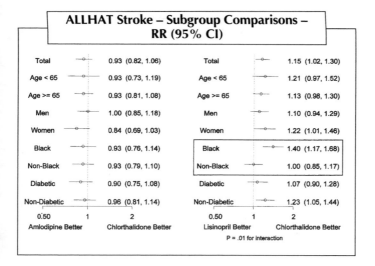

ALLHAT Stroke – Subgroup Comparisons – RR (95% CI)

Total	0.93 (0.82, 1.06)
Age < 65	0.93 (0.73, 1.19)
Age >= 65	0.93 (0.81, 1.08)
Men	1.00 (0.85, 1.18)
Women	0.84 (0.69, 1.03)
Black	0.93 (0.76, 1.14)
Non-Black	0.93 (0.79, 1.10)
Diabetic	0.90 (0.75, 1.08)
Non-Diabetic	0.96 (0.81, 1.14)

0.50 1 2
Amlodipine Better   Chlorthalidone Better

Total	1.15 (1.02, 1.30)
Age < 65	1.21 (0.97, 1.52)
Age >= 65	1.13 (0.98, 1.30)
Men	1.10 (0.94, 1.29)
Women	1.22 (1.01, 1.46)
Black	1.40 (1.17, 1.68)
Non-Black	1.00 (0.85, 1.17)
Diabetic	1.07 (0.90, 1.28)
Non-Diabetic	1.23 (1.05, 1.44)

0.50 1 2
Lisinopril Better   Chlorthalidone Better
P = .01 for interaction

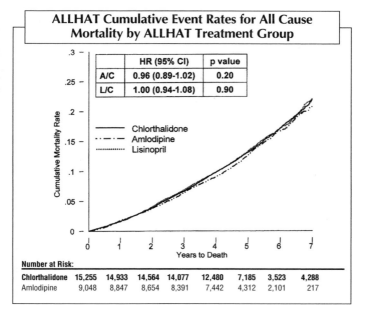

ALLHAT Cumulative Event Rates for All Cause Mortality by ALLHAT Treatment Group

	HR (95% CI)	p value
A/C	0.96 (0.89-1.02)	0.20
L/C	1.00 (0.94-1.08)	0.90

Chlorthalidone
Amlodipine
Lisinopril

Cumulative Mortality Rate

Years to Death

Number at Risk:

Chlorthalidone	15,255	14,933	14,564	14,077	12,480	7,185	3,523	4,288
Amlodipine	9,048	8,847	8,654	8,391	7,442	4,312	2,101	217

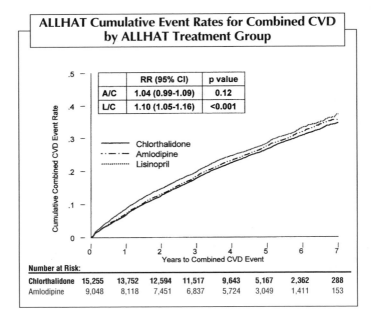

ALLHAT All Cause Mortality – Subgroup Comparisons – RR (95% CI)

Total	0.96 (0.89, 1.02)	Total	1.00 (0.94, 1.08)
Age < 65	0.96 (0.83, 1.10)	Age < 65	0.93 (0.81, 1.08)
Age >= 65	0.96 (0.88, 1.03)	Age >= 65	1.03 (0.95, 1.12)
Men	0.95 (0.87, 1.04)	Men	0.99 (0.91, 1.08)
Women	0.96 (0.86, 1.07)	Women	1.02 (0.91, 1.13)
Black	0.97 (0.87, 1.09)	Black	1.06 (0.95, 1.18)
Non-Black	0.94 (0.87, 1.03)	Non-Black	0.97 (0.89, 1.06)
Diabetic	0.96 (0.87, 1.07)	Diabetic	1.02 (0.91, 1.13)
Non-Diabetic	0.95 (0.87, 1.04)	Non-Diabetic	1.00 (0.91, 1.09)

0.50　　1　　2　　　　　　　　0.50　　1　　2
Amlodipine Better　Chlorthalidone Better　　Lisinopril Better　Chlorthalidone Better

ALLHAT Cumulative Event Rates for Combined CVD by ALLHAT Treatment Group

	RR (95% CI)	p value
A/C	1.04 (0.99-1.09)	0.12
L/C	1.10 (1.05-1.16)	<0.001

Cumulative Combined CVD Event Rate

—— Chlorthalidone
–·–·– Amlodipine
·········· Lisinopril

Years to Combined CVD Event

Number at Risk:

Chlorthalidone	15,255	13,752	12,594	11,517	9,643	5,167	2,362	288
Amlodipine	9,048	8,118	7,451	6,837	5,724	3,049	1,411	153

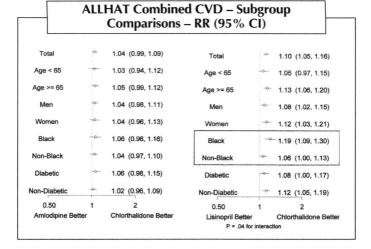

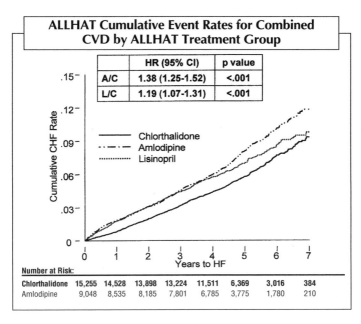

ALLHAT Heart Failure – Subgroup Comparisons – RR (95% CI)

Total	1.38 (1.25, 1.52)	
Age < 65	1.51 (1.25, 1.82)	
Age >= 65	1.33 (1.18, 1.49)	
Men	1.41 (1.24, 1.61)	
Women	1.33 (1.14, 1.55)	
Black	1.47 (1.24, 1.74)	
Non-Black	1.33 (1.18, 1.51)	
Diabetic	1.42 (1.23, 1.64)	
Non-Diabetic	1.33 (1.16, 1.52)	

0.50   1   2
Amlodipine Better   Chlorthalidone Better

Total	1.20 (1.09, 1.34)	
Age < 65	1.23 (1.01, 1.50)	
Age >= 65	1.20 (1.06, 1.35)	
Men	1.19 (1.03, 1.36)	
Women	1.23 (1.05, 1.43)	
Black	1.32 (1.11, 1.58)	
Non-Black	1.15 (1.01, 1.30)	
Diabetic	1.22 (1.05, 1.42)	
Non-Diabetic	1.20 (1.04, 1.38)	

0.50   1   2
Lisinopril Better   Chlorthalidone Better

STOP-2:[176]

Swedish Trial in Old Patients–2 (STOP-2)

6614 Patients 70-84 years – 5 years

SBP ≥ 1880 mm Hg, DBP ≥ 105 mm Hg

Diuretic or BB vs. CCB or ACEI

Equal BP Reduction

CV Morbidity and Mortality was Equal

Conventional	19.8 events/1000	ACEIs 20.5 events/1000
New Drugs	19.8 events/1000	ACEIs 19.2 events/1000
Last Visit:	46% on 2 drugs	
	61-66% on initial drugs	
Drug Combinations:	BB + Diuretic	
	CCB + BB	
	ACE + Diuretic	
Specific Drugs:	BBs: Atenolol, Metoprolol, Pindolol	
	Diuretics: Hydrochlorothiazide, Amiloride	
	ACEs: Enalapril, Lisinopril	
	CCBs: Felodipine, Isradipine	

Adapted from Hansson L, Lindholm LH, Ekbom T, et al, for the STOP-Hypertension-2 Study Group: Randomized trial of old and new antihypertensive drugs in elderly patients: Cardiovascular mortality and morbidity, the Swedish Trial in Old Patients with Hypertension-2 Study. Lancet 1999; 354: 1751-1756.

STOP-2
Relative Risk of CV Mortality and Morbidity for all Newer Drugs vs. Conventional Drugs[†]

	Relative Risk* (95% CI)	p	Newer Drugs better	Conventional drugs better
Cardiovascular mortality	0.99 (0.84-1.16)	0.8		
All myocardial infarction	1.04 (0.86-1.26)	0.6		
All stroke	0.89 (0.76-1.04)	0.1		
All major cardiovascular events	0.96 (0.86-1.08)	0.4		
Total mortality	1.01 (0.89-1.14)	0.9		
Frequency of diabetes mellitus	0.96 (0.75-1.23)	0.7		
Frequency of atrial fibrillation	1.09 (0.92-1.31)	0.3		
Frequency of congestive heart failure	0.95 (0.79-1.14)	0.5		

* Adjusted for age, sex, diabetes, diastolic blood pressure and smoking.
† Conventional drugs = atenolol, metoprolol, pindolol, hydrochlorothiazide, amiloride
CCBs = felodipine, isradipine

STOP-2
Relative Risk of CV Mortality and Morbidity for all ACE Inhibitors vs. Conventional Drugs[†]

	Relative Risk* (95% CI)	p	ACE Inhibitors better	Conventional drugs better
Cardiovascular mortality	1.01 (0.84-1.22)	0.8		
All myocardial infarction	0.90 (0.72-1.13)	0.3		
All stroke	0.90 (0.74-1.08)	0.2		
All major cardiovascular events	0.94 (0.82-1.07)	0.3		
Total mortality	1.02 (0.89-1.18)	0.7		
Frequency of diabetes mellitus	0.96 (0.72-1.27)	0.7		
Frequency of atrial fibrillation	1.15 (0.94-1.41)	0.1		
Frequency of congestive heart failure	0.83 (0.67-1.03)	0.09		

* Adjusted for age, sex, diabetes, diastolic blood pressure and smoking.
† Conventional drugs = atenolol, metoprolol, pindolol, hydrochlorothiazide, amiloride
CCBs = felodipine, isradipine

STOP-2
Relative Risk of CV Mortality and Morbidity for Calcium Antagonists vs. Conventional Drugs[†]

	Relative Risk* (95% CI)	p	Calcium antagonists better	Conventional drugs better
Cardiovascular mortality	0.97 (0.80-1.17)	0.72		
All myocardial infarction	1.18 (0.95-1.47)	0.13		
All stroke	0.88 (0.73-1.06)	0.16		
All major cardiovascular events	0.99 (0.87-1.12)	0.85		
Total mortality	0.99 (0.86-1.15)	0.90		
Frequency of diabetes mellitus	0.97 (0.73-1.29)	0.83		
Frequency of atrial fibrillation	1.04 (0.85-1.29)	0.68		
Frequency of congestive heart failure	1.06 (0.87-1.31)	0.56		

* Adjusted for age, sex, diabetes, diastolic blood pressure and smoking.
† Conventional drugs = atenolol, metoprolol, pindolol, hydrochlorothiazide, amiloride
CCBs = felodipine, isradipine

STOP-2
Relative Risk of CV Mortality and Morbidity for Ace Inhibitors vs. Calcium Antagonists[†]

	Relative Risk* (95% CI)	p	ACE inhibitors better	Calcium antagonists better
Cardiovascular mortality	1.04 (0.86-1.26)	0.72		
All myocardial infarction	0.77 (0.61-0.96)	0.018		
All stroke	1.02 (0.84-1.24)	0.84		
All major cardiovascular events	0.95 (0.83-1.08)	0.42		
Total mortality	1.03 (0.89-1.19)	0.71		
Frequency of diabetes mellitus	0.98 (0.74-1.31)	0.91		
Frequency of atrial fibrillation	1.10 (0.90-1.34)	0.37		
Frequency of congestive heart failure	0.78 (0.63-0.97)	0.025		

* Adjusted for age, sex, diabetes, diastolic blood pressure and smoking.
† Conventional drugs = atenolol, metoprolol, pindolol, hydrochlorothiazide, amiloride
CCBs = felodipine, isradipine

All five STOP-2 charts above are reprinted with the permission from Hansson L, Lindholm LH, Ekbom T, et al, for the STOP-Hypertension-2 Study Group: Randomized trial of old and new antihypertensive drugs in elderly patients: Cardiovascular mortality and morbidity the Swedish Trial in Old Patients with Hypertensive-2 Study. Lancet 1999; 354: 1751-1756.

Conclusions:

1. CV morbidity and mortality was equal among the drug combination groups, but the CCB + ACEI combinations were not studied in STOP-2.
2. ACEI vs. CCB results in a significantly reduced rate of all MI (p = 0.018) and CHF (p = 0.025).
3. ACEI & CCB was significantly better (25%) then diuretic/beta-blocker in preventing stroke in elderly patients with ISH. *(Blood Pressure 2004; 13:137-143).*

IDNT:[177]

1. 1,715 hypertensive patients with nephropathy due to type 2 diabetes with severe proteinuria (mean >1 gram per 24 hours)
2. Irbesartan vs. amlodipine vs. placebo
3. Mean treatment 2.6 years
4. Results
a. Irbesartan reduced risk of primary composite endpoint of doubling of creatinine ESRP or death by 20% vs. placebo (p=.02) and by 23% vs. amlodipine (p=.006).
   1) Risk of doubling of creatinine was 33% lower in irbesartan vs. placebo (p=.0030 and 37% lower in irbesartan vs. amlodipine (p< 0.001).
   2) ESRD risk was 23% lower with irbesartan vs. placebo or amlodipine (p=.07).
   3) Serum creatinine increased 24% more slowly in the irbesartan group than in the placebo group (p=0.008) and 21% more slowly than in the amlodipine group (p=0.02).
   4) Protection of renal function is independent of BP.
b. There were no significant differences in the rates of death from any cause or in the cardiovascular composite endpoint (CV mortality, non-fatal MI, CHF requiring hospitalization, CVA, or LE amputation).

AASK:[178]

1. 1094 African Americans age 18 to 70 years with non-diabetic hypertensive renal disease (GFR 20-65 ml/min/1.73 m)

2. Randomized DB prospective 3x2 factorial trial, 4 year

3. Compare 2 levels of BP and 3 antihypertensive drugs on GFR decline

4. BP levels MAP = 102 to 107 mm Hg or MAP < 92 mm Hg

5. Drugs: metoprolol vs. ramipril vs. amlodipine (open labels added drugs to BP control)

6. Outcomes measured
   a. Rate of change in GFR (GFR slope)
   b. Clinical composite outcome or reduction in GFR by 50% or more or > 25 ml/min from baseline
   c. ESRD
   d. CVD events
   e. Death

7. Results
   a. Mean GFR slope did not differ between 2 BP groups.
   b. Clinical composite outcome did not differ between 2 BP groups.
   c. No difference in GFR slope among the 3 drugs
   d. Ramipril reduced clinical composite outcomes by 22% vs. metoprolol (p=0.04) and by 38% vs. amlodipine (p=0.004). There was no difference between amlodipine and metoprolol.
   e. However, it was only in those patients with overt severe renal disease and 1gm protein / 24 hours (1/3 of patients) that the ACEI or BB were better at slowing rate of GFR decline and delaying time to renal events than amlodipine.
   f. In the remaining 2/3 of patients with mild to moderate renal disease and less than 1 gm of protein/ 24 hours, amlodipine was as effective as ACEI in delaying or slowing the progression of renal disease (GFR).
   g. BP was similar in all 3 arms.
   h. No difference in CVD events among the 3 arms.
   i. Finally, if one evaluates the effects in those patients

with < 300 mg protein/24 hours (urine protein/creatinine ratio < 0.22) then there was no difference between amlodipine and ramipril related to decline in GFR.

Only in those patients with >1gm protein/24 hours (urine protein/creatinine ratio > 0.66) (1/6 of total patients) was the overall change in GFR significantly less in the ACEI treated group.

ABCD:[179]

1. 470 patients with hypertension and diabetes type 2
2. 5.3 year follow-up. Endpoint: GFR by 24 hr CRC1
3. Nisoldipine vs. Enalapril
4. DBP > 90 mm Hg at baseline to goal DBP < 75 vs. DBP 80-89 mm Hg
5. Actual study mean BP
   Group I   132/78
   Group II   138/86
6. Results:
   a. BP control in both groups with either Nisoldipine or Enalapril-stabilized renal function in those without overt albuminuria.
   b. All cause mortality decreased.
   c. Despite an increase in CV events in the CCB group, this study was not powered or designed to determine this outcome, and is thus inconclusive.

ELSA:[181,207]

1. Prospective, randomized, double-blind, multinational trial
2. 2334 patients followed for 4 years. Ages 45-75 years
3. Treatment: Lacidipine vs. Atenolol (+ HCTZ)
4. BP levels at entry: 150-210/95-115 mm Hg
5. Endpoints: carotid atherosclerosis measured by maximal IMT with B-Mode ultrasound.
6. Results
   a. Lacidipine IMT progression rate = 0.0087 mm/year 40% reduction vs. atenolol (P=0.0073).

    b. Atenolol IMT progression rate=0.0145 mm/ year
    c. Lacidipine has less plaque progression and more
       plaque progression than atenolol.
    d. BP reductions were equal in clinical, but 24 hr arm
       showed atenolol to be more effective (-10 / 9 mm Hg
       vs. –7/5 mm Hg).
    e. Trend toward relative reduction in CVA, major CV
       events and mortality with lacidipine vs. atenolol (NS)
  7. Conclusions

Lacidipine has anti-atherosclerotic actions independent of BP
and is superior to atenolol despite the lacidipine group having
higher 24 hour BM, more smokers, and less use of statins and
anti-platelet drugs.

INVEST:[182, 183]

1. 27,000 CHD patients with hypertension in 1500 centers, mostly elderly > 60 yrs. Abnormal coronary angiogram or H/O or MI
2. Treatment: Verapamil/Trandolapril vs. Atenolol / HCTZ-(V/T vs. A/H).
3. Outcomes: All cause mortality, non-fatal MI, non-fatal CVA
4. Substudies on ABM, depression, QOL, genotyping
5. V/T treatment equals A/H treatment for BP control and all CV events
6. More D/M in A/H group. More CHF in V/T group *JAMA 2003; 290:2805-2816).*

SHELL:[184,208]

1. Open, blinded endpoint (probe), 4800 patients,
2. 1882 men and women age 60 years and over with ISH
3. ISH with SBP > 160 mm hg and DBP < 95 mm Hg
4. Treatment: Lacidipine vs. Chlorthalidone (L vs. C)
5. Endpoints: cardiovascular and cerebrovascular
6. Follow up 5 years in 115 centers in Italy
7. Substudies: 24 hr. ABM and ECHO
8. Equal BP reductions: Chlorthalidone: 36.8/8.1 mm Hg Lacidipine : 38.4/7.9 mm Hg
9. Total CV morbidity and mortality equal
10. L=C in reduction in SBP, CV events and total mortality. *(Blood Pressure 2003; 12:160-167).*

MIDAS: [185]

1. 883 patients with hypertension 149.7 + 16.6 / 96.5 + 5.1 mm Hg
2. Average age 58 years, 3 year study
3. Randomized, double-blind trial in 9 centers
4. Outcome: compare rate of progression of mean maximal IMT in carotid arteries with quantitative B-mode ultrasound
5. Treatment: Isradipine vs. HCTZ
6. Results
   a. No difference in rate of progression of mean maximum IMT between the two treatment groups
   b. HCTZ reduced BP more than isradipine 19.5 mm Hg vs. 16 mm Hg (p=0.002)
   c. DBP was reduced equally in the two groups.
   d. Higher incidence of vascular events CMI, CVD, CHF, angina, sudden death in isradipine vs. HCTZ group but it was not significant (p=.07)
   e. Higher increase in non-major vascular events and procedures, femoral-popliteal bypass graft in isradipine group (p=0.2)
7. Conclusions:
   The lack of power, study design and higher SBP in the Isradipine group make the IMT and CV outcome data inconclusive.

GLANT: [174, 175]

1. 1936 Japanese patients with mild to moderate essential hypertension. Mean age of 60 years
2. ACE inhibitor (Delapril) vs. CCB (various) such as short, intermediate and long acting CCB
3. 1 year study, prospective open trial
4. BP reduction greater with CCB vs. ACEI (p<0.001)
5. Cardiovascular and cerebrovascular morbidity and mortality were equal between groups.

FACET:[180]

1. 380 patients with NIDDM and hypertension
2. BP > 140/90 mm Hg
3. Amlodipine vs. Fosinopril
4. 3.5 year follow-up
5. Results
    a. BP control equal
    b. Metabolic parameters equal (lipids, Hg A_1,C, glucose)
    c. Despite a lower combined CV outcome (MI, CVA, angina) with Fosinopril, this study was not designed nor powered to evaluate clinical outcomes, thus the CV outcome data is *inconclusive*.

PRESERVE:[186]

- Nifedipine GITS vs. Enalapril
- 303 men and women with essential hypertension and increased LV mass by ECHO
- 48 week study
- BP reductions equal 22/12 mm Hg in 2 groups
- LV mass index reduction equal in 2 groups

ACTION:[160]

- 6000 patients with CHD over age 34 years
- Nifedipine GITS-DHP-CCB vs. placebo
- 5 year study

ASCOT:[160]

- 19,000 patients with hypertension and CVD risk
- Age 39-79 years
- BP > 139/89 mm HG
- Amlodipine ± Perindopril (DHP CCB ± ACEI) vs.
  BB ± Diuretic (Atenolol + Bendroflumethiazide)
  Cholesterol lowering vs. placebo ARM
- 5 year study
- Lipid arm stopped at 3 years (prematurely)
  Atorvastatin treated subjects had a 36% reduction in CHD
  and MI and a 27% reduction in CVA. These were hypertensive patients on a fixed dose of Atorvastatin (10 mg)
  daily. The reduction in CV events was independent of the
  initial LDL-C baseline level.
- The blood pressure part of the ASCOT trial was stopped
  in November 2004 because of cardiovascular benefits in
  favor of the newer calcium channel blocker plus angiotensin converting enzyme inhibitor treatment (am-
  lodipine+ perindopril) when compared with the beta-
  blocker, atenolol and the thiazide diuretic,
  bendroflumethiazide.
- The Steering Committee of ASCOT accepted on November 18, 2004 the recommendation of its Data Safety Monitoring Board that the blood pressure arm of the trial should
  be stopped and the majority of patients have now been informed. This announcement signals the end of the main
  clinical elements of the ASCOT trial, launched in 1997.
- The 19,000 patient Anglo-Scandinavian Cardiac Outcomes Trial (ASCOT) had been comparing a new treatment strategy for hypertension against an old one in order to discover which is better at preventing various
  cardiovascular events such as heart attacks and strokes.
  The complete results of the ASCOT trial will be made
  available when all data up to and including the last individual visit have been collected and analyzed. Investigators and patients will be informed of the final results of
  ASCOT when these data become available. The results
  will be published in the scientific press.

VALUE:[160]

- 15,313 patients with hypertension and CVD risk
- Age over 49 years
- BP> 210/115 mm Hg Valsartan (ARB) vs. DHP- CCB (Amlodipine)
- 6 year study
- Amlodipine reduced BP more than Valsartan
- Composite cardiac morbidity and mortality was equal with Amlodipine and Valsartan. *(Lancet 2004; 363:2022-2031)* (see page 194 for details)

CLEVER:[160]

- 10,000 patients with hypertension and CVD risk
- Age over 54 years
- BP 160/210 to 95-115 mm Hg
- DHP-CCB vs. placebo
- 3 year study

BENEDICT:[160]

- 2,400 patients with hypertension and DM
- Age over 39 years
- BP > 139 / 89 mm Hg
- ACEI vs. NDHP-CCB vs. placebo
- 3 year study

Summary of Published Hypertension Clinical Trials Involving Primarily Calcium Channel Blockers (CCBs)

1. The CCBs lower SBP and DBP as monotherapy equal to or better than all the other antihypertensive agents. This reduction is especially true in black and elderly hypertensive patients.

2. Both dihydropyridine and non-dihydropyridine CCB significantly reduce total mortality, cardiovascular, cerebrovascular and renal morbidity and mortality equal to or better than traditional conventional therapy with diuretics and beta-blockers. The combination of DHP-CCB with ACEI reduces CV events significantly better than a diuretic/BB combination (ASCOT Trial).

3. Coronary heart disease, fatal and non-fatal myocardial infarction are reduced significantly with CCB (Amlodipine) and this reduction is equal to that of diuretics (ALLHAT) and better than beta-blockers. However in the post-MI patient the non-DHP CCB may confer a survival advantage. The DHP-CCBs and diuretics are relatively contraindicated in the acute MI patient.

4. Cerebrovascular accidents including ischemic stroke and intracranial hemorrhage are reduced significantly more with CCBs (10-15% better) in most studies and there is a consistent trend in most other studies compared to diuretics, beta-blockers and ACEIs and ARBs. The DHP-CCB are superior to the none DHP-CCB in reducing ischemic CVA. Amlodipine is equal to Valsartan in reducing total cardiac events and mortality. Dementia may be prevented more with CCBs, particularly the DHP-CCB (SYST-EUR study), in the treatment of hypertension than with other antihypertensive agents. The CCBs reduce local cerebral resistance and correct the focal hypoperfusion without inducing a steal effect in patients with ICA stenosis, thus preserving total cerebral perfusion.

154

5. Congestive heart failure may not be prevented as well with DHP-CCB as it is with diuretics and beta-blockers, but study design, definitions of CHF, unmasking of asymptomatic CHF or masking of CHF in a prospective fashion, may confound the interpretation of the true incidence of CHF, thus making the literature inconclusive on this point. Non DHP-CCB should not be used in systolic CHF. However, CCBs improve diastolic relaxation and are excellent choices in the treatment of diastolic dysfunction and diastolic CHF.

6. Renal insufficiency (mild to moderate) with 24-hour urine protein less than 300 mg is prevented and treated as well with a dihydropyridine or non-dihydropyridine CCB compared to diuretics, beta-blockers, ACEIs and ARBs. However in severe renal insufficiency, if the 24-hour urine excretion is over 1000 mg per day, then an ACEI or ARB are preferred agents. Adding a CCB to an ACEI or ARB is very effective in reducing proteinuria and improving renal function. The combination of an ARB and CCB, in preliminary studies appears to be as effective as the ACEI and CCB combination. The non-DHP CCB would be the second preference agents. With mild to moderate renal insufficiency with 24 hour urine protein excretion between 300 mg and 1000 mg per 24 hours, either a CCB, ACEI, ARB, or beta-blocker may result in equivalent renoprotection, although the data with beta-blockers is less convincing and prospective clinical studies are fewer in number with lower numbers of subjects.

It should be noted, however, that certain diuretics, such as Hydrochlorothiazide, Chlorthalidone and other thiazide-like diuretics may promote nephrotoxicity, and increase the development of microalbuminuria, proteinuria and progression of renal insufficiency to ESRD. This nephrotoxicity etc. does NOT appear to be the case with the diuretic Indapamide, which is renoprotective.

7. The CCBs are metabolically neutral or favorable on all biochemical parameters including serum glucose, lipids, potassium, magnesium, sodium, homocysteine, uric acid and other blood tests. In addition, compared to diuretics, there is signfi-

cantly less new onset type 2 diabetes with the CCBs. CCBs improve insulin sensitivity, similar to ACEIs and ARBs.

8. The CCBs have anti-atherosclerotic effects in which they reduce progression and improve regression of IMT in carotid arteries and plaques in both carotid and coronary atereries that are independent of their antihypertensive effects. This includes the coronary arteries and carotid arteries in studies to date as evaluated by EBT, coronary arteriography, and B-mode ultrasound with measurement of maximum mean IMT. This is especially true when compared to thiazide and thiazide-like diuretics and beta-blockers.

9. There is NO increased incidence of GI bleeding or cancer with CCBs in any of the long-term comparative clinical trials. There is NO increased risk of CHD or MI with the long-acting CCB in any of the recent randomized prospective clinical hypertension or CV trials.

10. CCBs are very effective in reducing LV mass and are equivalent to ACEIs and ARBs but significantly better than diuretics or beta-blockers. In addition, they improve arterial compliance, C-1 (large arteries) and C-2 (small resistance and oscillitory arterioles) compliance, vascular structure and function, and endothelial dysfunction.

Clinical Hypertension Trials with Angiotensin Converting Enzyme Inhibitors: Published Trials (total 27 trials) and Trials in progress:[160]

1. CAPPP*
2. HOPE*
3. STOP-2*
4. PROGRESS*
5. AASK*
6. ABCD*
7. ALLHAT*
8. ANBP-2*
9. ASCOT**
10. BENEDICT
11. DIAB-HYCAR
12. EUROPA*
13. HDS
14. HYVET
15. IDNT*
16. PART-2
17. PEACE
18. PHYLLIS
19. QUIET
20. SCAT
21. ADVANCE
22. PRESERVE
23. PROTECT
24. FACET*
25. GLANT
26. PATE
27. ON-TARGET

Published trials.
**Lipid arm published. HBP arm unpublished.*

PEACE:[160]

- 8000 hypertensive patients + CHD
- Over age 50
- ACEI vs. placebo
- Any BP level
- 5 year follow-up

PHYLLIS:[160]

- 450 hypertensive patients with increased carotid intimal thickness
- Age 45-70 years
- BP 150-211/95-115 mm Hg
- ACEI vs. placebo
- 3 year follow-up

QUIET:[160]

- 1750 hypertensive patients with CHD.
- Ages 18-75
- Any BP level
- Quinipril ACEI vs. placebo
- ↓ PCTA only with ACE
- 3 year follow-up

SCAT:[160]

- 460 hypertensive patients with CHD
- Any BP level
- ACEI vs. placebo + Simvastatin
- 5 year follow up
- Showed fewer deaths, CVA, MI on Enalapril (p=0.043) but no angiographic CHD

ADVANCE:[160]

- 10,000 adults with type 2 DM + hypertension
- Any BP level, BS control 2 groups
- Perindopril-indapamide vs. placebo
- CV and renal end points
- 4.5 year follow-up

PROTECT:[160]

- 800 patients with hypertension + ↑ IM of common carotid artery
- Age 35-65 years
- Perindopril vs. HCTZ
- Follow carotid IMT
- 24 month follow-up

ANBP-2:[160, 209]

- 6000 elderly hypertensive patients
- PROBE design
- Ages 65 to 84 years
- BP: > 159 / 89 mm Hg.
- ACEI vs. diuretic. ACEI reduced MI better than diuretic by 17%.
- 5 year follow-up

DIAB-HYCAR:[160]

- 4000 Patients age 50 or older with hypertension and DM, any BP level
- Low dose Ramipril- ACEI vs. placebo
- 3 year follow-up

EUROPA: [160]

- 10,500 patients with hypertension and CHD
- Age 18 or more
- Any BP level
- ACEI vs. placebo
- 3 year follow-up
- ACEI reduced recurrent MI 25%

HDS: [160]

- 1,148 patients with hypertension and DM
- Age 25-75 years
- BP >149 / 84 mm Hg
- ACEI vs. beta-blocker
- 8.2 year follow-up

HYVET: [160]

- 2,100 patients with hypertension
- Age > 80 years
- BP 159-220/ 89-110 mm Hg
- Perindopril ACEI vs. diuretic (Indapamide) vs. placebo
- 5 year follow-up

PART-2: [160]

- 617 patients with hypertension and atherosclerosis
- Age 18-75
- Any BP level
- Ramipril-ACEI vs. placebo
- 4 year follow-up
- Carotid IMT: same by B-mode ultrasound LVMI reduced
  with Ramipril

On Target and Transcend

- 28,400 patients, men and women, high risk CVD
- Randomized, double–blind, multicentered trial
- Telimisartan vs. ramipril vs. combination of both
- Primary endpoints:
  Composite CV death, MI, CVA or hospitalization for CHF
- Secondary endpoints
  New CHF, revascularization, New DM, cognitive decline, dementia and atrial fibrillation
- Other endpoints
  All cause mortality
  Non CV death
  LVH
  BP changes
  Acute ischemic syndrome
  TIA
  Nephropathy
  Microvascular DM complications
- Follow-up 3.5–5.5 years

CAPPP: 188, 133

- 10,985 patients in 536 centers in Scandinavia
- Prospective, randomized, open trial with blinded endpoint evaluation
- Ages 25-66 years
- DBP > 100 mm Hg
- Treatment: captopril vs. diuretics, beta-blockers (conventional therapy) *Note that captopril was given only 50 mg OD or BID.*
- Primary endpoint: composite of fatal and non-fatal MI CVA and other CV events.
- Follow-up 6.1 years (mean). Only 0.25% lost follow-up.

Results:
1. Primary endpoint composite was equal.
2. Captopril 363 patients (11.1 per 1000 patient years)
3. Conventional treatment (10.2 per 1000 patient years) Relative risk = 1.05 (95% CI 0.90-1.22) p=0.52
- Cardiovascular mortality was lower with Captopril than with conventional treatment (76 vs. 95 events) relative risk= 0.77 (0.57-1.04) p=0.092 (23% reduction).
- Rate of fatal and non-fatal MI was simple in both groups (0.96, p=0.68).
- Total mortality was equal (0.93, p=0.49).
- Fatal and non-fatal CVA were equal in DM patients.
- Fatal and non-fatal CVA were more common with captopril (189 vs. 148) in non-diabetic patients only relative risk 1.25(1.01-1.55) p=0.044 (25% increase).
- Rates of all other cardiac events were equal (0.94; p=0.30)
- Initial SBP, DBP, creatinine, cholesterol and, DM and glucose were significantly higher in the captopril vs. conventional therapy. This indicates an overall higher baseline CV risk in the Captopril patients.

SBP/DBP differences:

	P	Captopril	Conventional
Untreated	<0.0001	166.6/103.6	163.3/101.2
Treated	0.025	157.4/96.2	156.2/95.4

This initial BP was 3.3/2.4 mm Hg higher in the Captopril previously untreated group and 1.2/0.8 mm Hg higher in the captopril previously treated patients.

- Reduced incidence for new onset DM in Captopril group (0.86 p=0.039)
- BP remained significantly higher in the Captopril treated patients compared to conventional therapy.
- Target BP was achieved more rapidly with conventional therapy in the first 6-12 months.
- Captopril was superior to conventional therapy in patients with DM in all CV endpoints (22% reduction) (.78; p=0.041).

Conclusions
- Captopril is superior to conventional beta-blocker and di-uretic therapy in reducing all of the following:
  1. Fatal cardiovascular events
  2. Prevention of new-onset DM
- Captopril is equal to diuretics and beta-blockers in CVA reduction when BP levels are corrected between groups. A difference of 3.3/2.4 mm Hg accounts for about a 21% difference in CVA incidence.
- Captopril is superior to conventional therapy in hyperten-sive diabetic patients in reducing all cardiovascular events.
- Captopril decreases the incidence of new-onset DM.
- Captopril has fewer adverse effects and higher compliance rate than conventional therapy.

CAPPP[188][133] Baseline Characteristics

Table 1

Characteristic	Captopril Treatment (n=5492)	Conventional Treatment (n=5493)
Demographics		
Male/Female	3016/2476	2858/2635
Age (years)*	52.4 (8.3)	52.7 (8.4)
Clinical		
Weight (kg)*	81.6 (15.2)	80.6 (15.1)
Height (cm)*	170.8 (9.0)	170.1 (9.1)
Supine systolic blood pressure (mm Hg)	161.8 (19.9)	159.6 (20.1)
Supine diastolic blood pressure (mm Hg)	99.8 (9.9)	98.1 (10.1)
Serum creatinine (μmol/L)*	86.5 (15.2)	86.1 (15.0)
Serum cholesterol (mmol/L)	6.20 (1.19)	6.16 (1.16)
Fasting blood glucose (mmol/L)*	5.22 (1.38)	5.23 (1.36)
Previously untreated	2640	2605
Smokers	1217	1214
Medical History		
Myocardial infarction	40	55
Ischemic heart disease	64	81
Stroke	50	39
Transient ischemic attacks	43	35
Atrial fibrillation	36	34
Congestive heart failure	19	10
Cardiovascular complications	219	213
Diabetes mellitus	309	263

Data are number of patients or *mean (SD).

CAPPP[188][133] Blood Pressure During Study

Table 2

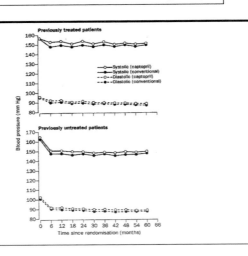

CAPPP[188][133] Patients with Events During Follow-up Treatment Group

Table 3

Event	Captopril Group	Conventional Group
Fatal myocardial infarction	27	35
Fatal Stroke	20	22
Other cardiovascular deaths	23	24
Sudden death	6	14
Non-fatal myocardial infarction	137	128
Non-fatal stroke	173	127
Ischemic heart disease	258	251
Atrial fibrilation	117	135
Congestive heart failure	75	66
Diabetes mellitus	337	380
Transient ischemic attacks	31	25

CAPPP[188][133] On-treatment Analysis: Relative Risk of Captopril vs. Conventional Therapy

Table 4

	Relative Risk (95% CI)	p
Primary endpoint	1.12 (0.94-1.32)	0.20
Fatal cardiovascular events	0.88 (0.62-1.25)`	0.47
Stroke, fatal and non-fatal	1.43 (1.12-1.82)	0.004
Myocardial infarction, fatal and non-fatal	0.94 (0.73-1.20)	0.61
All fatal events	1.04 (0.82-1.32)	0.75
All cardiac events	0.94 (0.82-1.07)	0.33
Diabetes mellitus	0.79 (0.67-0.94)	0.007

* Adjusted for age, sex, diabetes, systolic blood pressure, and previous treatment.

Relative Risk of Captopril vs. Conventional Therapy

Figure 1

	Relative risk* (95% CI)	p	Favors Captopril / Favors Conventional
Primary endpoint	1.05 (0.90–1.22)	0.52	
Fatal cardiovascular events	0.77 (0.57–1.04)	0.092	
Stroke, fatal and non-fatal	1.25 (1.01–1.55)	0.044	
Myocardial infarction, fatal and non-fatal	0.96 (0.77–1.19)	.68	
All fatal events	0.93 (0.76–1.14)	0.49	
All cardiac events	0.94 (0.83–1.06)	0.30	
Diabetes mellitus	0.86 (0.74–0.99)	0.039	

Scale: 0.5 — 1.0 — 2.0

* Adjusted for age, sex, diabetes, systolic blood pressure

Relative Risk in Previously Untreated Patients (n=5245)

Figure 2

	Relative risk* (95% CI)	p	Favors Captopril / Favors Conventional
Primary endpoint	0.92 (0.72–1.16)	0.47	
Fatal cardiovascular events	0.54 (0.33–0.89)	0.015	
Stroke, fatal and non-fatal	1.18 (0.84–1.65)	0.34	
Myocardial infarction, fatal and non-fatal	0.84 (0.59–1.21)	0.35	
All fatal events	0.89 (0.64–1.23)	0.48	
All cardiac events	0.93 (0.77–1.13)	0.48	
Diabetes mellitus	0.78 (0.62–0.99)	0.041	

Scale: 0.5 — 1.0 — 2.0

* Adjusted for age, sex, diabetes, systolic blood pressure

Relative Risk in Patients with Diabetes Mellitus at Baseline (n=572)

Figure 3

	Relative risk* (95% CI)	p	Favors Captopril / Favors Conventional
Primary endpoint	0.59 (0.38–0.91)	0.019	
Fatal cardiovascular events	0.48 (0.21–1.10)	0.085	
Stroke, fatal and non-fatal	1.02 (0.55–1.88)	0.95	
Myocardial infarction, fatal and non-fatal	0.34 (0.17–0.67)	0.002	
All fatal events	0.54 (0.31–0.96)	0.034	
All cardiac events	0.67 (0.46–0.96)	0.030	

Scale: 0.25 — 0.5 — 1.0 — 2.0

* Adjusted for age, sex, diabetes, systolic blood pressure and previous treatment.

Heart Outcomes Prevention Evaluation Study
(HOPE)

9297 High-risk Patients Over Age 55 with:
Vascular Disease
Diabetes Mellitus + One CV Risk Factor

Ramipril	10 mg qd vs. placebo x 5 years		
Ramipril:	653 patients reached 1 endpoint	14.1%	P=<.001
Placebo:	824 patients reached 1 endpoint	17.1%	Primary endpoints

	Ramipril	Placebo	P
CV Death	6.1%	8.1%	<. 001
MI	9.9%	12.2%	<. 001
CVA	3.4%	4.9%	<. 001
CHF	7.4%	9.4%	<. 001

BP Reduced 3/2 mm Hg 40% of CVA and 25% of MI

Adapted from The Heart Outcomes Prevention Evaluation Study Investigators: Effects of angiotensin-converting-enzyme inhibitor, ramipril, on cardiovascular events in high-risk patients. New Engl J Med 2000;342:145-153.

Objective
Randomized trial of the ACE inhibitor ramipril and vitamin E in patients at high risk for cardiovascular events versus placebo. Primary end point of the study was composite of myocardial infarction, stroke, or death from cardiovascular causes.

Inclusion Criteria
Patients aged >55 years at high risk for cardiovascular events because of: any evidence of vascular disease (CHD, stroke, PVD). diabetes plus 1 other coronary risk factor.

Exclusion Criteria
Heart failure or low ejection fraction; patient already on ACE inhibitor therapy or vitamin E.

Study Design
A total of 9297 patients were randomly assigned to receive ramipril (10 mg per day) or placebo for a mean of 5 years. In addition, all patients were randomly assigned to receive vitamin E, 400 IU/day, or placebo.

Patient Characteristics
Mean age was 66 years, with just over 25% female; 80.6% had
any evidence of coronary artery disease, 52.8% a previous MI,
43.4% peripheral vascular disease, 38.3% diabetes, 46.5% hypertension, 65.8% an elevated cholesterol. Antiplatelet therapy (aspirin or other) was being taken by 76% at the time of enrollment,
beta-blockers by 40%, and lipid-lowering agents by 28.9%.

Results
The data safety monitoring board recommended termination of
the study in early, March 1999, owing to an overwhelming benefit of ramipril.

Vitamin E vs Placebo: There were no significant differences in
the primary outcome of death, MI, stroke (16.2% in vitamin E
group vs 15.5% in placebo; P= .35). All-cause mortality was not
different between the 2 groups, either.

Ramipril vs Placebo: In the ramipril group, there was a significant
reduction in the primary end point from 17.7% in placebo to
14.1% in the treatment group (relative risk reduction of 22%; P =
.000002). There was also a significant reduction in MI, stroke,
and cardiovascular death. In addition, all-cause mortality was significantly reduced by 16% in the ramipril group (P = .0058).
Regarding blood pressure reduction, there was an average reduction in systolic blood pressure of 3.3 mm Hg in patients taking
ramipril. The benefits on stroke and MI reduction achieved in the
HOPE trial (31% and 20%, respectively) appear to be far greater
than what would be expected from blood pressure reduction
alone. Moreover, the benefits were sustained across various quar-
tiles of systolic and diastolic blood pressure, including those in
the normal range.

Conclusions
There is overwhelming evidence that, in a broad range of high-risk patients, ramipril prevents cardiovascular death, stroke, and MI heart failure, revascularization development of diabetes diabetic microvascular complications including nephropathy The benefits of ramipril are incremental to existing therapy. The beneficial effects of ramipril are independent of blood pressure lowering. Vitamin E does not have any significant protective effect.

Progress: 187

- 6105 subjects from 172 centers
- Hypertensive and non-hypertensive subjects with a history of CVA or TIA (1 month to 5 years)
- Treatment with perindopril or perindopril with indapamide vs. placebo against a background of standard care
- Mean BP 147/86 mm Hg (hypertensive group 159/94 mm Hg) (Non-hypertensive group 136/79)
- 4 year follow-up
- Average age 64 years, 11% were DM
- **Primary outcome:** Total stroke (fatal or non-fatal)
- **Secondary outcomes:**
  - Fatal or disabling stroke
  - Total major vascular events comprising the composite of non-fatal stroke, non-fatal myocardial infarction or death from any vascular cause
  - Total and cause specific deaths and hospital admissions
  - Dementia and cognitive function

Results:

1. BP reduction
   - Overall: 9/4 mm Hg active vs. placebo
   - Combination therapy: 12.3/5 mm Hg
   - Single drug therapy: 4.9/2.8 mm Hg
   - Hypertensive group: 9.5/3.9 mm Hg
   - Non-hypertensive group: 8.8/4.2 mm Hg
2. CVA reduction in all CVA subtypes
   - Combination therapy: reduced 43% (perindopril plus indapamide)
   - Active treatment vs. placebo: reduced 28% (95% CI 17-38, $p < 0.0001$)
   - Single drug treatment: NS (perindopril)
   - Active treatment group CVA had fewer fatal disabling or severe CVA vs. placebo
   - Similar reductions in risk of stroke in hypertensive and non-hypertensive patients ($p < 0.01$)
   - Cumulative CVA risk curves diverged early.

- Annual rate of new CVA 2.7 % in treatment
  group vs. 3.8% in control group
3. Total major vascular events
   - Active treatment reduced 26% (p < 0.0001)
   - Decreased non-fatal CVA by 42% (p< 0.0001)
   - Decreased non-fatal MI by 38%-42%(p,0.001)
   - Vascular death was same in active or placebo group
   - Decreased total major coronary events (non-fatal MI
     or death from CHD) by 26% (95% CI 6-42)
     (p< 0.0001)
4. Total deaths or deaths from vascular or non-vascular
   causes: NS
5. Hospital admissions reduced 9%
6. Dementia reduced 34% (p<0.0001) and severe cognitive
   decline reduced 45% (p<0.0001) in those with CVA

Conclusions

- Perindopril (ACEI) + indapamide reduce all CVA in
  both hypertensive and non-hypertensive patients.
- Major coronary events are reduced twice as much
  compared to previous diuretic beta-blocker based trials.
- Dementia is reduced and cognitive decline is reduced.
- The reduction in non-fatal MI is greater than expected
  from the BP reduction suggesting an independent ACEI
  or indapamide effect.
- BP reductions (mean BP) down to 124/74 mm Hg
  showed continued benefit without any "J shaped" curve.
- Very low adverse effects and withdrawal rate.

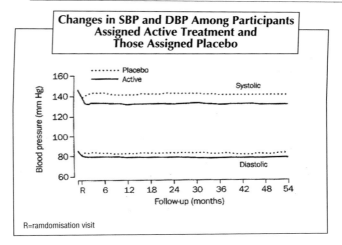

Changes in SBP and DBP Among Participants Assigned Active Treatment and Those Assigned Placebo

R=ramdomisation visit

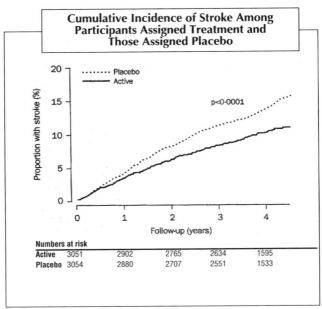

Cumulative Incidence of Stroke Among Participants Assigned Treatment and Those Assigned Placebo

Effects of Study Treatment on Stroke Subtypes, Major Vascular Events and Deaths

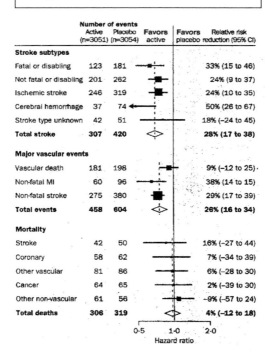

	Number of events				
	Active (n=3051)	Placebo (n=3054)	Favors active	Favors placebo	Relative risk reduction (95% CI)
Stroke subtypes					
Fatal or disabling	123	181			33% (15 to 46)
Not fatal or disabling	201	262			24% (9 to 37)
Ischemic stroke	246	319			24% (10 to 35)
Cerebral hemorrhage	37	74			50% (26 to 67)
Stroke type unknown	42	51			18% (−24 to 45)
Total stroke	307	420			28% (17 to 38)
Major vascular events					
Vascular death	181	198			9% (−12 to 25)
Non-fatal MI	60	96			38% (14 to 15)
Non-fatal stroke	275	380			29% (17 to 39)
Total events	458	604			26% (16 to 34)
Mortality					
Stroke	42	50			16% (−27 to 44)
Coronary	58	62			7% (−34 to 39)
Other vascular	81	86			6% (−28 to 30)
Cancer	64	65			2% (−39 to 30)
Other non-vascular	61	56			−9% (−57 to 24)
Total deaths	306	319			4% (−12 to 18)

0·5   1·0   2·0
Hazard ratio

Black squares=point estimates (with area proportional to number of events); horizontal lines=95% CIs. Diamonds=point estimate and 95% CI for overall effects. Vertical broken line=point for overall effect. MI=myocardial infarction.

Effects of Study Treatment on Stroke and Major Vascular Events in Subgroups of Patients

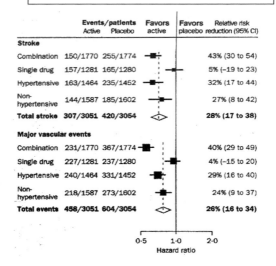

	Events/patients		Favors	Favors	Relative risk
	Active	Placebo	active	placebo	reduction (95% CI)
Stroke					
Combination	150/1770	255/1774			43% (30 to 54)
Single drug	157/1281	165/1280			5% (−19 to 23)
Hypertensive	163/1464	235/1452			32% (17 to 44)
Non-hypertensive	144/1587	185/1602			27% (8 to 42)
Total stroke	307/3051	420/3054			28% (17 to 38)
Major vascular events					
Combination	231/1770	367/1774			40% (29 to 49)
Single drug	227/1281	237/1280			4% (−15 to 20)
Hypertensive	240/1464	331/1452			29% (16 to 40)
Non-hypertensive	218/1587	273/1602			24% (9 to 37)
Total events	458/3051	604/3054			26% (16 to 34)

```
                   0·5      1·0      2·0
                        Hazard ratio
```

Hazard rations (and 95% CIs) for hypertensive and non-hypertensive subgroups standardised to study-wide proportions of patients for whom combination or single drug therapy was planned, p values for homogeneity (combination therapy vs. single drug therapy) both <0.001; p values for homogeneity (hypertensive vs. non-hypertensive) both >0.6

Combination Therapy (12/5mm Hg) & Single Drug Therapy (5/3 mm Hg)

	Events		Hazard Ratio (95% CI)	RR(%)
	Active	Placebo		
Stroke				
Combination	150	255	0.57 (0.46-0.70)	43%
Single Drug	157	165	0.95 (0.77-1.19)	5%
Total	**307**	**420**	**0.72 (0.62-0.83)**	**28%**
Major Vascular Events*				
Combination	231	367	0.60 (0.50-0.71)	40%
Single Drug	227	237	0.96 (0.80-1.15)	4%
Total	**458**	**604**	**0.74 (0.66-0.80)**	**26%**

Presented during the 11th Meeting of European Sociey of Hypertension. June 16, 2001, Milan, Italy

Dementia (DSM IV) and Severe Cognitive Decline (MMSE)

	Events		Odds Ratio (95% CI)	RR(%)
	Active	Placebo		
With Stroke	43	65	0.66 (0.45-0.97)	34%
Without Stroke	150	152	0.99 (0.78-1.24)	1%
Total	**193**	**217**	**0.88 (0.72-1.08)**	**12%**
With Stroke	48	86	0.55 (0.38-0.78)	45%
Without Stroke	228	248	0.90 (0.75-1.09)	10%

ANBP-2: [209]

Key points:

- Comparison of ACEI based therapy with diuretic based therapy
- A community physician-based trial
- Prospective, randomized, open label study with blinded assessment of endpoints (PROBE design)
- 6083 subjects aged 65-84 in 1594 family practices followed for median 4.1 yrs.

Findings: Figure 3

Conclusion: ACE inhibition therapy, particularly in older men, leads to better outcomes than treatment with diuretics despite similar BP reductions, MI reduced 17% in men ($p<0.02$).

(N Engl. J Med 2003; 348: 583-92)

ACE Inhibitors vs. Diuretics for Hypertension

Figure 3. Primary Endpoints Among All Subjects, Male Subjects and Female Subjects

All Subjects

EndPoint	Hazard Ratio (95% CI)	P Value
All cardiovascular events or death from any cause	0.89 (0.79-1.00)	0.05
First cardiovascular event or death from any cause	0.89 (0.79-1.01)	0.06
Death from any cause	0.90 (0.75-1.09)	0.27

Male Subjects

EndPoint	Hazard Ratio (95% CI)	P Value
All cardiovascular events or death from any cause	0.83 (0.71-0.97)	0.02
First cardiovascular event or death from any cause	0.83 (0.71-0.97)	0.02
Death from any cause	0.83 (0.66-1.06)	0.14

Female Subjects

EndPoint	Hazard Ratio (95% CI)	P Value
All cardiovascular events or death from any cause	1.00 (0.83-121)	0.98
First cardiovascular event or death from any cause	1.00 (0.83-1.20)	0.98
Death from any cause	1.01 (0.76-1.35)	0.94

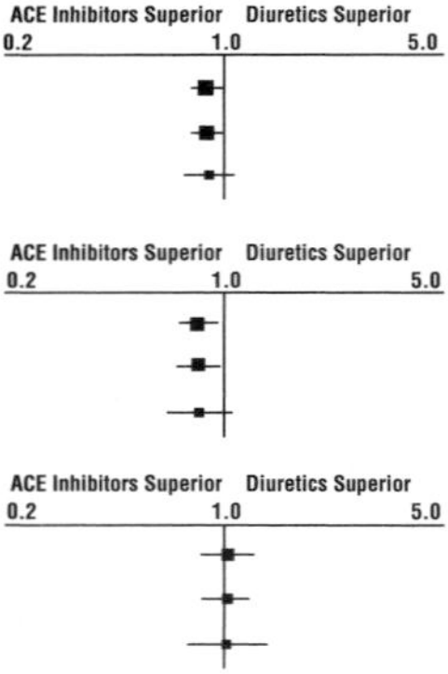
ACE Inhibitors Superior
Diuretics Superior
0.2
1.0
5.0
ACE Inhibitors Superior
Diuretics Superior
0.2
1.0
5.0
ACE Inhibitors Superior
Diuretics Superior
0.2
1.0
5.0

ACE denotes angiotensin-converting enzyme, and CI–confidence interval.

Summary of the Clinical Hypertension Trials Using Primarily Angiotensin Converting Enzyme Inhibitors (ACEIs)

1. ACEIs are effective in reducing BP when administered at correct doses and dosing intervals in all patients regardless of age, gender or race. Reductions in BP are equal to diuretics, beta-blockers, calcium channel blockers and angiotensin receptor antagonists as well as other classes of antihypertensive agents.

2. The role of tissue selectivity in clinical outcome studies remains to be proven, although surrogate endpoints suggest possible advantages of the tissue selective ACEIs.

3. ACEIs should be administered in higher doses to achieve BP control. There is evidence that they have beneficial vascular effects that are both due to the antihypertensive effect as well as the non-antihypertensive effect.

4. Coronary heart disease and myocardial infarction morbidity and mortality have been significantly reduced. They are equal to (ALLHAT, STOP 2, CAPPP) or better than diuretic ANBP-2 and beta-blockers (PROGRESS) equal to CCB (ALLHAT) but superior to beta-blockers as monotherapy, especially in the elderly hypertensive. In addition, they are effective in reducing recurrent MI in patients who have already had a MI (HOPE and others).

5. Cerebrovascular accidents are significantly reduced with ACEIs in all clinical trials (STOP 2, CAPPP, PROGRESS, HOPE, SCAT), with the possible exception of ALLHAT. However, the ALLHAT results are controversial due to the higher BP in the ACEI group, improper dosing, as was done in CAPPP, and the unfavorable results were limited to black hypertensive patients. Corrections for these factors indicate that ACEIs in ALLHAT were almost as effective as diuretics.

6. Congestive heart failure is significantly reduced. Systolic and diastolic dysfunction is improved. CHF is reduced equal to or better than diuretics (STOP 2, CAPPP, PROGRESS, HOPE). The ALLHAT data on CHF is controversial related to ACEI vs. diuretic due to higher BP levels on the ACEI, study design, potential masking of CHF symptoms on diuretics and many other factors. (see ALLHAT discussion).

7. Renal insufficiency, ESRD, microalbuminuria, and proteinuria are signficantly reduced compared to diuretics and beta-blockers. They are preferred drugs in CRI and proteinuric states.

8. New onset DM is reduced significantly (HOPE, CAPPP, ALLHAT, STOP 2). They are preferred initial agents in hypertensive diabetes along with ARBs and CCBs. They are superior to diuretics and beta-blockers in reducing CV events in the diabetic hypertensive (SYST-EUR, CAPPP).

9. Adverse effects are low and compliance with continuation of therapy is high. Initial rise in serum creatinine up to 20% above baseline is normal and expected in patients with any renal impairment and does not require treatment cessation.

10. Anti-atherogenic effects on the coronary and carotid arteries have been demonstrated (QUIET, SCAT, PART 2).

11. Improvement of vascular biology related to endothelial function and arterial compliance (both function and structure).

12. Reduce dementia and cognitive dysfunction (PROGRESS).

13. Neutral metabolic and biochemical changes, improve insulin sensitivity.

14. Reduce LVMI and LVH.

Clinical Trials in Hypertension with Angiotensin Receptor Blockers (ARBs) (total of 8 trials): [160]

1. **LIFE:** Losartan Intervention For Endpoint reduction in hypertension (discussed in detail in following sections)
2. **IDNT:** Irbesartan Diabetes Nephropathy Trial (see renal and diabetes sections)
3. **RENAAL:** Randomized Evaluation of NIDDM with the Ang-II antagonist Losartan
4. **SCOPE:** Study of cognition and prognosis in elderly patients with hypertension (in progress)
   - 4000 patients with hypertension
   - Age 70-89 with 2.5 year follow-up
   - BP 160-179/90-99 mm Hg
   - Endpoints of CVA, CHD, dementia
   - ARB vs. placebo
   - In progress
5. **VALUE:** Valsartan Antihypertensive Long Term Use Evaluation
   - 15,313 patients
   - Age >49 years with 6 year follow-up
   - BP <210/115 mm Hg
   - Endpoints of CHD, CVA, CV death
   - ARB = DHP-CCB
6. **On-Target and Transcend:** (see clinical trials section on ACEIs)
7. **MARVAL:** (see renal section)
8. **MOSES:** eprosartan (concluded, see page 194)

Clinical trials in hypertension with Angiotensin Receptor Blockers (ARBs): [189, 190]

LIFE Study[190]

- Double-masked, randomized, parallel-group trial
- 9,193 subjects aged 55 to 80 years
- BP: 160-200/95-115 mm Hg
- LVH by ECG
- Follow-up 4 years

Results:

- BP fell   30.2 / 16.6 in Losartan group
              29.1 / 16.8 in Atenolol group
- Primary composite endpoint of CV death, CVA or MI
  Losartan 23.8/1000 patient years
  Atenolol 27.9/1000 patient years
  RR 0.87, 95% CI 0.77-0.98
  P=0.021
  13% reduction favoring Losartan
- CV disease deaths were equal
  RR 0.89, 95% CI 0.73-1.07
  P=0.206
- Fatal and nonfatal CVA reduced by Losartan
  RR 0.75, 95% CI 0.63-0.89
  P=0.001
  25% reductions favoring Losartan
- Myocardial infarction (non-fatal and fatal): equal
  RR 1.07; 0.88-1.31
  P=0.491
- New-onset DM less frequent with Losartan
- Losartan is better tolerated, has fewer adverse effects and a better compliance rate.
- Losartan reduced composite CV endpoints significantly more than Atenolol in the diabetic subgroup (24.5%; P=0.031).
- Losartan reduced total mortality 39% (P=0.002) compared to Atenolol.

Conclusion:

1. Losartan prevents more CV morbidity and mortality than atenolol, for a similar reduction in BP.

2. Losartan prevents more CVA morbidity and mortality than atenolol, for a similar reduction in BP.

3. Losartan confers benefits in vascular disease independent of, and beyond BP reduction. These benefits may be related to complete blockade of the RAS, improvement in endothelial function, arterial compliance, vascular function and structure, or other factors.

4. Losartan prevents more new-onset DM than Atenolol.

5. In the hypertensive diabetic patients, Losartan is superior to Atenolol in reductions.
   - CV death
   - CVA
   - MI
   - Total mortality

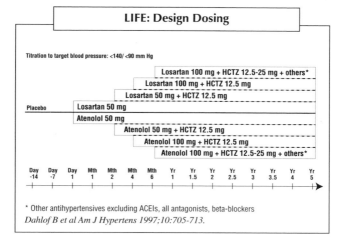

LIFE: Design Dosing

Titration to target blood pressure: <140/ <90 mm Hg

Losartan 100 mg + HCTZ 12.5-25 mg + others*
Losartan 100 mg + HCTZ 12.5 mg
Losartan 50 mg + HCTZ 12.5 mg
Placebo   Losartan 50 mg
Atenolol 50 mg
Atenolol 50 mg + HCTZ 12.5 mg
Atenolol 100 mg + HCTZ 12.5 mg
Atenolol 100 mg + HCTZ 12.5-25 mg + others*

| Day -14 | Day -7 | Day 1 | Mth 1 | Mth 2 | Mth 4 | Mth 6 | Yr 1 | Yr 1.5 | Yr 2 | Yr 2.5 | Yr 3 | Yr 3.5 | Yr 4 | Yr 5 |

* Other antihypertensives excluding ACEIs, all antagonists, beta-blockers
Dahlof B et al Am J Hypertens 1997;10:705-713.

LIFE: Blood Pressure Results – Follow-up

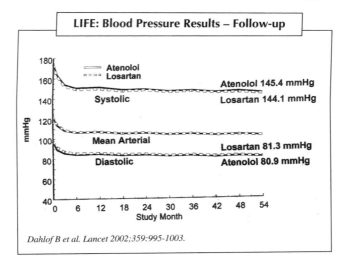

Dahlof B et al. Lancet 2002;359:995-1003.

LIFE: Blood Pressure and Responder Rates

	Losartan (n=4605)	Atenolol (n=4588)
SBP ≤ 140 mm Hg, %	49.5	46.2
DBP ≤ 90 mm Hg, %	87.6	89.4
MAP last vist, mm Hg	102.2	102.4

B Dahlof et al. Lancet 2002;359:995-1003.

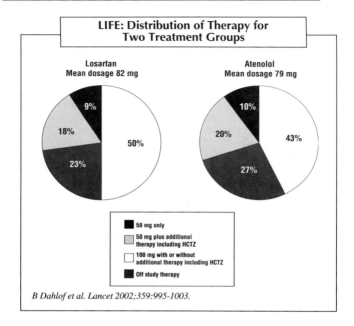

LIFE: Distribution of Therapy for Two Treatment Groups

Losartan
Mean dosage 82 mg

Atenolol
Mean dosage 79 mg

- ■ 50 mg only
- ▨ 50 mg plus additional therapy including HCTZ
- □ 100 mg with or without additional therapy including HCTZ
- ▨ Off study therapy

B Dahlof et al. Lancet 2002;359:995-1003.

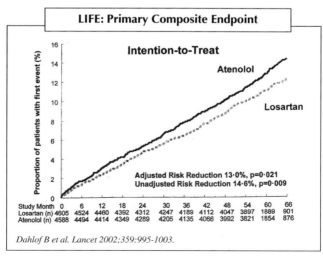

LIFE: Primary Composite Endpoint

Intention-to-Treat

Atenolol

Losartan

Adjusted Risk Reduction 13·0%, p=0·021
Unadjusted Risk Reduction 14·6%, p=0·009

Study Month	0	6	12	18	24	30	36	42	48	54	60	66
Losartan (n)	4605	4524	4460	4392	4312	4247	4189	4112	4047	3897	1889	901
Atenolol (n)	4588	4494	4414	4349	4289	4205	4135	4066	3992	3821	1854	876

Dahlof B et al. Lancet 2002;359:995-1003.

LIFE: Components of Primary Endpoint

CV Mortality
Fatal/Non-fatal Stroke
Fatal/Non-fatal MI

**Each category including only first event patients
may appear in more than one category.**

Dahlof B et al. Lancet 2002;359:995-1003.

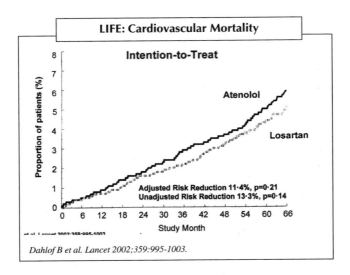

LIFE: Cardiovascular Mortality

Dahlof B et al. Lancet 2002;359:995-1003.

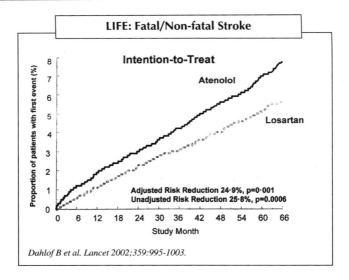

Dahlof B et al. Lancet 2002;359:995-1003.

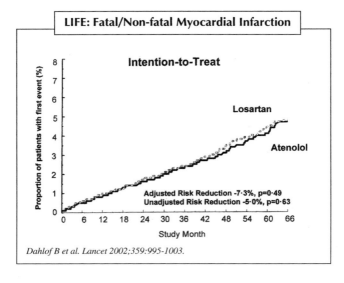

Dahlof B et al. Lancet 2002;359:995-1003.

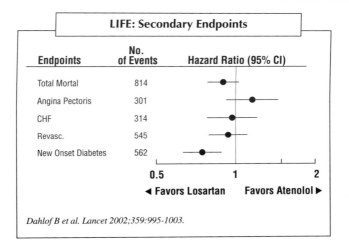

LIFE: Secondary Endpoints

Endpoints	No. of Events	Hazard Ratio (95% CI)
Total Mortal	814	
Angina Pectoris	301	
CHF	314	
Revasc.	545	
New Onset Diabetes	562	

◄ Favors Losartan   Favors Atenolol ►

Dahlof B et al. Lancet 2002;359:995-1003.

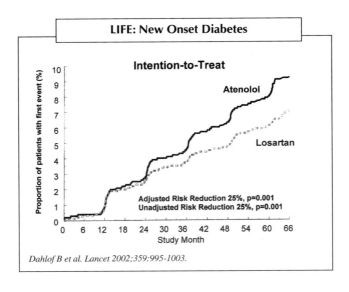

LIFE: New Onset Diabetes

Intention-to-Treat

Atenolol

Losartan

Adjusted Risk Reduction 25%, p=0.001
Unadjusted Risk Reduction 25%, p=0.001

Dahlof B et al. Lancet 2002;359:995-1003.

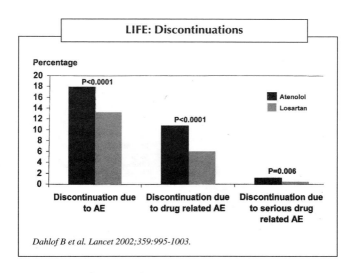

LIFE: Primary and Secondary Outcomes

	Losartan (n=4605)	Atenolol (n=4588)	Adjusted RR (%)	p	Unadjusted RR (%)	p
Primary composite	508	588	-13	0.021	-15	0.009
CV Mortality	204	234	-11	0.21	-13	0.14
Stroke	232	309	-25	0.001	-26	0.0006
MI	198	188	+7	0.49	+5	0.63
Total Morality	**383**	**431**	**-10**	**0.13**	**-12**	**0.08**
New Onset DM	241	319	-25	<0.001	-25	<0.001

B Dahlof et al. Lancet 2002;359:995-1003.

LIFE: Discontinuations

Percentage

- Atenolol
- Losartan

P<0.0001 — Discontinuation due to AE
P<0.0001 — Discontinuation due to drug related AE
P=0.006 — Discontinuation due to serious drug related AE

Dahlof B et al. Lancet 2002;359:995-1003.

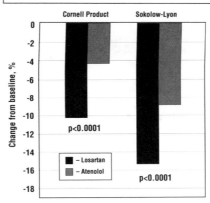

LIFE: ECG-LVH Regression from Baseline

Dahlof B et al. Lancet 2002;359:995-1003.

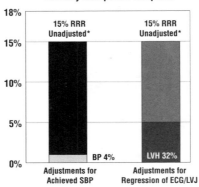

LIFE: Adjustments for Difference

Conclusion: Adjusting for differences in achieved BP
and degree of LVH regression only explains part of the
study outcome.

* Unadjusted for Framingham risk score and LVH
Adjusted for Framingham and LVH-=130% RRR

Clinical Trials in Hypertension with Angiotensin Receptor Blockers (ARBs): [189]

LIFE Study[189] (ISH Substudy)

- Double-blind, randomized, parallel-group study
- 1326 men and women ages 55 to 80 years (mean 70)
- SBP > 160-200 mm HG
  DBP < 90 mm HG (mean 174 / 83 mm Hg)
- ECG-LVH present
- Treatment: Lorsartan vs. Atenolol + HCTZ in either group
- Main outcome measure: composite endpoint of CV death, CVA or MI
- Mean follow-up 4.7 years

Results

1. BP reduction equal in both groups 28 /9 mm Hg but last BP was 146 / 75 mm Hg in Losartan group and 146 / 74 mm Hg on Atenolol group (p=0.04 for DBP)
2. Main outcome reduced by 25% with Losartan vs. Atenolol 25.1 vs. 35.4 events / 1000 patient year Relative risk 0.75 95% CI 0.56-1.01; (P=.06 adjusted risk and LVH degree unadjusted RR 0.71, 95% CI 0.53-0.95, P=.02)
3. MI: no difference
4. CV mortality: 8.7 vs. 16.9 events / 1000 pts year RR 0.54 95% CI 0.34-0.87 P=.01 46% reduction
5. Non-fatal and fatal CVA: 10.6 vs. 18.9 events/1000 pts year RR 0.60 95% CI 0.38-0.92 P=0.02 40% reduction
6. New-onset DM 12.6 vs. 16.9 events / 1000 pts year RR 0.62 95% CI 0.40-0.97 P=.04 38% reduction

7. Total mortality: 21.2 vs 30.2 events / 1000 pts year
   RR 0.72 95% CI 0.53-1.00
   P=0.046
8. LVH reduction: Losartan better than Atenolol P<0.001
9. Curves for CV mortality and CVH separated early in
   favor of Losartan
10. Losartan was better tolerated

Conclusion

1. Losartan is superior to Atenolol for treatment of patients
   with isolated systolic hypertension in reducing CVA, CV
   mortality, composite CV morbidity and mortality, total
   mortality, new-onset DM and LVH.
2. The reduction in these events was independent of BP
   levels suggesting other beneficial effects of Losartan on
   vascular events, possibly related to blockade of the RAS
   and favorable effects on vascular biology.

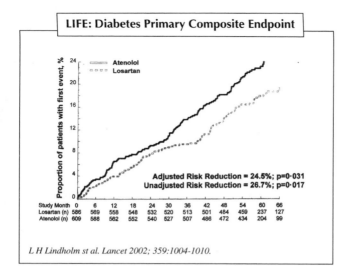

LIFE: Diabetes Primary Composite Endpoint

Adjusted Risk Reduction = 24.5%; p=0·031
Unadjusted Risk Reduction = 26.7%; p=0·017

Study Month	0	6	12	18	24	30	36	42	48	54	60	66
Losartan (n)	586	569	558	548	532	520	513	501	484	459	237	127
Atenolol (n)	609	588	562	552	540	527	507	486	472	434	204	99

L H Lindholm st al. Lancet 2002; 359:1004-1010.

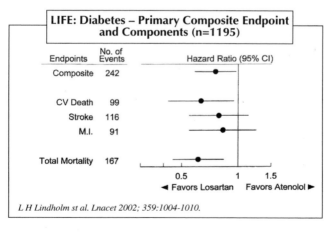

**LIFE: Diabetes – Primary Composite Endpoint
and Components (n=1195)**

Endpoints	No. of Events	Hazard Ratio (95% CI)
Composite	242	
CV Death	99	
Stroke	116	
M.I.	91	
Total Mortality	167	

◄ Favors Losartan   Favors Atenolol ►

L H Lindholm st al. Lnacet 2002; 359:1004-1010.

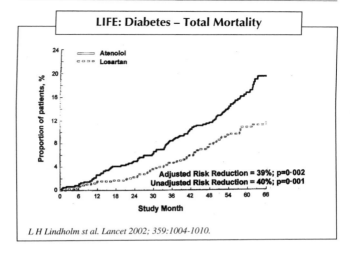

LIFE: Diabetes – Total Mortality

L H Lindholm st al. Lancet 2002; 359:1004-1010.

LIFE: Public Health Implications

- Based on NHANES III, 3.9 million persons in the U.S. are over age 55 with high blood pressure, LVH and without CHF (2.7 million without diabetes).
- Assuming these patients experience events similar to LIFE participants randomized to atenolol, then over 4.8 years use of losartan would lead to:
  - 70,000 avoided CV morbidity/mortality clinical endpoints and 66,000 fewer first strokes
  - 54,000 less new-onset diabetes cases

B Dahlof, ACC, Atlanta, March 20, 2002.

LIFE: Summary

- Compared with atenolol-based therapy, losartan-based antihypertensive therapy was associated with:
  - Less cardiovascular morbidity and mortality (13%)
  - Less stroke (25%)
  - Less onset of diabetes (25%)
  - Better regression in LVH
  - Better tolerability with significantly fewer discontinuations for adverse events for similar blood pressure reduction

LIFE: Summary 2

- Following adjustment for effects on BP and LVH the primary outcome seemed to be explained only partially by the effect on these parameters.
- In the diabetic subgroup:
  - Losartan provided better protection against cardiovascular morbidity and mortality, a reduction of 24%.
  - Losartan reduced total mortality by 39%.

LIFE: Conclusions

- Losartan offers better protection against cardiovascular morbidity and death (including stroke) compared to atenolol with benefits beyond blood pressure reduction.
- Losartan was protective in the higher (e.g. DM) as well as the lower (e.g. non-vascular) risk group.
- Losartan reduces the rate of new onset of diabetes compared to Atenolol.
- Losartan is significantly better tolerated than Atenolol.
- These results are directly applicable in clinical practice.

Morbidity and Mortality After Stroke – Eprosartan Compared with Nitrendipine for Secondary Prevention (MOSES Study)

Schrader J. et al. European Society of Cardiology Congress 2004; August 28 – September 1, 2004; Munich, Germany.

Overview

- First study which compared 2 antihypertensive drugs
- Investigator created, initatied and performed study
- Blinded endpoint committee
- 100% monitoring of all centers and all patients
- Well defined hypertensive stroke patients
- Previous and study medication well balanced
- Very tight clinical control
- Early and comparable blood pressure control

Objective: to compare efficacy of Eprosartan and Nitrendipine in secondary stroke prevention and the reduction of cardiovascular and cerebrovascular morbidity and mortality.

MOSES: Rationale
  1. Why Eprosartan?
  - Effectively reduces blood pressure and is well tolerated
  - Reduces SNS activity
  - Increases post-stroke survival in animal models

  2. Why Nitrendipine?
  - In the Syst-Eur study, Nitrendipine reduced the frequency of stroke and dementia

MOSES: Study design
1. PROBE design
   • Prospective, randomized, open-label, blinded endpoint
2. Primary endpoints
   • Total mortality + total number of cardiovascular and cerebrovascular events
3. Secondary endpoints
   • Functional status (Barthel's index, Rankin scale)
   • Cognitive Function
4. Follow-up
   • Mean: 2.5 years
5. prior to randomization: qualifying event documented by CCT or MRI and diagnosis of hypertension
6. Randomisation
   • At entry: office BP, ABPM, MMS, Rankin, Barthel
   • Pretreated patients: rolled over directly to study medication
7. Initital treatment dosage
   • Eprosartan 600 mg
   • Nitrendipine 10 mg
   • During the study, dosage was increased or combination:
      a. Diuretics b. beta-blockers c. Alpha-blockers/other

MOSES: Assessments

1. Procedures regularly performed
   - Sitting and ambulatory blood pressure measurements (ABPM)
   - Mini Mental Status Examination (MMSE) score
   - Documentation of all drugs taken
   - Barthel Index and Rankin scale
   - Electrocardiogram
   - Adverse event reporting

MOSES: Trial profile

1. 1405 patients eligible for randomization
2. 710 assigned to Eprosartan-based regimen; 685 assigned to Nitrendipine-based regimen
3. 29 patients withdrew consent prior to first intake of study drug (Eprosartan)
4. 24 withdrew consent prior to first intake of study drug (Nitrendipine)

MOSES: Inclusion criteria

1. Hypertension (confirmed by ABPM) + cerebral ischemia (TIA, PRIND, complete stroke)

OR

2. Cerebral hemorrhage during the last 24 month prior to study commencement (cerebral scan or MRI was necessary to confirm)

MOSES: Baseline characteristics of patients

	Eprosartan	Nitrendipine
Total number of Eligible patients	681	671
Sex		
number % male	365 (53.6%)	368 (54.8%)
number % female	316 (46.4%)	303 (45.2%)
Age (years)	67.7	68.1
BMI	27.7	27.4
Time between qualifying event and allocation	347.6	349.8

MOSES: baseline characteristics of patients with anti-hypertensive pretreatment: 84%

	Eprosartan	Nitrendipine
Systolic office blood pressure mm Hg	139.7	140.0
Diastolic office blood pressure (mm Hg)	87.0	87.2
Heart rate	74.7	75.7

Qualifying Disease

	Eprosartan	Nitrendipine
Stroke	418 (61.4%)	407 (60.7%)
TIA	186 (27.3%)	184 (27.4%)
PRIND	36 (5.3%)	47 (7%)
Intracerebral hemorrhage	41 (6.0%)	33 (4.9%)

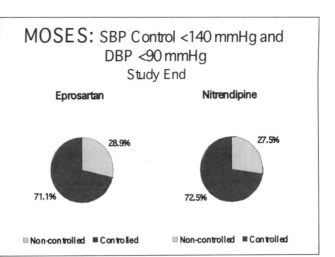

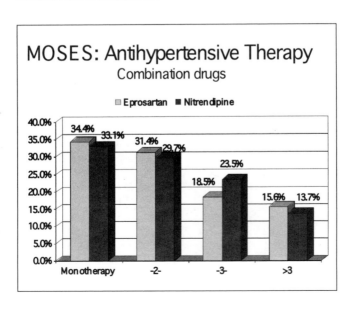

MOSES: SBP Control <140 mmHg and DBP <90 mmHg
Study End

Eprosartan

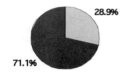

28.9%

71.1%

▨ Non-controlled   ■ Controlled

Nitrendipine

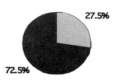

27.5%

72.5%

▨ Non-controlled   ■ Controlled

MOSES: Antihypertensive medication (final visit)

▨ Eprosartan   ■ Nitrendipine

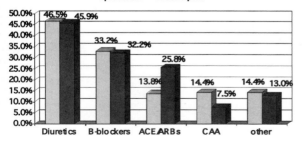

MOSES: Primary and secondary outcomes

Outcome	Eprosartan (n)	Nitrendipine (n)	p
All deaths and CV and CE events, recurrent (n=461)	206	255	0.014
All CE events, recurrent (n=236)	102	134	0.02
All CV events, recurrent (n=178)	77	101	0.06
First event, all (n=320)	149	171	0.15
First event, CE (n=169)	80	89	0.42
First event, CV (n=144)	60	84	0.03

Schrader J. European Society of Cardiology Congress 2004;
August 28–September 1, 2004; Munich, Germany.

MOSES: mini mental status score; Rankin Scale; Barthel Index

	Eprosartan	Nitrendipine
MMSE mean score	25.6	25.5
Modified Rankin Scale (score)	1.4	1.5
Barthel Index (score)	88.8	88.1

MOSES: Conclusion 1

1. First comparison of 2 antihypertensive drugs in stroke patients
2. Well defined hypertensive post-stroke patients
3. Previous and study medications well balanced
4. Early an dcomparable blood pressure control
5. High number of normotensive patients at study end
6. Blood pressure values confirmed by ABPM

MOSES: Conclusion 2

1. Advantages for Eprosartan with regard to:
   - 20% fewer primary endpoints including recurrent events
   - 25% fewer cerebrovascular events including recrurrent events
   - 30% fewer first cardiovascular events

2. No difference between the groups with regard to:
   - First primary endoints in each category
   - First cerebrovascular events
   - Cardiovascular events including recurrent events
   - Dementia

Valsartan Antihypertension Long-term Use Evaluation Trial (VALUE)

VALUE Trial Design

Objective

VALUE was designed to test the hypothesis that, for the same BP control, valsartan would reduce cardiac morbidity and mortality more than amlodipine in hypertensive patients at high CV risk.

Design

VALUE was a prospective, multinational, multicenter trial utilizing a double-blind, randomized, active-controlled, 2-arm, parallel-group comparison. Patients were randomized to either Valsartan or Amlodipine-based therapy. Additional antihypertensive medications were added in a 5-step, response-dependent dose titration scheme to achieve a target BP goal of <140/90 mm HG.

- Step 1: Patients were randomized to receive either Valsartan (80 mg qd) or Amlodipine (5 mg qd).
- Step 2: Doses were up-titrated to valsartan 160 mg or amlodipine 10 mg, depending on BP response.
- Steps 3 and 4: Addition of HCTZ 12.5 mg and 25 mg, respectively, based on achieved BP response
- Step 5: Free add-on of antihypertensive agents other than ACEs, CCBs, ARBs, or diuretics other than HCTZ. The only exception was replacement of loop diuretics in patients with impaired renal function or CHF.

Study Population

15,313 patients aged ≥50 years with treated or untreated hypertension who were at high CV risk. BP entry criteria were 160-210/95-115 mm HG for untreated patients and 210/115 mm HG for those already receiving antihypertensive therapy.

Baseline Characteristics

	Valsartan (n=7649)	Amlodipine (n=7596)
Demographics		
Sex (number % women)	3240 (42.4%)	3228 (42.5%)
Men (number %)	4409 (57.6%)	4368 (57.5%)
Age (years)	67.2	67.3
BMI (kg/m^2)	28.6	28.7
SBP (mm Hg)	154.5	154.8
DBP (mm Hg)	87.4	87.6
Heart Rate (beats per min)	72.3	72.5
Race		
White	6821 (89.2%)	6796 (89.5%)
Black	325 (4.3%)	314 (4.1%)
Oriental	272 (3.6%)	261 (3.4%)
Other	231 (3.0%)	225 (3.0%)
Antihypertension medication taken at time of randomization		
Previously treated for hypertension	7088 (92.7%)	6989 (92.0%)
ACE inhibitors	3148 (41.3%)	3135 (41.4%)
ARBs	812 (10.7%)	800 (10.6%)
a-blockers	540 (7.1%)	495 (6.5%)
b-blockers	2496 (32.7%)	2551 (33.7%)
CCBs	3181 (41.7%)	3048 (40.2%)
Diuretics as monotherapy	2047 (26.9%)	2020 (26.7%)
Fixed-dose diuretic combinations	686 (9.0%)	634 (8.4%)
Qualifying disease factors		
CHD	3490 (45.6%)	3491 (46.0%)
PAD	1052 (13.8%)	1062 (14.0%)
Stroke or TIA	1513 (19.8%)	1501 (19.8%)
LVH with strain pattern (including left bundle branch block)	454 (5.9%)	462 (6.1%)

Study Endpoints (Value Trial)

Primary: Time to first cardiac event (composite of morbidity and/or mortality events):

- Cardiac morbidity: new or chronic CHF requiring hospital management, non-fatal acute MI, emergency procedures performed to prevent MI

- Cordiac mortality: sudden cardiac death, fatal MI, death during or after percutaneous transluminal coronary angioplasty (PTCA) or coronary artery bypass graft (CABG), death due to CHF, death associated with evidence of recent acute MI on autopsy

Secondary: fatal and non-fatal MI, fatal and non-fatal CHF, fatal and non-fatal stroke.

- Worsening of chronic stable angina or unstable angina, routine interventional procedures, potentially lethal arrhythmias, syncope or near-syncope, silent MI, and end-stage renal failure

Prescribed Analysis:

- New-onset diabetes mellitus
- All-cause mortality—previously specified as a secondary endpoint

BP Results

The most consistent and statistically significant difference between the 2 groups was in BP control. BP was substantially lower (4.0 mm Hg/2.1 mm HG) in the amlodipine group in the early months starting from the end of month 1, when the patients were predominantly treated with monotherapy. The BP decrease observed favored amlodipine throughout the trial: on average, the BP difference between the 2 groups remained at least 2.0 mm Hg/1.5 mm HG. At the end of the study, BP reductions from baseline were 17.3/9.9 mm HG for the Amlodipine group and 15.2/8.2 mm HG for the Valsartan group (p<.0001). The target BP (<140/90 mm Hg) was achieved in the 56% of patients in the Valsartan group and 62% in the Amlodipine group. Fewer patients required add-on therapy with Amlodipine (41%) than with Valsartan (48%).

EndPoint Results (Value Trial)

Primary endpoint results	**Time to first cardiac morbidity or mortality:** No significant difference between treatment groups, HR for valsartan 1.04 (0.94-1.15), p=.49
Results for components of primary endpoint	**Cardiac morbidity:** No significant difference between treatment groups, HR 1.02 (0.91-1.15), p=.71
	Cardiac mortality: No significant difference between treatment groups, HR 1.01 (0.86-1.18), p=.90
Secondary endpoint results	**Fatal and non-fatal MI:** Significant difference between treatment groups favoring amlodipine, HR 1.19 (1.02-1.38), p=.02
	Fatal and non-fatal stroke: No significant difference between treatment groups, HR 1.15 (0.98-1.35), p=.08
	Fatal and non-fatal CHF: No significant difference between treatment groups, HR 0.89 (0.77-1.03), p=.12
	All-cause mortality: No significant difference between treatment groups, HR 1.04 (0.94-1.14), p=.45
Other analyses	**New-onset diabetes:** Significant difference between treatment groups favoring valsartan, OR 0.77 (0.69-0.86), p<.0001

Other Results (Value Trial)

Serum creatine	Baseline: valsartan = 101.2; amlodipine = 100.9 End of study: valsartan = 108.1; amlodipine = 103.2
Safety and tolerability	Both treatment strategies were well tolerated with few severe adverse events. The discontinuation rates due to AEs were 11.9% for valsartan and 12.9% for amlodipine. Peripheral edema and hypokalemia were more common on valsartan: dizziness, headache, diarrhea, fatigue, serious angina, and syncope.

Clinical Hypertension Trials in Hypertension with Angiotensin Receptor Blockers (ARBs): Summary

1. Only one large clinical trial has compared an ARB (Losartan) with a beta-blocker (Atenolol) in hypertensive patients in regard to total CV endpoints. This is the LIFE trial. The results indicated significant superiority of Losartan over atenolol in all of the following endpoints:

   a. Reduction in composite CV morbidity and mortality including CV death, CVA, MI, and total mortality.

   b. Reduction in fatal and non-fatal CVA

   c. Reduction in new onset diabetes mellitus

   d. In the diabetic hypertensive, Losartan signficantly reduced (more than atenolol)

      1. CV death

      2. MI

      3. CVA

      4. Total mortality

2. VALUE demonstrated equal reduction in composite cardiac morbidity and mortality with an ARB and DHP-CCB.

3. Renal endpoint clinical trials such as RENAAL, IDNT, IRMA indicate reductions in progression to ESRD and decreased proteinuria with ARBs (Lorsartan and Irbesartan), in patients with diabetes mellitus and proteinuria.

4. ARBs reduce LVH signficantly and better than beta-blockers.

5. ARBs improve endothelial dysfunction and arterial compliance, improve vascular biologic parameters of function and structure.

6. The side effect profile is low and they are well tolerated with high compliance rate.

7. The metabolic and biochemical profile is neutral or favorable.

Coronary Heart Disease: Risk Factors[53–55]

1. Hypertension—SBP and DBP*
2. Hyperlipoproteinemia:*
   a. Hypercholesterolemia: increased LDL cholesterol (especially oxidized LDL, small dense LDL), and increased number of LDL particles by NMR
   b. Decreased HDL cholesterol and abnormal paraoxanase activity
      (1) High HDL_2 subfraction is associated with low incidence of CHD
      (2) HDL_3 subfraction: less CHD association.
   c. Hypertriglyceridemia: VLDL elevation and increased number of VLDL particles by NMR (often seen with low HDL) (especially those with increased total cholesterol). Remnant particles increased CHD risk.
   d. Apolipoprotein A-I and A-II: low levels
   e. Apolipoprotein B: high levels
   f. Lipoprotein A (Lp[a]): high levels
   g. Increased APO-CII
   h. Serum free fatty acids
3. Smoking*
4. Hyperglycemia, (FBS over 90 mg%), diabetes mellitus, elevated hemoglobin A_1C and ACEs (Advanced glycosylation end products)
5. Insulin resistance*
6. Family history of premature cardiovascular disease
7. Physical inactivity (lack of aerobic exercise)*
8. LVH*
9. Stress, anxiety and depression
10. Type A personality (aggressive subtype)

12. Obesity (central)*, BMI>25, increased waist size, increased neck circumference, ↑ WHR, ↑ % body fat
13. Male gender
14. Hyperuricemia*
15. Caffeine abuse (controversial)
16. Age
17. Elevated HS-CRP (high sensitivity C-reactive protein)

---

* Factors modified by antihypertensive therapy.

Coronary Heart Disease: More Potential Risk Factors[55–67]

1. Excessive intake of alcohol: May increase risk; however, small quantities of alcohol increase HDL_3 subfraction and have anti-inflammatory effects that are associated with decreased risk of CHD.[55,58] Low levels of carbohydrate deficient transferrin (CDT) and high levels of GGTP increase CHD risk

2. Increased platelet adhesion or aggregation (or both) and abnormal thrombogenic potential (TPA/PAI-1 ratio)*[59,60]

3. Hemodynamic effects that alter arterial flow disturbances and induce endothelial damage, which enhances atherosclerosis (blood velocity, surfaces)*[61]

4. Renin and angiotensin II: Vasculotoxic and induce LVH*[62,63] and endothelin

5. Sympathetic nervous system overactivity, elevated catecholamines, vasculotoxic (NE and epinephrine [EPI] levels): Induces LVH*[64]

6. Elevated blood viscosity*[65]

7. Hyperinsulinemia*[66,67] and increased proinsulin

8. Hyperfibrinogenemia* increased VWF and increased clotting factors (Factor V, VII, IX, X, XII), protein C, S deficiency

9. Elevated homocysteine levels.

10. Low vitamin C, E, lycopene, and reduced fruits and vegetables in diet (antioxidants)

11. Leukocytosis

12. Corneal arcus, diagonal earlobe crease, and hairy earlobes

13. Linoleic acid deficiency, and reduced intake of omega-3 fatty acids

14. Short stature

15. Low levels of dehydroepiandrosterone sulfate (DHEAS)

16. Nonspecific ST-T wave changes on ECG

17. Lower socioeconomic status

18. Increased plasma levels of PAI-I

19. Elevated serum estradiol in men
20. Chromium deficiency
21. Lean hypertensive men (bottom 20% of IBW)
22. Polycythemia
23. Hypomagnesemia[5]
24. Male pattern baldness
25. Elevated serum creatinine[5]
26. Microalbuminuria and proteinuria[5]
27. Chronic tachycardia, and slow heart rate recovery after TMT
28. Elevated serum iron
29. Chronic infections (HSV, CMV, EBV, H. Flu, Chlamydia, pneumoniae, H. pylori) (mycoplasma)
30. Chronic periodontal infection
31. Osteoporosis at menopause
32. Chronic cough or chronic inflammatory lung disease
33. Hypochloremia
34. Elevated intracellular adhesion molecules (ICAM-1) (V-CAM, p-selectin etc.)
35. Low vitamin K levels
36. Increased Myeloperoxipase levels (MPO)
37. Increased APO-E4
38. Low serum folate and MTHFR 677C T $\rightarrow$ polymorphism
39. Increased CD-14 monocytes and NK T cells
40. Low serum copper
41. Increased phospholipase A_2
42. Increased serum leptin
43. Increased desaturated lecithin
44. Increased interleukin 6 (IL-6), IL-B, TNF-Alpha, LPA
45. Genetic increase in certain SNP (single nucleotide polymorphisms) such as TSP-1 and TSP-4 (thrombospondins)
46. Hostility
47. Aortic calcifications
48. Elevated serum TNF-α (Tumor Necrosis Factor-alpha)
49. Elevated HSP (Heated Shock Protein) in serum
50. Low serum calcitonin gene-related peptide (CGRP)
51. Low sex hormone binding globulin (SHBG)
52. Increased serum amyloid A (SAA)
53. Low levels of serum coenzyme Q-10
54. Low glutathione and glutathione peroxidase activity
55. Low intravascular SOD

---

* Factors modified by antihypertensive therapy.

Coronary Heart Disease Risk Factors: Influence of Diuretic and Beta-Blocker Therapy

	Diuretic (Thiazide and Thiazide-like)	Beta-Blocker (without ISA)
Hypokalemia	Yes	No
Hypomagnesemia	Yes	No
Dyslipidemia	Yes	Yes
Hypercholesterolemia	Yes	Yes or no
Hypertriglyceridemia	Yes	Yes
Elevated LDL cholesterol change	Yes	Yes or no
Lowered HDL cholesterol	Yes or no change	Yes
Elevated apolipoprotein B	Yes	Yes
Lowered apolipoprotein A	Yes	Yes
Elevated Lp(a)	Yes	Yes
Glucose intolerance (hyperglycemia) and onset DM	Yes	Yes
Insulin resistance	Yes	Yes
Hyperuricemia	Yes	Yes
Impaired aerobic exercise	Yes— minimal	Yes
LVH regression	No change	Inconsistent
Improved diastolic dysfunction	No	Inconsistent
Increased blood viscosity	Yes	No
Increased catecholamines	Yes	Yes
Increased angiotensin II	Yes	No
Potentiated arrhythmias	Yes	No
Acid-base abnormalities and other electrolyte disorders	Yes	No
Blood velocity and arterial turbulence abnormalities	Yes	No
Hyperfibrinogenemia	Yes	No
Abnormal platelet function (aggregation and adhesion)	Yes	No
Increased thrombogenic potential increased PAI-1 and PAI-1/TPA ratio	Yes	No
Homocysteinemia	Yes	No
Proteinuria/MAU	Yes	No
Increased creatinine	Yes	No
Reduced GFR	Yes	No

Antihypertensive Drugs and Serum Lipids[5,68,77]

Antihypertensive Drugs with Known Unfavorable Effects on Serum Lipids

1. Diuretics: thiazides, chlorthalidone, loop diuretics, thiazide-like diuretics (not indapamide), metolazone
2. Beta-blockers (without ISA):
   a. Atenolol (Tenormin)
   b. Betaxolol (Kerlone)
   c. Metoprolol (Lopressor, Toprol XL)
   d. Nadolol (Corgard)
   e. Propranolol (Inderal LA)
   f. Timolol (Blocadren)
   g. Bisoprolol (Zebeta)
3. Methyldopa (Aldomet)
4. Reserpine

Antihypertensive Drugs with Potentially Favorable Effects on Serum Lipids

1. Alpha-blockers:
   a. Doxazosin (Cardura)
   b. Prazosin (Minipress)
   c. Terazosin (Hytrin)
2. Calcium channel blockers:
   a. Amlodipine (Norvasc)
   b. Diltiazem (Cardizem SR, CD, LA Dilacor XR, Tiazac)
   c. Felodipine (Plendil)
   d. Isradipine (DynaCirc)

    e. Nicardipine (Cardene and Cardene SR)

    f. Nifedipine (Adalat CC, Adalat Oros, Procardia XL)

    g. Verapamil (Calan SR, Isoptin SR, Verelan, Covera HS)

    h. Nisoldipine (Sular)

3. Central alpha-agonists:

    a. Clonidine (Catapres and Catapres-TTS)

    b. Guanabenz (Wytensin)

    c. Guanfacine (Tenex)

Antihypertensive Drugs with Neutral Effects on Serum Lipids

1. ACE inhibitors:

    a. Benazepril (Lotensin)

    b. Captopril (Capoten)

    c. Enalapril (Vasotec)

    d. Fosinopril (Monopril)

    e. Lisinopril (Prinivil, Zestril)

    f. Quinapril (Accupril)

    g. Ramipril (Altace)

    h. Moexipril (Univasc)

    i. Trandolapril (Mavik)

    j. Perindopril (Aceon)

2. Direct vasodilators:

    a. Hydralazine (Apresoline)

    b. Minoxidil (Loniten)

3. Beta-blockers with ISA:

    a. Acebutolol (Sectral)

    b. Penbutolol (Levatol)

    c. Pindolol (Visken)

    d. Carteolol (Cartrol)

4. Beta-blockers with alpha blocking activity:
    a. Labetalol (Trandate, Normodyne)
    b. Carvedilol (Coreg)
5. Indapamide (Lozol)
6. Angiotensin II inhibitors:
    a. Losartan (Cozaar)
    b. Valsartan (Diovan)
    c. Irbesartan (Avapro)
    d. Telmisartan (Micardis)
    e. Candesartan cilexetil (Atacand)
    f. Eprosartan (Teveten)
    g. Olmesartan (Benicar)

Serum Lipids and Antihypertensive Therapy with Diuretics and Beta-Blockers: *Summary*

1. Dose related: Higher doses of beta-blockers have more adverse effects, but even low doses of thiazide diuretics and thiazide-like diuretics (hydrochlorothiazide). [HCTZ] 12.5 mg, chlorthalidone 12.5 mg) have adverse effects. However, indapamide does *not* adversly affect glucose or lipids.

2. Elevations blunted but *not* prevented by:
   a. Nutritional restriction of fats, carbohydrates and weight loss.
   b. Exercise and reduction of smoking.

3. Duration: Adverse effects persist with long-term therapy well above initial serum lipid levels.

4. Diuretics plus beta-blockers cause additive adverse effects.

5. Thiazide and thiazide-like diuretics have similar adverse lipid effects in equipotent doses except for indapamide, which has neutral effects on lipids.

6. Beta-blockers may differ depending on several factors:
   a. Nonselective: Greatest adverse alteration in serum lipids.
   b. Cardioselective: Less adverse alteration in serum lipids.
   c. ISA: Least alteration in lipids (neutral effect).

7. Diuretic effects on serum lipids appear to be more pronounced in postmenopausal women, men, and obese patients.

8. Increase in lipids is more marked in patients with higher baseline values (average change is about 10% to 20%).

9. Abnormal lipid levels reverse to normal after cessation of therapy (takes 2 to 4 months).

Effects of Antihypertensive Drugs on Coronary Heart Disease Risk Factors[5,78–84]

	Thiazide and Thiazide-like Diuretics	Indapamide	Beta-Blockers without ISA	Beta-Blockers with ISA	Labetalol	Guanthidin Guanad
Hypertension	↓	↓	↓	↓	↓	↓
Dyslipidemia	↑	→	↑	→	→	→
Glucose intolerance	↑	→	↑	↑	↑	→
Insulin resistance	↑	→	↑	↑	?	?
LVH	→	↓	→/↓	↑	↓	↓
Exercise	→/↓	→	↓	↓	→/↓	↓
Potassium	↓	↓*	→/↑	→	→	→
Magnesium	↓	↓*	→	→	→	→
Uric acid	↑	↑*	↑	↑	↑	→
Blood viscosity	↑	→	→	→	→	→
Blood velocity	→/↑	→	↓	→	→	→
Catecholamines	↑	↓	↑	↑	→	↓
Angiotensin II	↑	→	↓	→	↓	↑
Arrhythmia potential	↑	→	↓	→/↑	→	↑
Fibrinogen	↑	→	?	?	?	?
Platelet function	↑	↓	→/↓	?	?	?
Thrombogenic potential	↑	↓	?	?	?	?
Antiatherogenic	→	→	↑†	?	?	↑
Homocysteinemia	↑	→	→	→	→	?
Renal dysfunction						
Proteinuria, MAU	↑	→/↑	→/↑	→/↑	→/↑	?
CHD relative risk ratio	17:20	3:20	6:20	7:20	3:20	3:2

*Minimal.

†Animal studies.

‡Animal and human studies.

↓, Reduced; ↑, increased; →, no change; ?, unknown.

Continues on opposite page

tral pha- nists	Methyl-dopa	Direct Vasodilators	Alpha-Blockers	ACE Inhibitors	Ang-II Inhibitors	Calcium Blockers	Reserpine
↓	↓	↓	↓	↓	↓	↓	↓
↓	↑	→	↓	→	→	↓	↑
↓	→	→	↓	↓	↓	↓	→
↓	→	→	↓	↓	↓	→/↓	?
↓	↓	↑	↓	↓	↓	↓	↓
→	→	→	→	→	→	→	↓
→	→	→	→	↑	↑	→	→
→	→	→	→	→/↑	→/↑	→	→
→/↓	→/↓	→	→	↓	↓	→/↓	→
→	→	↓	↓	→	→	?	?
↓	↑	↑	↓	↓	↓	↓	↓
↓	↓	↑	→/↓	↓	↓	↓	↓
↓	↓	↑	→/↓	↓	↓	↓	↓
↓	↓	↑	→	↓	↓	↓	↑
?	?	?	↓	?	?	?	?
↓	→	?	?	↓	↓	↓	?
?	?	?	?	?	?	↓	?
?	?	?	?	↓[†]	↓[†]	↓[‡]	↑[†]
?	?	?	?	→	→	→	?
→/↑	→/↑	→/↑	→/↑	→/↑	↓	↓	→
20	2:20	5:20	0:20	0:20	0:20	0:20	3:20

Antihypertensive Drugs and Coronary Heart Disease Risk Factors: *Summary*

Favorable Effects (0:20 CHD Relative Risk Ratio)

1. *Calcium channel blockers:*
   a. Amlodipine (Norvasc)
   b. Diltiazem (Cardizem SR, CD and LA, Dilacor XR, Tiazac)
   c. Felodipine (Plendil)
   d. Isradipine (DynaCirc)
   e. Nicardipine (Cardene, Cardene SR)
   f. Nifedipine (Adalat CC, Adalat Oros, Procardia XL)
   g. Verapamil (Calan SR, Isoptin SR, Verelan, Covera HS)
   h. Nisoldipine (Sular)
2. *Alpha-blockers:*
   a. Doxazosin (Cardura)
   b. Prazosin (Minipress)
   c. Terazosin (Hytrin)
3. *Central alpha-agonists:*
   a. Clonidine (Catapres and Catapres-TTS)
   b. Guanabenz (Wytensin)
   c. Guanfacine (Tenex)
4. *ACE inhibitors:*
   a. Benazepril (Lotensin)
   b. Captopril (Capoten)
   c. Enalapril (Vasotec)
   d. Fosinopril (Monopril)
   e. Lisinopril (Prinivil, Zestril)
   f. Quinapril (Accupril)
   g. Ramipril (Altace)
   h. Moexipril (Univasc)
   i. Trandolapril (Mavik)
   j. Perindopril (Aceon)
5. *Angiotensin II blockers:*
   a. Losartan (Cozaar)
   b. Valsartan (Diovan)
   c. Irbesartan (Avapro)
   d. Telmisartan (Micardis)
   e. Candesartan cilexetil (Atacand)

    f. Eprosartan (Teveten)

    g. Olmesartan (Benicar)

Neutral Effects (0–5:20 CHD Relative Risk Ratio)

1. *Diuretics (selected):*
   a. Amiloride (Midamor)
   b. Indapamide (Lozol)
   c. Spironolactone (Aldactone)
   d. Eplerenone (INSPRA)
   e. Triamterene (Dyrenium)
2. *Direct vasodilators:*
   a. Hydralazine (Apresoline)
   b. Minoxidil (Loniten)
3. *Central alpha-agonist:*
   a. Methyldopa (Aldomet)
4. *Alpha-blocker and beta-blocker:*
   a. Labetalol (Trandate, Normodyne)
   b. Carvedilol (Coreg)
5. *Neuronal-inhibiting drugs:*
   a. Guanadrel (Hylorel)
   b. Guanethidine (Ismelin)
   c. Reserpine (Serpasil)

Unfavorable Effects (Over 5:20 CHD Relative Risk Ratio)

1. *Diuretics (selected):*
   a. Chlorthalidone (Hygroton, Thalitone)
   b. Loop diuretics (furosemide, bumetanide, ethacrynic acid, torsemide)
   c. Quinazolines (metolazone)
   d. Thiazides (HCTZ, chlorothiazide, cyclothiazide, poly-thiazide, methyclothiazide)
2. *Beta-blockers without ISA:*
   a. Atenolol (Tenormin)
   b. Betaxolol (Kerlone)
   c. Metoprolol (Lopressor, Toprol XL)
   d. Nadolol (Corgard)
   e. Propranolol (Inderal, Inderal LA)
   f. Timolol (Blocadren)
   g. Bisoprolol (Zebeta)

3. *Beta-blockers with ISA:*
   a. Acebutolol (Sectral)
   b. Penbutolol (Levatol)
   c. Pindolol (Visken)
   d. Carteolol (Cartrol)

Calcium Channel Blockers and Atherosclerosis (Coronary Heart Disease Reduction) Trials

Nifedipine vs. propranolol vs. isosorbide[85]	CHD/angina
Nifedipine vs. placebo (INTACT)[86]	Mild CHD/angina
Nifedipine vs. placebo (INTACT2)[125]	Mild CHD/angina
Verapamil vs. non–calcium channel blocker[87]	CHD/angina
Verapamil vs. placebo (FIPS)[87]	CHD/angina
Isradipine vs. HCTZ (MIDAS)[88]	Carotid artery
Nicardipine vs. placebo[89]	CHD
Verapamil vs. chlorthalidone (VHAS)	CHD/CVD/carotid
Amlodipine vs. placebo (PREVENT)	CHD/CVD/carotid
Nifedipine vs. co-amilozide (INSIGHT)	CHD by EBT
Lacidipine vs. atenolol (ELSA)	Carotid IMT

Hypertension and Renal Damage*

Classification of Chronic Kidney Disease[1]

Stage	Description	GFR (ml/min/1.73m2)
1	Kidney damage with normal or ↑GFR.	>90
2	Kidney damage with mild ↓ GFR	60-89
3	Moderate ↓ GFR	30-59
4	Severe ↓ GFR	15-29
5	Kidney failure (ESRD)	<15 (or dialysis)

Classification of Urinary Protein Excretion

Urinary Protein Excretion Rate per Day	Description/Nomenclature
< 30 mg albumin per day	Not identified as disease state
30-300 mg albumin per day	Microalbuminuria
> 300 mg albumin per day	Macroalbuminuria
> 330 mg total protein per day	Overt proteinuria
>1000 mg total protein per day	Macroproteinuria
> 3500 mg total protein per day	Nephrotic range proteinuria

Hypertension and Renal Damage

1. Hypertensive nephrosclerosis accounts for 23% of the prevalent end-stage renal disease in the U.S. and 26% of incident new cases in 2000. In consideration of the critical role of blood pressure control on renal disease progression, hypertensive nephrosclerosis and diabetic nephrosclerosis together accounted for 57.5% of prevalent end-stage renal disease and 69% of incident new cases of end-stage renal disease in 2000.[2]

2. It is estimated that 11% of the American adult population over age 20 have evidence of chronic kidney disease with at least Stage 1 nephropathy.[3] Furthermore, while 32% of the US adult population has hypertension, 58% of the hypertensive adult American population is estimated to have at least mild reduction of glomerular filtration rate

*(References for this section are found on pages 233 - 235) 221

GFR (Stage 2). The proportion of patients with treated hypertension with impaired renal function is 64%, and the proportion of patients with untreated hypertension with impaired renal function is 52%. At least one study is supportive of the hypothesis that patients with primary hypertension are born with fewer functioning nephrons.[4]

3. Although no data show a reduction in end-stage renal disease related to the treatment of stage I-II mild to moderate hypertension, elevations of blood pressure have been shown to be a strong independent risk factor for end-stage renal disease.[5]

4. Clinical trials, both prospective and retrospective, suggest that 15% to 35% of patients with mild to moderate hypertension progress to renal insufficiency on stepped care therapy (diuretics and beta-blockers) despite adequate BP control. This progression particularly true for African American hypertensive patients.[6]

5. It is postulated that chronic elevations of intraglomerular capillary pressure (Pgc) accelerate the loss of glomeruli and nephron function seen with normal aging. The relative difference in the resistance to flow between the afferent (preglomerular) and efferent (postglomerular) arterioles determines the glomerular capillary pressure.

6. As BP increases, there is a progressive rise in renal vascular resistance (RVR), decreases in effective renal blood flow (RBF) and renal plasma flow (RPF), and a later decrease in GFR. Decline in GFR is initially hemodynamic (reversible) but becomes irreversible due to accelerated glomerulosclerosis and nephron loss. Once the functioning global number of nephrons falls by more than 50%, autoregulation becomes impaired and afferent (preglomerular) arteriolar dilatation induces structural hypertrophy and functional hyperfiltration of each remaining intact "remnant" nephron. Hyperperfusion and hyperfiltration result in glomerular hypertension, which accelerates further global loss of remnant nephrons.

7. Antihypertensive therapy that normalizes both systemic BP and intraglomerular pressure while preserving the autoregulatory ability of the afferent arteriole would be ex

pected to provide protection of glomerular filtration function.

8. Angiotensin II, catecholamines and vasopressin regulate efferent (post-glomerular) arteriolar vasoconstriction. Drugs that interfere with or attenuate angiotensin II, catecholamines, or vasopressin actions (ACE inhibitors, angiotensin receptor antagonists, and calcium channel blockers) may offer renal protection beyond blood pressure reduction alone, whereas drugs that increase angiotensin II, catecholamines and vasopressin (diuretics) may promote glomerular injury despite systemic blood pressure reduction. Drugs that cause regression of glomerular and renal vascular hypertrophy may improve renal function or prolong renal survival (ACE inhibitors, angiotensin receptor antagonists, calcium channel blockers).

9. Clinical trials have demonstrated that different drug categories have different abilities to prevent the decline of GFR in hypertensive patients. ACE inhibitors have been demonstrated to be beneficial in kidney diseased patients with both diabetic[7] and non-diabetic nephropathy with both microalbuminuria and macroproteinuria.[8, 9] ARBs have been demonstrated to be beneficial in patients with type II diabetes mellitus, with microproteinuria or with macroproteinuria. Calcium channel blockers have been shown to be renoprotective in patients with nephropathy that is either diabetic or hypertensive, but calcium channel blocker monotherapy has limited application for renal protection when macroproteinuria is present. Combining calcium channel blockers with either ACE inhibitors or ARBs is very effective. Combination therapy of ACE inhibitors with ARBs is also showing considerable benefit in nondiabetic primary nephropathies.[10]

10. Both SBP and DBP correlate with the development and progression of renal insufficiency and end-stage renal failure, but SBP is more important than DBP as a risk factor. Any degree of hypertension can promote acceleration of renal disease progression.

11. Meta-analysis demonstrates that hypertensive
nephrosclerosis is reduced proportionately with the reduction in blood pressure. Target BP should be 110-
120/70-75 mm Hg in hypertensive patients with renal
impairment and macroproteinuria and in hypertensive
diabetics. Target blood pressure in the absence of
macroproteinuria and diabetes is less clear; results of
the MDRD trial show that there is benefit of aggressive
blood pressure reduction below 130/85, but the AASK
trial did not demonstrate significant benefit in preventing adverse renal outcomes in a population of high-risk
African Americans with Stage 3 and Stage 4 nephropathy without macroproteinuria or diabetes in lowering
BP from group mean of 141/85 to a group mean of
128/78. Other investigators have demonstrated that
while intensive BP lowering (MAP 92) does not slow
the rate of GFR decline in Type I diabetics compared to
usual therapy (MAP 100 to 107), that intensive therapy
does confer the benefit of significant proteinuria reduction compared to usual therapy.[11]

Hypertension-Related Renal Damage: Postulated Mechanisms[4,5,90–93]

↑ PGC
- Glomerular hyperfiltration
- Glomerular hypertension
- Glomerular hyperperfusion
- Efferent arteriolar constriction
- Afferent arteriolar dilation (↑ flow)

Structural changes
- Mesangium
- Glomerular hypertrophy
- Renal tubular hypermetabolism
- Smooth muscle arteriolar hypertrophy and hyperplasia
- Ischemia

Glomerular injury
Glomerular sclerosis

Renal insufficiency
Glomerulosclerosis

Microalbuminuria
Proteinuria

Coagulation disorders
Nephrocalcinosis
Lipids/lipoproteins
Ammonia
Sodium
Protein

Is Thiazide Diuretic-Based Antihypertensive Therapy Associated With Increased Risk of Renal Injury?

1. Despite the fact that most antihypertensive trials in North America incorporating a diuretic arm in the study design have been designed to use the diuretic chlorthalidone, the thiazide diuretic hydrochlorothiazide remains the most commonly prescribed diuretic for blood pressure control in North America.

2. Hydrochlorothiazide has been shown in laboratory animals to increase renal vascular resistance, increase intraglomerular pressure, and increase the production of vasotoxic cytokines including transforming growth factor beta (TGFβ) and plasminogen activator inhibitor (PAI-1) as well as stimulating production of renin, angiotensin II, aldosterone, and homocysteine, all of which have been associated with increased vascular injury. Hydrochlorothiazide has been shown to accelerate glomerular injury in the L-NAME model of glomerulosclerosis, whereas ACE inhibitors, ARBs and CCBs have all been shown to retard renal injury in that model.

3. The National Health and Nutrition Evaluation Survey III (NHANES III) gave a valuable cross-section sampling of the presence of hypertension, adequacy of hypertension therapy and the use of various antihypertensive agents in the United States during data sampling from 1988-94. An analysis of this data has shown that in patients with hypertension, the presence of elevated creatinine level was 1.7 –fold increased (nearly doubled) with the prescription of diuretics (after adjusting for the number of medications prescribed, age, sex, race and diabetes).[12]

4. A number of clinical trials lend evidence in support of the contention that thiazide based antihypertensive therapy is either nephrotoxic or fails to exert discernible

renoprotection. The European Working Party on High Blood Pressure in the Elderly trial (EWPHE)[13], the Hypertension in Elderly Patients in Primary Care trial (HEP)[14] and the Swedish Trial in Old Patients with Hypertension (STOP)[15] all demonstrated significant increases in serum creatinine level in the patients receiving step-care therapy with thiazide diuretics either alone or in combination with beta-blockers (HEP, STOP) or with alpha methyldopa (EWPHE).

5. In the Systolic Hypertension in the Elderly Program (SHEP) trial, after 3 years of follow-up, serum creatinine level had not changed in the placebo group but had significantly increased in the actively treated group (chlorthalidone).[16] The incidence of mild renal insufficiency was similar in placebo and active treatment group regardless of the absence or presence of diabetes. This suggests that chlorthalidone therapy does not confer renal benefit even while cardiovascular and stroke endpoints are significantly reduced.

6. Analysis[17] of the Syst-EUR trial studying changes in renal function in untreated and treated patients showed that serum creatinine levels did not change over 5 years in patients randomized to nitrendipine monotherapy, whereas patients receiving hydrochlorothiazide either alone or in combination with study medication showed a significant increase in serum creatinine level.

7. The International Nifedipine GITS study: Intervention as a Goal in Hypertension Treatment (INSIGHT)[18] demonstrated that when compared with CCB therapy that the diuretic co-amilozide conferred approximately 2.5-fold increased risk of impaired renal function developing during four years of follow-up (4.6% vs. 1.8%).

8. The Antihypertensive and Lipid Lowering treatment to prevent Heart Attack Trial (ALLHAT)[19] found that therapy based upon the diuretic chlorthalidone was associated with a significantly lower glomerular filtration rate at 2 year and 4 years of follow-up compared to both therapies based upon the CCB amlodipine or the ACE inhibitor lisinopril.

9. Analysis of diuretic prescribing practices in the United States show that a direct relationship exists between total American spending for all diuretic therapy and the rate of increase in the incidence rate of ESRD four years later. Renal failure incidence attenuates following reductions of diuretic distribution in the United States. Given that total Medicare spending for ESRD in 2000 approached $14 billion and is rising at approximately 6% annually, further study of the economic impact of expanded diuretic use in the United States is warranted.

Major Clinical Trials Showing Renoprotection

Clinical Trial	Primary Renal Disease	No. Participants	Design and Therapy	Outcome Description
REIN-1[20]	Non-diabetic renal disease with macroproteinuria between 1 Gm and 3 Gm daily	78 active treatment 88 placebo	Ramipril up to 5mg daily vs. placebo	Ramipril reduced macroproteinuria and slowed GFR decline by 56%, greater than expected by BP control alone.
REIN-2[21]	Non-diabetic renal disease with nephrotic range proteinuria above 3 Gm daily	117 patients	Ramipril up to 5mg daily vs. placebo	52% reduction in rate of GFR decline
IRMA-2[22]	Hypertensive type II DM	590 patients	Double blind placebo controlled trial of Irbesartan 150mg daily, 300mg daily and placebo	70% risk reduction of renal endpoints seen in 300mg dose group; risk reduction for 150mg group was not significant
IDNT[23]	Hypertensive type II DM	1715 patients	Double blind placebo controlled Irbesartan vs. Amlodipine vs. conventional BP therapy	Irbesartan reduced risk of renal endpoints by 20% compared to placebo and 23% compared to amlodipine
RENAAL[24]	Type II DM with nephropathy	15 13 patients	Losartan vs. placebo	16% risk reduction in Active treatment group
COOPERATE[25]	Nondiabetic adult patients with Stage 2 to Stage 4 nephropathy, with or without hypertension	336 patients	Losartan vs. Trandolapril vs. combination therapy of both drugs	Combination therapy reduced risk of doubling creatinine or ESRD by 62% compared to trandolapril monotherapy and 60% compared to losartan monotherapy

Major Clinical Trials Showing Renoprotection

Clinical Trial	Primary Renal Disease	No. Participants	Design and Therapy	Outcome Description
AASK[26]	Non-diabetic hypertensive African-Americans with mild to severe renal impairment (Stage 2 to 4 nephropathy)	1094 patients	Amlodipine vs. Metoprolol vs. Ramipril based therapy; BP goals assigned either 102-107 MAP "usual" goal or less than 92 MAP	ACE inhibitor reduced risk of achieving the composite endpoint by 22% compared to BB and 38% compared to CCB. No difference between BB and CCB; no added advantage of achieving aggressive BP target
MARVAL[27]	Type II DM with microalbuminuria, with or without HTN	332 patients	Valsartan 80mg/d vs. Amlodipine 5mg/d for 24 weeks	Valsartan treated patients had significant 44% reduction in Albumin excretion compared to baseline, amlodipine treated patients had non-significant 8% reduction
CALM[28]	Type II DM with hypertension and microalbuminuria	199 patients	Randomized to receive Candesartan or Lisinopril monotherapy for the first 12 weeks; then half the patients were randomized to receive combination therapy of both drugs for the second 12 week period.	At 12 weeks both Candesartan and lisinopril monotherapy significantly reduced proteinuria; at 24 weeks the combination therapy achieved lower blood pressure control than either monotherapy but proteinuria was not significantly further reduced.
MICRO-HOPE[29]	Diabetic patients with at least one other CV risk factor, no proteinuria	3577 patients (subset of HOPE trial)	Randomized to Ramipril 10mg/d or placebo	24% risk reduction of overt nephropathy after 4.5 years independent of BP reduction
EUCLID[30]	Normotensive nonalbuminuric Type I DM patients	530 patients	Placebo controlled Lisinopril therapy trial with 2 year followup	Lisinopril therapy in normotensive nonalbuminuric diabetics reduces the excretion of urinary albumin by 18% after 2 years of follow-up.

Major Clinical Trials Showing Renoprotection

Clinical Trial	Primary Renal Disease	No. Participants	Design and Therapy	Outcome Description
AIPRI[31]	All chronic nephropathies but predominantly nondiabetic	583 patients	Benazepril vs. placebo	53% risk reduction
MDRD[32]	Study 1: Stage 3 nephropathy including diabetic and nondiabetic Study 2: Stage 4 nephropathy including diabetic and nondiabetic	Study 1: 585 patients Study 2: 255 patients	Study 1: Patients assigned usual or low dietary protein intake; BP randomized to "usual" 107 MAP or "low" 92 MAP using any medications Study 2: Patients assigned to low or very low dietary protein intake; BP randomized as in Study 1	Patients in Study 1 had no change in rate of GFR decline regardless of protein intake or BP control. Pooled results of both study arms showed that patients with proteinuria treated to lower BP target MAP 92 had slower decline in GFR.
UKPDS[33]	Type II DM and hypertension	758 patients	Captopril vs. Atenolol	No significant difference between medications; all benefits were ascribed to magnitude of BP lowering
ABCD[34]	Hypertensive type II DM with various degrees of proteinuria	470 patients	Randomized to either CCB Nisoldipine or ACE inhibitor Enalapril; randomized to two levels of BP control "intensive (132/78)" or "moderate (138/86)"	No difference observed between levels of BP control for renal function decline. Both CCB and ACE inhibitor were equally protective of GFR and proteinuria
Collaborative Study Group (Lewis EJ et al.),[35]	Type I DM with overt proteinuria	207 active treatment 202 placebo	Captopril 25 mg TID vs. placebo. 3 year median follow-up	Captopril associated with 50% decline in death, dialysis and transplantation independent of BP difference.

Effects of Antihypertensive Drugs on Renal Function[4,5]

	Diuretics	Beta-Blockers	Beta-Blockers with ISA	Beta-Blockers + Alpha Blockers	Direct Vasodilators	Neuronal Inhibitors	Calcium Channel Blockers	A-II Inhibitors + ACE Inhibitors	Central Alpha-Agonists	Alpha Methyldopa	Alpha-Blockers
GFR	→	→/↓	↑	↑	→/↑	→	←	→	↑/→	↑/→	→/↑
ERPF	→	→/↓	↑	↑	→/↑	→	←	←	↑	↑	↑/↑
GFR/ERPF	↑	↑	↑	↑	↑	→	↑	↑	↑	↑	↑
RBF	→	→/↓	→/↑	→/↑	→/↑	→	↑/→	→/→	↑/→	↑/→	→/↑
RVR	←	→/↑	↑	↑	→	?	→/↓	→	→	→	→
IGCP	←	?	?	?	←	?	→/→	→	?	?	?
Urinary albumin	←	?	?	?	←	→	→/→	→	?	?	?
Urinary Na+	←	→/↓	→/↓	↑	→	↑/↓	↑/→	→/↓	↑/←	→/↓	→/↓
Urinary K+	←	→/↓	↑	↑	↑	↑	↑	→	↑	↑	↑
Urinary Mg2+	←	→/↓	↑	↑	↑	↑	↑	→	↑	↑	↑
Plasma volume	→	→/↑	→/↑	→/↑	←	→/↓	→	↑/↓	→/↑	←	↑

ERPF, Effective renal plasma flow.

↓ Reduced; ↑ increased; → no change; ? unknown.

References
Hypertension and Renal Damage - pgs. 221- 228.

1 National Kidney Foundation: K/DOQI Clinical Practice Guidelines for Chronic Kidney Disease: Evaluation, Classification and Stratification. Am J Kidney Dis 2002; 39 (suppl 1):S1-S266.

2 US Renal Data System: USRDS 2002 Annual Data Report. The National Institutes of Health, National Institute of Diabetes and Digestive and Kidney Diseases, Bethesda, MD, 2002.

3 Coresh J et al. Prevalence of Chronic Kidney Disease and Decreased Kidney Function in the Adult US Population: Third National Health and Nutrition Examination Survey. Am J Kidney Dis 2003;41:1-12.

4 Keller G et al. Nephron Number in Patients with Primary Hypertension. N Engl J Med 2003 348(2): 101-108.

5 Klag, MJ et al. Blood Pressure and End-Stage Renal Disease in Men. N Engl J Med 1996;334:8-13.

6 Rostand SG et al. Renal insufficiency in treated essential hypertension. N Engl J Med 1989;320:684-688.

7 Bakris GL et al. Preserving Renal Function in Adults with Hypertension and Diabetes: A Consensus Approach. Am J Kidney Dis 2000;36(3):646-661.

8 Jafar TH et al. Angiotensin-Converting Enzyme Inhibitors and Progression of Nondiabetic Renal Disease. Ann Intern Med 2001;135:73-87.

9 Kshirsagar AV et al. Effect of ACE Inhibitors in Diabetic and Nondiabetic Chronic Renal Disease: a systematic overview of randomized placebo-controlled trials. Am J Kidney Dis 2000;35(4):695-707.

10 Russo D et al. Coadministration of Losartan and Enalapril Exerts Additive Antiproteinuric Effect in IgA Nephropathy. Am J Kidney Dis 2001;38: 18-25.

11 Lewis JB et al. Effect of Intensive Blood Pressure control on the Course of Type I Diabetic Nephropathy. Am J Kidney Dis 1999;34(5): 809-817.

12 Coresh J et al. Prevalence of High Blood Pressure and Elevated Serum Creatinine Level in the United States. Arch Intern Med 2001;161: 1207-1216.

13 Fletcher A et al. Risks and benefits in the trial of the European Working Party on High Blood Pressure in the Elderly. J Hypertens 1991;9:225-230.

14 Coope J et al. Randomised trial of treatment of hypertension in elderly patients in primary care. BMJ 1986;293:1145-1151.

15 Ekbom T et al. Antihypertensive efficacy and side effects of three beta-blockers and a diuretic in elderly hypertensives: a report from the STOP-Hypertension study. J Hypertens 1992;10:1525-1530.

16 Savage PJ et al. Influence of long-term low-dose diuretic-based antihypertensive therapy on glucose, lipid, uric acid and potassium levels in older men and women with isolated systolic hypertension. The Systolic Hypertension in the Elderly Program. Arch Intern Med 1999;158:741-751.

17 Voyaki SM et al. Follow-up of renal function in treated and untreated older patients with isolated systolic hypertension. J Hypertens 2001;19:511-519.

18 Brown MJ et al. Morbidity and mortality in patients randomized to double-blind treatment with a long-acting calcium-channel blocker or diuretic in the International Nifedipine GITS study: Intervention as a Goal in Hypertension Treatment (INSIGHT). Lancet 2000;356:366-372.

19 The ALLHAT Study Group. Major Outcomes in High-Risk Hypertensive Patients Randomized to Angiotensin-Converting Enzyme Inhibitor or Calcium-Channel Blocker vs. Diuretic. JAMA 2002;288:2981-1997.

20 Ruggenenti P et al. Renoprotective properties of ACE-inhibition in non-diabetic nephropathies with non-nephrotic proteinuria. Lancet 1999;354:359-364.

21 The GISEN Group: Randomised placebo-controlled trial of effect of ramipril on decline in glomerular filtration rate and risk of terminal renal failure in proteinuric, non-diabetic nephropathy. Lancet 1997;349:1857-1863.

22 Parving, H et al. The Effect of Irbesartan on the Development of Diabetic Nephropathy in Patients with Type 2 Diabetes. N Engl J Med 2001;345(12): 870-878.

23 Lewis EJ et al. Renoprotective Effect of the Angiotensin-Receptor Antagonist Irbesartan in Patients with Nephropathy Due to Type 2 Diabetes. N Engl J Med 2001;345(12):851-860.

24 Brenner BM et al. Effects of Losartan on Renal and Cardiovascular Outcomes in Patients with Type 2 Diabetes and Nephropathy. N Engl J Med 2001;345(12): 861-869.

25 Nakao N et al. Combination treatment of angiotensin-II receptor blocker and angiotensin-converting-enzyme inhibitor in non-diabetic renal disease (COOPERATE): a randomized controlled trial. Lancet 2003;361:117-124.

26 Wright JT et al. Effect of Blood Pressure Lowering and Antihypertensive Drug Class on Progression of Hypertensive Kidney Disease. JAMA 2002;288:2421-2431.

27 Viberti G et al. Microalbuminuria Reduction with Valsartan in Patients with Type 2 Diabetes Mellitus. Circulation 2002;106:672-678.

28 Mogensen CE et al. Randomised controlled trial of dual blockade of renin-angiotensin system in patients with hypertension, microalbuminuria and non-insulin dependent diabetes: the candesartan and lisinopril microalbuminuria (CALM) study. BMJ 2000 Dec 9;321(7274):1440-1444.

29 Heart Outcomes Prevention Evaluation (HOPE) Study Investigators: Effects of ramipril on cardiovascular and microvascular outcomes in people with diabetes mellitus: Results of the HOPE study and MICRO-HOPE substudy. Lancet 2000; 355:253-259, 2000.

30 The EURODIAB Contolled Trial of Lisinopril in Insulin-Dependent Diabetes Mellitus (EUCLID) Study Group. Randomised placebo-controlled trial of lisinopril in normotensive patients with insulin-dependent diabetes and normoalbuminuria or microalbuminuria. Lancet 1997 Jun 21;349(9068):1787-92.

31 Maschio G et al. Effect of the angiotensin-converting enzyme inhibitor benazepril on the progression of chronic renal insufficiency. The Angiotensin-Converting Enzyme Inhibition in Progressive renal insufficiency study group. N Engl J Med 1996;334:939-945.

32 Klahr S et al. The Effects of Dietary Protein Restriction and Blood Pressure Control on the Progression of Chronic Renal Disease. N Engl J Med 1994; 330(13):877-884.

33 UK Prospective Diabetes Study Group: Efficacy of atenolol and captopril in reducing risk of macrovascular and microvascular complications in patients with hypertension and type 2 diabetes: UKPDS 39. BMJ 1998; 317:713-720.

34 Estacio RO et al. Effect of blood pressure control on diabetic microvascular complications in patients with hypertension and type 2 diabetes. Diabetes Care 2000 Apr;23 (suppl) 2:B54-64.

35 Lewis EJ et al. The effect of angiotensin-converting enzyme inhibition on diabetic nephropathy. N Engl J Med 1993;329:1456-1462.

Hypertension and Diabetes Mellitus

Causes of Death Among People with Diabetes

Cause	% of Deaths
Ischemic heart disease	40
Other heart disease	15
Diabetes (acute complications)	13
Cancer	13
Cerebrovascular disease	10
Pneumonia/influenza	4
All other causes	5

From Geiss LS, et al. Mortality in non-insulin–dependent diabetes. Diabetes in America, 2nd ed. Bethesda, MD. National Diabetes Data Group, 1995,233-257.

Major CV Events in Patients with Diabetes in Relation to Target Blood Pressure Groups.

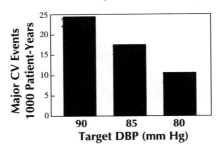

JNC-7 Recommendations for Patients with Diabetes Mellitus

- Combination of 2 or more drugs to achieve BP<130/ 80 mm Hg
- ACEI and ARB slow progression and reduce albuminuria
- ARBs reduce progression to macroalbuminuria

Large Clinical Trials in Hypertension and Type 2 Diabetes or Impaired Glucose Metabolism[191]

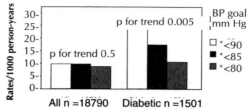

HOT — Rate of Major CV Events According to Randomized Groups

From Hanson L, Zanchelli A, Carruthers SG, et al. Effects of intensive blood-pressure lowering and low-dose aspirin in patients with hypertension: Principal results of the Hypertension Optimal Treatment (HOT) randomised trial. Lancet. 1998;351:1755-1762, with permission.

UK Prospective Diabetes Study

Tight vs. less tight BP control

Endpoint	RR	9-5% CI
Any endpoint	0.76	0.62 - 0.92
Diabetes death	0.68	0.49 - 0.94
Any death	0.82	0.63 - 1.08
MI	0.79	0.59 - 1.07
Stroke	0.56	0.35 - 0.89
PAD	0.51	0.19 - 1.37
Microvascular disease	0.63	0.44 - 0.89

n = 758 vs. 390.

From UK Prospective Diabetes Study Group. Tight blood pressure control and risk of macrovascular and microvascular complications in type 2 diabetes. UKPDS 38. BMJ. 1998;317:703-713, with permission.

UK Prospective Diabetes Study

Captopril vs Atenolol		
Endpoint	RR	95% CI
Any endpoint	1.10	0.86–1.41
Diabetes death	1.27	0.82–1.97
Any death	1.14	0.81–1.61
MI	1.20	0.82–1.76
Stroke	1.12	0.59–2.12
PAD	1.48	0.35–6.19
Microvascular disease	1.29	0.80–2.10

n = 400 vs 358.

From UK Prospective Diabetes Study Group. Efficacy of atenolol and
captopril in reducing risk of macrovascular and microvascular complications
in type 2 diabetes: UKPDS 39. BMJ. 1998;317:713–720, with permission.

SYST-EUR
Systolic Hypertension in Europe Trial:
Effect of active treatment in diabetic (n=492)
and nondiabetic (n=4203) hypertensive patients (n=4695)
Median follow-up was 2 years

CCB treatment reduced stroke 69% and cardiac events
57% in diabetic hypertensives

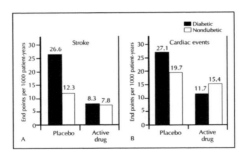

Benefit of active treatment began soon after randomization, when
most patients were still on monotherapy with nitrendipine.

Prisant LM, Louard RJ: Controversies surrounding the treatment of the hypertensive
patient with diabetes. Current Hypertension Reports 1999, 1:512–520, with permission.

CAPPP — Patients with Diabetes[133*]

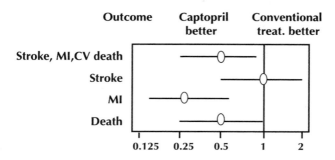

SHEP
Systolic Hypertension in the Elderly Program:
**Relative risk reduction of endpoints by active treatment versus placebo for diabetic (n=583) and nondiabetic (n=4149) patients by treatment group
Mean follow-up was 4.5 years**

Diuretic with beta-blocker treatment reduced cardiac events 54% but did *not* alter CVA morbidity or mortality compared to placebo.

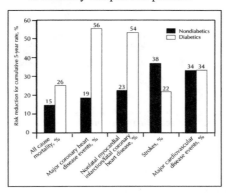

Prisant LM, Louard RJ: Controversies surrounding the treatment of the hypertensive patient with diabetes. Current Hypertension Reports 1999, 1:512-520, with permission.

Hypertensive Diabetics: Mortality, CHD and Antihypertensive Therapy[94]

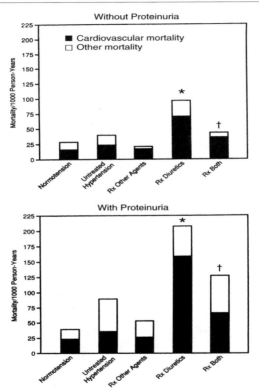

Mortality per 1000 person-years in diabetic patients without proteinuria and with proteinuria according to hypertension status and type of antihypertensive treatment (Rx) during each year of follow-up. Diuretics increased cardiovascular mortality and total mortality compared to other antihypertensive drugs or no treatment. *P < 0.025; †P < 0.025 vs. treatment with diuretics alone. (From Warram JH, Laffel LMB, Valsania P, et al. Excess mortality associated with diuretic therapy in diabetes mellitus. *Arch Intern Med* 1991; 151:1350–1356, with permission).

SHEP and Syst-Eur in Diabetic and Nondiabetic Patients

	Diabetics		Nondiabetics	
	SHEP	Syst-Eur	SHEP	Syst-Eur
N (% of Total)	590 (12.3)	492 (10.5)	4,149 (87.7)	4,203 (89.5)
Mean blood pressure reduction corrected for placebo				
Systolic (mmHg)	-9.8	-8.6	-12.5	-10.3
Diastolic (mmHg)	-2.2	-3.9	-4.1	-4.6
Risk in placebo group (events/1000 patient-years)				
Total mortality	35.6	45.1	21.8	21.6
Cardiovascular endpoints	63.0	55.0	36.8	28.9
Stroke	28.8	26.6	15.0	12.3
Coronary events	32.2	23.1	15.2	12.4
Percent change with active treatment (95% confidence interval)				
Mortality	-26 (-54, 18)	-64 (-83, -25)	-15 (-32, 6)	-18 (-40, 13)
All cardiovascular endpoints	-34 (-54, -6)	-68 (-84, -35)	-34 (-45, -21)	-30 (-47, -8)
Stroke	-22 (55, 34)	-86 (-96, -58)	-38 (-54, -17)	-39 (-60, -7)
Coronary events	-56 (-75, -23)	-58 (-87, 37)	-19 (-38, 5)	-22 (-47, 17)

The combinatin of a CCB and ACEI is more effective than a
diuretic and beta-blocker in reducing all of the following:
1. Total Mortality
2. CV events
3. CVA
4. Coronary events

(See Syst-Eur vs. SHEP)

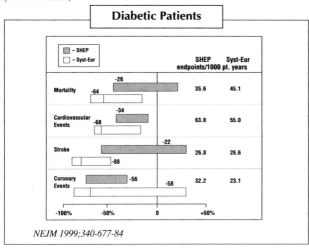

NEJM 1999;340-677-84

Trials Comparing More with Less Intensive or Active with Placebo Treatment: Effects on Renal Function[191]

Trial	Renal variable	Patients (n)	BP	A	Treatment (Comparison)	Years	BP Difference mm Hg	More Intensive or active	Less Intensive or placebo	p
SHEP[31]	SCr (Δ μmol/l)	583	HT	—	D versus Pl	3	-9.8/-2.2	+4.8	+0.7	NS
UKPDS[15]	SCr (Δ)	1148	HT	—	More versus less	9	-10/-5	—	—	NS
HOT[9]	SCr (Δ μmol/l)	1501	HT	—	More versus less	3.8	-3/-3	+2.2	+2.7	NS
Syst-Eur[10]	SCr (Δ μmol/l)	492	HT	—	CA versus Pl	2	-8.6/-3.9	+3.3	+4.4	NS
IDNT[12]	SCr (Δ μmol/l per year)	1148	HT	OA	AIIA versus Pl	3	-4/-3	+40	+53	0.008
IDNT[12]	SCr (Δ μmol/l per year)	1136	HT	OA	CA versus Pl	3	-3/-3	+51	+52	NS
Ravid et al.[28]	100/SCr (Δ)	94	NT	MA	ACEI versus Pl	5	-0.01	-0.12	<0.05	-0.47
Lebovitz et al.[27]	GFR (Δ ml/min/1.73 m^2 per month)	121	HT	MA	ACEI versus Pl	2	-0.47	-2.2	-0.13	0.012
Ahmad et al.[28]	GFR (Δ ml/min/1.73 m^2 per month)	103	NT	MA	ACEI versus Pl	5	0/-3	-5	-5	NS
Ravid et al.[28]	CrCl (Δ ml/min per year)	156	NT	NA	ACEI versus Pl	6	-4	-1.5	-2.4	0.040
ABCD-HT[24]	CrCl (Δ ml/min/1.73 m^2 per year)	470	HT	—	More versus less	5	-6/-8	-7	-11	NS
ABCD-NT[9]	CrCl (Δ ml/min/1.73 m^2 per year)	480	NT	—	More versus less	5	-9/-6	-8	-8	NS
IRMA[14]	CrCl (Δ ml/min/1.73 m^2 per year)	590	HT	MA	AIIA versus Pl	2	-2/0	-8.5	-4.8	NS
RENAAL[13]	est CrCl (Δ ml/min/1.73 m^2 per year)	1513	HT	OT	AIIA versus Pl	3.4	-2.5/-0.5	-4.4	-5.2	0.01

SCr–Serum creatinine; GFR– glomerular filtration rate; CrCl– estimated creatinine clearance; HT–hypertensives; NT–normotensives; A– albuminuria; NA–no albuminuria; MA–microalbuminuria; OA–overt albuminuria; D–diuretics; CA–calcium antagonists; ACEI–ACE inhibitors; AIIA–angiotensin II receptor antagonists; Pl–placebo; NS–non-significant. The blood pressure (BP) differences (diff) between treatment groups are expressed as systolic BP/diastolic BP or (single figure) as mean BP.

Trials Comparing More with Less Intensive or Active with Placebo Treatment: Effects on Renal Dysfunction or Failure[191]

Trial	Renal variable	Comparison	Years	More Intensive or active	Less Intensive or placebo	P	RR	95% CI
SHEP[31]	% Patients with SCr≥176.8 µmol	D versus Pl	3	18	29	NS		
HOT[6]	% Patients with SCr≥176.8 µmol	More versus less	3.8	9.8	12.2	NS		
UKPDS[15]	n renal failure per 1000 patients yrs	More versus less	9	1.4	2.3	NS		
Syst-Eur[10]	n renal failure per 1000 patients yrs	CA versus Pl	2	5.7	5.7	NS		
IDNT[12]	% Patients with 2x SCr + ESRD + death	AIIA versus Pl	3	32.6	39.0	0.02	0.80	0.66-0.97
	% Patients with 2x SCr	AIIA versus Pl	3	16.9	23.7	0.003	0.67	0.52-0.87
	% Patients with ESRD	AIIA versus Pl	3	14.2	17.8	0.07	0.77	0.57-1.03
	% Patients with 2x SCr + ESRD + death	CA versus Pl	3	41.1	39.0	NS	1.04	0.86-1.25
	% Patients with 2x SCr	CA versus Pl	3	25.4	23.7	NS	1.06	0.84-1.35
	% Patients with ESRD	CA versus Pl	3	18.3	17.8	NS	1.00	0.76-1.32
RENAAL[13]	% Patients with 2x SCr + ESRD + death	AIIA versus Pl	3.4	15.9	18.1	0.02	0.84	0.72-0.98
	% Patients with 2x SCr	AIIA versus Pl	3.4	7.9	10.0	0.006	0.75	0.61-0.92
	% Patients with ESRD	AIIA versus Pl	3.4	6.9	9.1	0.002	0.72	0.58-0.89

SCr–Serum creatinine; D–diuretics; AIIA–angiotensin II receptor antagonists; Pl–placebo; NS–non-significant; ESRD–end-stage renal failure; RR–relative risk; CI–confidence intervals.

Trials Comparing More with Less Intensive or Active with Placebo Treatment: Effects on Urinary Albumin Excretion[191]

Trial	Renal variable	Treatment Comparison	Years	More Intensive or active	Less Intensive or placebo	P
Ravid et al.[26]	ΔUAE (mg/24 h)	ACEI versus PI	5	−3	+187	<0.05
Lebovitz et al.[26]	ΔUAE (mg/24 h)	ACEI versus PI	2	−310	+470	NR
Ahmad et al.[28]	ΔUAER (μg/min)	ACEI versus PI	5	−35	+32	<0.001
Ravid et al.[29]	ΔUAE (mg/24 h)	ACEI versus PI	6	−4.2	−15.7	0.001
MICROHOPE[11]	ΔUA/Cr ratio	ACEI versus PI	4.5	+1.35	−1.9	0.02
ABCD-HT[34]	% ΔUAE	More versus less	5	+0.1	+0.2	NS
ABCD-NT[9]	% ΔUAE	More versus less	5	+0.36	+.066	0.001
IDNT[12]	% ΔUAE % ΔUAE	AIIA versus PI CA versus PI	3 3	−33 −6	−10 −10	NS NS
RENAAL[13]	ΔlogUAE	AIIA versus PI	3.4	−35	+5	0.0001
IRMA[14]	ΔlogUAE	AIIA versus PI	2	−31	−2	<0.001

CA–Calcium antagonists; ACEI–angiotensin -converting enzyme inhibitors; AIIA–angiotensin II receptor antagonists; PI–placebo; NS–non-significant; UAE– urninary albumin excretion; NR– not reported. The data of Lebovitz et al 27 are from the subgroup of patients with baseline overt albuminuria.

Trials Comparing More with Less Intensive or Active with Placebo Treatment: New or Worsening Proteinuria[191]

Trial	Renal variable	Treatment Comparison	Years	More Intensive or active	Less Intensive or placebo	P	RR or OR* (95% CI)
Ravid et al.[26]	From MA to OA (%)	ACEI versus PI	5	12	42	< 0.001	
Lebovitz et al.[26]	From MA to OA (%)	ACEI versus PI	3	7	21	NR	
Ahmad et al.[28]	From MA to OA (%)	ACEI versus PI	5	7.7	23.5	< 0.001	
Ravid et al.[29]	From MA to MA (%)	ACEI versus PI	6	6.5	19.0	< 0.042	
Gaede et al.[29]	From MA to OA (%)	More versus less multi-management	3.8	10.4	24.4	0.01	0.27* (0.10–0.75)
UKPDS[15]	New MA (n/1000 pt year) New OA (n/1000 pt year)	More versus less More versus less	6 6	20.3 5.3	28.5 8.6	0.009 NS	0.76 (0.51–0.99) 0.61 (0.31–1.21)
MICROHOPE[11]	New MA	ACEI versus PI	4.5	-	-	NS	0.91 (0.80–1.04)
Syst-Eur[10]	New OA (n/1000 pt year)	CA versus PI	2	18.8	58.0	0.008	0.29 (0.12–0.69)
ABCD-HT[34]	From NA to MA (%) From MA to OA (%)	More versus less More versus less	5 5	25 16	18 23	NS NS	
ABCD-NT[8]	From NA to OA (%) From MA to OA (%)	More versus less More versus less	5 5	lower lower	higher higher	0.012 0.028	
IRMA[14]	From MA to OA (%)	AHA versus PI	2	5.2	14.9	< 0.001	0.30 (0.14–0.61)

MA– Microalbuminuria; OA– overt albuminuria; CA–calcium antagonists; ACEI–angiotensin-converting enzyme inhibitors; PI– placebo; pt– patient; NS– non-significant; NR– not reported; NA– no albuminuria; AHA– angiotensin II receptor antagonists; RR– relative risk; CI– confidence intervals; OR– odds ratio

Trials Comparing Regimens Based on Different Drug Classes: *Renal Effects*[191]

Trial	Treatment Comparison	Patients Years	n	BP	A	Change in CrCL ml/min/1.73m² 1	2	P	Renal Failure % patients 1	2	P	Change in UAE % 1	2	P	New MA % patients 1	2	P	New OAH % patients 1	2	P
UKPDS[23]	ACEI versus βB	9	758	HT	–				1.3	1.4	NS				31*	26*	NS	5*	10*	NS
INSIGHT[20]	CA versus D	3.5	1302	HT	–				0.6	1.1	NS									
ABCD-HT[34]	ACEI versus CA	5	470	HT	–	-10	-8	NS				-0.3	+0.2	<0.05**	20	23	NS	19	20	NS
ABCD-NT[8]	ACEI versus CA	5	354	NT	–	-7	-7	NS						NS			NS			NS
IDNT[72]	AIIA versus CA	3	1146	HT	OA	-5.5†	-6.8†	NR	32.6	41.1	0.006	-33	-6	NR						
LIFE[25]	AIIA versus βB	5	1195	HT	–													7	13	0.002

CrCl, Creatinine clearance; HT, hypertensives; NT, normotensives; OA, overt albuminuria; MA, microalbuminuria; D, diuretics; CA, calcium antagonists; ACEI, angiotensin-converting enzyme inhibitors; AHA, angiotensin II receptor antagonists; NS, non-significant; NR, not reported; UAE, urinary albumin excretion; _B, beta-blockers. 1 and 2 indicate the first and the second treatment, respectively, of the column treatment comparison. * MA and OA at the end of the study, independently of baselines. **Significance lost after 3.5 years. †Changes in creatinine clearance per year.

Trials Comparing Different Antihypertensive Regimens: Worsening of Diabetes[191]

Trial	n	Treatment Comparison	Years	Variable	Treatment 1	Treatment 2	P
UKPDS [15]	1148	More versus less	4	Final HbA1c (%)		7.2	7.2	NS
			8	Final HbA1c (%)		8.3	8.3	NS
MiCROHOPE[11]	3577	ACEI versus PI	4.5	ΔHbA1c(%)		2.2	2.0	NS
ABCD-HT [34]	470	More versus less	5	Final HbA1c (%)		10.2	9.9	NS
ABCD-NT [8]	480	More versus less	5	Final HbA1c (%)		10.5	10.5	NS
IRMA[14]	590	AHA versus PI	2	ΔHbA1c (%)		0.4	0.3	NS
UKPDS [23]	758	ACEI versus βB	4	Final HbA1c (%)		7.0	7.5	< 0.01
			8	Final HbA1c (%)		8.3	8.4	NS
			4	Added antidiabetics (%)		53	66	< 0.005
			8	Added antidiabetics (%)		71	81	<0.05
ABCD-HT [34]	470	ACEI versus CA	5	final HbA1c (%)		10.0	10.0	NS
ABCD-NT [8]	480	ACEI versus CA	5	final HbA1c(%)		10.8	10.2	NS

CA–Calcium antagonists; ACEI–angiotensin-converting enzyme inhibitors; βB–beta-blocker; AIIA–angiotensin II receptor antagonists; PI–placebo; NS, non-significant.

Trials Comparing Different Antihypertensive Regimens: New Onset Diabetes[191]

Trial	n	Treatment Comparison	Years	New Onset Diabetes % Patients 1	2	n/1000 pt year 1	2	P	RR (95% CI)
SHEP [29]	3209	D versus PI	3	8.6	7.5			NS	
HOPE [4]	5720	ACEI versus PI	4.5	3.6	5.4			< 0.001	0.66 (0.51-0.85)
NORDIL [21]	10881	CA versus D/βB	4.5			9.4	10.8	NS	0.87 (0.73-1.04)
STOP-2 [45]	1409	CA versus D/βB	5			9.9	10.0	NS	0.97 (0.73-1.29)
INSIGHT [20]	6321	CA versus D	3.5	4.3	5.6			< 0.05	
NICS-EH [46]	414	CA versus D	5	0	1.9			NS	
CAPPP [47]	10985	ACEI versus D/βB	6.1					0.039	0.86 (0.74-0.99)
STOP-2 [45]	4418	ACEI versus D/βB	5			9.6	10.0	NS	0.96 (0.72-1.27)
STOP-2 [45]	4401	ACEI versus CA	5			9.6	9.9	NS	0.98 (0.74-1.31)
LIFE [48]	7998	AHA versus βB	4.8	6	8	13.0	17.4	0.001	0.75 (0.63-0.88)

D–Diuretics; CA–calcium antagonists; ACEI–angiotensin-converting enzyme inhibitors; AIIA– angiotensin II receptor antagonists; βB, beta-blockers; PI– placebo; NS–non-significant; pt–patient; RR–relative risk; CI–confidence interval.

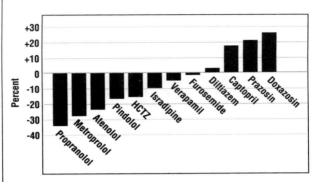

Insulin Sensitivity and Antihypertensive Drugs

The effects on insulin sensitivity index of 3 to 6 months of antihypertensive monotherapy given to groups of hypertensive patients.

Lithell HO. Effect of antihypertensive drugs on insulin, glucose, and lipid metabolism. Diabetes Care 1991;14:203-209.

Primary Trials of Hypertension Control in Diabetes*

Trial	Intervention and Primary Agents	Primary Subgroup Analysis	Total Cardiovascular Events		Total Mortality		Microvascular EndPoints	
			Relative Risk	Absolute Risk	Relative Risk	Absolute Risk	Relative Risk	Absolute Risk
SHEP	Thiazide diuretic vs. usual care	Subgroup	0.66 (0.46 to 0.94)	0.08(0.01 to 0.14)	0.74 (0.46 to 1.18)	0.02 (-0.04 to 0.08)	Not reported	Not reported
Syst-Eur	Calcium-channel blocker vs. placebo	Subgroup	0.38 (0.20 to 0.81)	0.08 (0.03 to 0.13)	0.59 (0.31 to 1.09)	0.03 (-0.01 to 0.09)	Not reported	Not reported
HOPE	ACE inhibitor vs. placebo	Subgroup	0.75 (0.64 to 0.88)	0.05 (0.02 to 0.07)	0.76 (0.63 to 0.92)	0.03 (0.01 to 0.05)	0.84 (0.71 to 0.99)	0.03 (0.00 to 0.05)‡
RENAAL	Angiotensin II receptor blocker vs. placebo	Primary	0.90†	0.02 (-0.03 to 0.07)	1.02 (0.73 to 1.19)	-0.01 (-0.05 to 0.03)	0.79 (0.66 to 0.95)‡	0.04 (0.00 to 0.09)‡
IPDM	Angiotensin II receptor blocker vs. placebo	Primary	Not reported	Not reported	Not reported	Not reported	0.30 (0.14 to 0.61)§	0.10 (0.04 to 0.16)§
HOT	Target diastolic blood pressure <80 mm Hg or <90 mm Hg; agents = felodipine, then ACE inhibitor or β-blocker	Subgroup	0.49 (0.14 to 0.78)	0.05 (0.02 to 0.08)	0.56(0.31 to 1.02)	0.03 (0.00 to 0.05)	Not reported	Not reported
UKPDS	Target blood pressure <180/105 mm Hg vs. <150/85 mm Hg; agents = captopril or atenolol	Primary	0.66‖	Not reported	0.82 (0.63 to 1.08)	0.04 (-0.01 to 0.09)	0.63 (0.44 to 0.89)	0.05 (0.01 to 0.09)
ABCD	Target diastolic blood pressure 75 mm Hg vs. 80-89 mm Hg; agent = nisoldipine or enalapril	Primary	No difference	Not reported	0.51 (0.27 to 0.97)	0.05 (0.00 to 0.10)	No difference¶	No difference

* Values in parentheses are 95% CIs. ABCD = Appropriate Blood Pressure Control in Diabetes; ACE = angiotensin-converting enzyme; HOPE = Heart Outcomes and Prevention Evaluation study; HOT = Hypertension Optimal Treatment; IDPM = Irbesartan in Patients with Type 1 Diabetes and Microalbuminuria; RENAAL = Reduction of Endpoints in NIDDM with the Angiotensin II Antagonist Losartan; SHEP = Systolic Hypertension in the Elderly Program; Syst-Eur = Systolic Hypertension in Europe; UKPDS = United Kingdom Prospective Diabetes Study.

† P>0.2; ‡Renal outcomes (doubling of serum creatinine concentration and risk for end-stage renal disease).

§ Comparison for 300-mg dose of Irbesartan; 150-mg dose did not significantly reduce risk; risk is for progression of nephropathy.‖ P = 0.019.

¶ No combined endpoint reported. Relative risks for individual endpoints comparing intensive with moderate blood pressure control were as follows; progression from normoalbuminuria to microalbuminuria, 1.38 (CI, 0.84 to 2.27); progression from microalbuminuria to overt albuminuria, 0.70 (CI, 0.36 to 1.36); retinopathy progression, 0.88 (CI, 0.68 to 1.15); and neuropathy progression, 1.30 (CI, 1.01 to 1.66).

Vijan S, Hayward RA, treatment of hypertension in type 2 diabetes mellitus: Blood Pressure goals, choice of agents and setting priorities in diabetes care. Ann Intern Med 2003; 138: 593-602.

Effects of Different Drug Classes in Treatment of Hypertension in Diabetes

Trial	Intervention and Primary Agents	Primary Subgroup Analysis	Total Cardiovascular Events		Total Mortality		Microvascular EndPoints	
			Relative Risk	Absolute Risk	Relative Risk	Absolute Risk	Relative Risk	Absolute Risk
ABCD	Enalapril vs. nisoldipine	Primary	0.43 (0.25 to 0.73)	0.09 (0.04 to 0.13)	0.77 (0.36 to 1.67)	0.02 (-0.03 to 0.06)	Not reported	Not reported
FACET	Fosinopril vs. amlodipine	Primary	0.49 (0.26 to 0.95)	0.07 (0.01 to 0.13)	0.81 (0.22 to 3.02)	0.01 (-0.03 to 0.04)	Not reported	Not reported
CAPPP	Captopril vs. thiazide diuretic or β-blocker	Subgroup	0.59 (0.38 to 0.91)	Not reported	0.54 (0.31 to 0.96)	Not reported	Not reported	Not reported
UKPDS	Captopril vs. atenolol	Primary	1.29 (0.92 to 1.81)	Not reported	1.14 (0.81 to 1.61)	-0.02 (-0.08 to 0.03)	1.29 (0.80 to 2.10)	-0.02 (-0.06 to 0.02)
NORDIL	Diltiazem vs. β-blocker or diuretics	Subgroup	1.01 (0.66 to 1.53)	-0.01 (-0.06 to 0.04)	1.07 (0.63 to 1.84)	-0.01 (-0.05 to 0.03)	Not reported	Not reported
INSIGHT	Nifedipine GITS vs. coamilozide	Subgroup	0.99 (0.69 to 1.42)	0.00 (-0.03 to 0.03)	0.75† (0.52 to 1.09)	Not reported	Not reported	Not reported
STOP-2 (3 groups)								
	Calcium-channel blocker vs. diuretics or β-blocker	Subgroup	0.91 (0.66 to 1.26)	0.03 (-0.06 to 0.11)	0.79 (0.54 to 1.14)	0.05 (-0.03 to 0.12)	Not reported	Not reported
	ACE inhibitor vs. diuretics or β-blocker		0.85 (0.62 to 1.18)	0.04 (-0.04 to 0.12)	0.88 (0.62 to 1.26)	0.03 (-0.05 to 0.10)	Not reported	Not reported
	ACE inhibitor vs. calcium-channel		0.94 (0.67 to 1.32)‡	0.01 (-0.07 to 0.10)	1.14 (0.78 to 1.67)	-0.02 (-0.10 to 0.05)	Not reported	Not reported
IDNT (3 groups)								
	Irbesartan vs. placebo	Primary	0.91 (0.72 to 1.14)	0.02 (-0.04 to 0.07)	0.92 (0.69 to 1.23)	0.01 (-0.03 to 0.06)	0.80 (0.66 to 0.97) §	0.06 (0.01 to 0.12)
	Amlodipine vs. placebo		0.88 (0.69 to 1.12)	0.03 (-0.02 to 0.08)	0.88 (0.66 to 1.19)	0.00 (-0.03 to 0.06)	1.04 (0.86 to 1.25) §	-0.02 (-0.08 to 0.04)
	Irbesartan vs. amlodipine		1.03 (0.81 to 1.31)	-0.01 (-0.06 to 0.04)	1.04 (0.77 to 1.40)	0.00 (-0.05 to 0.04)	0.77 (0.63 to 0.93)§	0.09 (0.03 to 0.14)
LIFE	Losartan vs. atenolol	Secondary	0.76 (0.58 to 0.98)	0.05 (0.01 to 0.10)	0.61 (0.45 to 0.84)	0.06 (0.02 to 0.10)	‖	‖
ALLHAT (3 groups)								
	Lisinopril vs. chlorthalidone	Secondary	1.08 (1.00 to 1.17)	Not reported	1.02 (0.91 to 1.13)	Not reported	Not reported	Not reported
	Amlodipine vs. chlorthalidone		1.06 (0.98 to 1.15)	Not reported	0.96 (0.86 to 1.07)	Not reported	Not reported	Not reported

*Values in parentheses are 95% CIs. ABCD = Appropriate Blood Pressure Control in Diabetes; ACE = angiotensin-converting enzyme; ALLHAT = Antihypertensive and Lipid-Lowering treatment to prevent Heart Attack Trial; CAPPP = Captopril Prevention Project; FACET = Fosinopril versus Amlodipine Cardiovascular Events Trial; GITS = gastrointestinal therapeutic system; IDNT = irbesartan Diabetic Nephropathy Trial; INSIGHT = International Nifedipine GITS Study: Intervention as a Goal in Hypertension Treatment; LIFE = Losartan Intervention for Endpoint Reduction; NORDIL = Nordic Diltiazem; STOP-2 = Swedish Trial in Old Patients with Hypertension-2; UKPDS = United Kingdom Prospective Diabetes Study.

Brown M. Personal communication.

‡The risk for myocardial infarction in the ACE inhibitor group was 0.51 (CI, 0.28 to 0.92) compared with the calcium-channel blocker group.

§ Composite microvascular endpoint = doubling of serum creatinine concentration + development of end-stage renal disease + all-cause mortality; individually, only doubling of the serum creatinine concentration was statistically significantly lower with irbesartan compared with either placebo or amlodipine. ‖ Risk for microalbuminuria was lower in the losartan group, although the risk/hazard ratio is not presented (P = 0.002).

Vijan S, Hayward RA. treatment of hypertension in type 2 diabetes mellitus: Blood Pressure goals, choice of agents and setting priorities in diabetes care. Ann. Intern Med 2003; 138: 593-602.

BP Level Effects on Type II-DM Nephropathy

- **Blood pressure analysis of RENAAL Trial**
  (Losartan vs. Placebo)

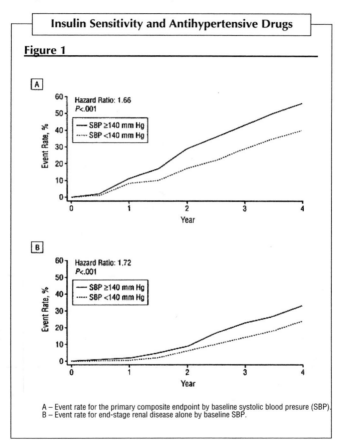

Insulin Sensitivity and Antihypertensive Drugs

Figure 1

A – Event rate for the primary composite endpoint by baseline systolic blood presure (SBP).
B – Event rate for end-stage renal disease alone by baseline SBP.

RENAAL

Design

- Losartan vs placebo
- 1513 pts with diabetic nephropathy
- 2 x s-Cr, ESRD, CV mortality/morbidity

losartan 50 - 100 mg

®

placebo

Results

- Losartan superior to placebo on primary endpoint
- Less hospitalisation for CHF on losartan

RENNAL:
Impact of Losartan on Primary Composite Endpoint*

	Losartan[+] Group n = 751		Placebo[+] Group n = 762			% Relative Risk Reduction
	n	%	n	%	Pvalue	(95%CI)
Primary composite end point*	327	43.5	359	47.1	0.02	16 (2 to 28)
Doubling of serum creatinine	162	21.6	198	26.0	0.006	25 (8 to 39)
ESRD	147	19.6	194	25.5	0.002	28 (11 to 42)
Death	158	21.0	155	2.03	0.88	-2 (-27 to 19)
ESRD or death	255	34.0	300	39.4	0.01	20 (5 to 32)
Doubling of serum creatinine and ESRD	226	30.1	263	34.5	0.01	21 (5 to 34)

*Composite of a doubling of SCr, ESRD, or death;
+In combination with open-label diuretic, CCB, β-blocker, α-blocker, and/or centrally acting agent.
Brenner et al. *N Engl J Med*. 2001;345:861-869.

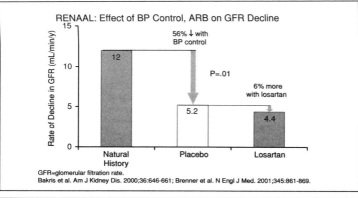

RENAAL: Effect of BP Control, ARB on GFR Decline

GFR=glomerular filtration rate.
Bakris et al. Am J Kidney Dis. 2000;36:646-661; Brenner et al. N Engl J Med. 2001;345:861-869.

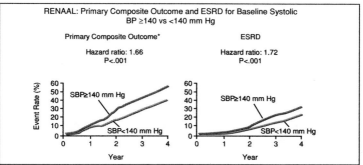

RENAAL: Primary Composite Outcome and ESRD for Baseline Systolic BP ≥140 vs <140 mm Hg

RENAAL: Concurrent Use of DHP CCB With ARB

- 66% of patients in losartan group were using DHP CCB
- Risk of primary outcome ↓ 16.1% with DHP CCB + losartan vs 16% with losartan alone*
- Concurrent DHP CCB + ARB is safe in patients with diabetic nephropathy
  - Provides benefit of additional BP lowering and does not have negative renal effects

* Doubling of baseline SCr, ESRD, or death. Bakris et al. *Arch Intern Med*. 2003;163:1555-1565.

Insulin Sensitivity and Antihypertensive Drugs

Figure 1

BP, mm Hg	Losartan*	Placebo*	P value	Favors Losartan	Favors Placebo
SBP					
<140	45/361	54/317	.03		
≥140	102/390	140/4445	.05		
DBP					
<90	119/660	165/673	<.001		
≥90	29/91	29/89	.54		
<140/90	43/353	54/307	.02		

0.25   0.50   0.75   1   1.25   1.50   1.75
Relative Risk (95% Confidence Interval)

Comparison of end-stage renal disease outcomes in the groups randomized to losartan (given as losartan potassium) vs. placebo at different achieved mean blood pressures (BPs) up until primary composite event. SBP indicates systolic BP; DBP – diastolic BP. Asterisk indicates data are number of events/total number of patients.

Key Points
- In Type II diabetes and HTN, baseline SBP is a stronger predictor of nephropathy than DBP.
- Those diabetics with highest baseline pulse pressure (SBP-DBP) have the highest risk of nephropathy and derive the greatest benefit from lowering SBP to less than 140 mmHg.

Diabetic Nephropathy Meta-analysis: [221]

Key points:
- One study in type I DM (Lewis et al) demonstrates albuminuria reduction and renal function protection with ACEI vs. placebo.
- One study in type II DM demonstrates renal function protection with ACEI vs. placebo (Lebovitz et al).
- Two studies in type II DM demonstrate renal function protection ARB vs. placebo or versus CCB and placebo (RENAAL, IDNT respectively).

Trials Comparing Intensive vs. Regular or Active vs. Placebo Blood Pressure Control: Effect on Albuminuria and Renal Function[221]

Table 1.

Trial	n	Years	Condition*	BP Treatment	Difference	P Value	Albuminuria	Renal Value	Function	P Value
Lewis et al[19]	409	3	DM1 ON	ACEI v Pl	-3/-1		-0.3/NRII	<.001	-43%§	<.007
Lebovitz et al[123]	121	3	DM2 ON	ACEI v Pl	-4,-9	<.001	7%/21%¶	NR	0.20/-0.33*	.004
Nielsen et al[24]	43	3	DM2 ON	ACEI v/βB+D	-4/-1		-55%/-15%**	<.01	-0.59/-0.54#	ns
UKPDS 38[26]	1148	9	DM2	Tight v regular	-10/-5		7%/6.6%¶	ns	No difference	
UKPDS 39[27]	1148	9	DM2	ACEI v βB	1/2		5%/9%¶	ns	No difference	
Gaede et al[31]	149	3.8	DM2 MA	Intensive v regular	-7/-3		10.9%/25%¶	<.01	—	
ABCD[32]	470	5.0	DM2 MA ON	Intensive v moderate	-6/-8		16%/23%¶	ns	No difference	
ABCD[32]	470	5	DM2 MA ON	ACEI v CCB	No difference		19%/20%¶	ns	No difference	
MICRO-HOPE[33]	3577	4.5	DM2 MA	ACEI v Pl	-2.5/-1		6%/7%¶	.07	—	
IRMA4[44]	590	2	DM2 MA	ARB 300 v 150 v Pl	141/144/144‡‡		5.2%/9.7%/14.9%¶	<.001		
IDNT[45]	1715	2.6	DM2 ON	ARB v CCB v Pl	98.0/98.3/101.3‡‡	.001	-33%/-6%/-10%**		23%/20%§§	.006/0.02
RENAAL[46]	1513	3.4	DM2 ON	ARB v Pl	98.6/99.9‡‡		-35%/No change**	<.001	16%§§	.02

BP = blood pressure; DBP = diastolic BP; MBP = mean BP; SBP = systolic BP; IND = Renoprotective Effect of the Angiotensin Antagonist Irbesartan in Patients With Nephropathy Due to Type 2 Diabetes; IRMA = Effect of Irbesartan in the Development of Diabetic Nephropathy in Patients With Type 2 Diabetes; NR = not reported; ns = not significant.

*DM1/DM2 = diabetes mellitus type I/or 2; MA = microalbuminuria, subclinical nephropathy; ON = overt nephropathy;

† ACEI = angiotensin converting enzyme inhibitors; βB = (β-blockers, D = diuretics, CCB = calcium channel blockers, Pl = placebo plus nonstudy drugs if needed, ARB = angiotensin receptor blockers (for IRMA the two doses of 300 mg and 150 mg are shown, for IDNT the groups of active drugs are two). ‡ – Difference of SBP/DBP mm Hg of the first treatment from the second is shown, (-) = less BP in the first treatment, if one number is shown it represents MBP. § – Percent reduction in risk of doubling of serum creatinine. II Absolute decrease in g/day during follow-up. ¶ – Percentage of patients progressing to overt nephropathy. # – Decrease in glomerular filtration rate mL/min/1.73 m2/month. ** – Percentage reduction of proteinuria. †† – Median SBP during follow-up. ‡‡ – Median MBP during follow-up. §§ – Percent reduction in risk of approaching the composite endpoints of the first treatment versus second or third.

Renal function deterioration was not an endpoint in these trials.

Diabetes Mellitus and Hypertension Summary: 191, 192

1. The aggregate of major CV, renal events and total mortality was lowest in more actively treated patients with lower BP. The recommended BP goal is 110/ 70 mm Hg. Thus more intensive BP lowering is recommended.

2. Approximately 4 antihypertensive drugs will be required to reach these goal levels for BP.

3. ACEIs (CAPPP) and ARBs (losartan-LIFE) showed better reduction in CV events compared to conventional diuretic or beta–blocker therapy especially in CHD, CHF and CVA events.

4. ACEI + CCB is superior to diuretic and beta-blocker in combination treatment to reduce CV events (Syst-Eur vs. SHEP).

5. Renal insufficiency, microalbuminuria and proteinuria are best prevented by ACEIs and ARBs as initial therapy. Selective use of CCBs depending on the level of proteinuria (ie < 1 gram/ 24 hrs) :[192] is also renoprotective and reduces proteinuria. ACEIs, ARBs and CCBs are superior to diuretics and beta-blockers. (IDNT, IRMA, RENAAL, CAPPP, ABCD-HT, LIFE, AASK, HOPE, MICROHOPE).

6. New onset Type 2 DM is more common with diuretics and beta-blockers than other drug classes (HOPE, CAPPP, STOP-II, LIFE, UKPDS, SHEP, MICRO-HOPE, INSIGHT, NORDIL, NICS-EH, ARICS and ALLHAT).

Additional References on Hypertension
and Diabetes Mellitus

K/DOQI clinical practice guidelines for chronic kidney disease: evaluation, classification and stratification. Kidney Disease Outcome Quality Initiative. Am J Kidney Dis 2002;39(suppl 2):S46-S75.

Miettinen H, Haffner SM, Lehto S, Ronnemaa T, Pyorala K, Laakso M: Proteinuria predicts stroke and other atherosclerotic vascular disease events in nondiabetic and non-insulin-dependent diabetic subjects. Stroke 1996;27:2033-2039.

Weir MR: Diabetes and hypertension: blood pressure control and consequences. Am J Hypertens 1999;12(suppl):170S-178S.

Bidani AK, Schwartz MM, Lewis EJ: Renal autoregulation and vulnerability to hypertensive injury in remnant kidney. Am J Physiol 1987;252:F1003-F1010.

Ritz E, Keller C, Bergis K, Strojek K: Pathogenesis and course of renal disease in IDDM/NIDDM: differences and similarities. Am J Hypertens 1997;10(suppl):202S-207S.

Ismail N, Becker B, Strzelczyk P, Ritz E: Renal disease and hypertension in non-insulin-dependent diabetes mellitus. Kidney Int 1999;55:1-28.

Waeber B, Feihl F, Ruilope LM: Diabetes and hypertension. Blood Press 2001;10:311-321.

Parving HH: Hypertension and diabetes: the scope of the problem. Blood Press 2001;10(Suppl 2):25-31.

US Renal Data System: USRDS 1999 annual data report. Bethesda, MD: National Institute of Diabetes and Digestive and Kidney Disease 1999:25-38.

Bretzel RG: Effects of antihypertensive drugs on renal function in patients with diabetic nephropathy. Am J Hypertens 1997; 10(suppl):208S-217S.

Lewis EJ, Hunsicker LG, Bain RP, Rohde RD: The effect of angio-tensin-converting-enzyme inhibition on diabetic nephropathy. The Collaborative Study Group. N Engl J Med 1993;329:1456-1462.

Kasiske BL, Kalil RS, Ma JZ, Liao M, Keane WF: Effect of antihypertensive therapy on the kidney in patients with diabetes: a meta-regression analysis. Ann Intern Med 1993;118:129-138.

Weidmann P, Schneider M, Bohlen L: Therapeutic efficacy of different antihypertensive drugs in human diabetic nephropathy: an updated meta-analysis. Nephrol Dial Transplant 1995;10:39-45.

Maki DD, Ma JZ, Louis TA, Kasiske BL: Long-term effects of antihypertensive agents on proteinuria and renal function. Arch Intern Med 1995; 155:1073-1080.

257

Lebovitz HE, Wiegmann TB, Cnaan A, Shahinfar S, Sica DA, Broadstone V, Schwartz SL, Mengel MC, Segal R, Versaggi JA, Bolton WK. Renal protective effects of enalapril in hypertensive NIDDM: role of baseline albuminuria. Kidney Int 1994;45(suppl): S150-S155.

Nielsen FS, Rossing P, Gall MA, Skott P, Smidt UM, Parving HH. Long-term effect of lisinopril and atenolol on kidney function in hypertensive NIDDM subjects with diabetic nephropathy. Diabetes 1997;46:1182-1188.

UK Prospective Diabetes Study (UKPDS) Group. Intensive blood-glucose control with sulphonylureas or insulin compared with conventional treatment and risk of complications in patients with type 2 diabetes (UKPDS 33). Lancet 1998;352:837-853.

UK Prospective Diabetes Study Group. Tight blood pressure control and risk of macrovascular and microvascular complications in type 2 diabetes: UKPDS 38. Br Med J 1998:317:703-713.

UK Prospective Diabetes Study Group: Efficacy of atenolol and captopril in reducing risk of macrovascular and microvascular complications in type 2 diabetes. UKPDS 39. Br Med J 1998;317:713-720.

Hansson L, Zanchetti A, Carruthers SG, Dahlof B, Elmfeldt D, Julius S, Menard I, Rahn KH, Wedel H, Westerling S. Effects of intensive blood pressure lowering and low-dose aspirin in patients with hypertension: principal results of the Hypertension Optimal Treatment (HOT) randomized trial. Lancet 1998;351:1755-1762.

Guidelines Subcommittee: 1999 World Health Organization-International Society of Hypertension Guidelines for the Management of Hypertension. J Hypertens 1999;17:151-183.

Kjeldsen SE, Os I, Farsang C, Mallion JM, Hansson L, Sleight P. Treatment of hypertension in patients with type-2 diabetes mellitus. J Hypertens 2000;18:1345-1346.

Gaede P, Vedel P, Parving HH, Pedersen O. Intensified multifactorial intervention in patients with type 2 diabetes mellitus and microalbuminuria: the Steno type 2 randomized study. Lancet 1999; 353:617-622.

Estacio RO, Jeffers BW, Gifford N, Schrier RW. Effect of blood pressure control on diabetic microvascular complications in patients with hypertension and type 2 diabetes. Diabetes Care 2000;23(suppl 2):B54-B64.

Heart Outcomes Prevention Evaluation (HOPE) Study Investigators. Effects of ramipril on cardiovascular and microvascular outcomes in people with diabetes mellitus: results of the HOPE study and MICRO-HOPE substudy. Lancet 2000;355:253-259.

Velussi M, Brocco E, Frigato F, Zolli M, Muollo B, Maioli M, Carraro A, Tonolo G, Fresu P, Cernigoi AM, Fioretto P, Nosadini R. Effects of cilazapril and amlodipine on kidney function in hypertensive NIDDM patients. Diabetes 1996;45:216-222.

Bakris GL, Copley JB, Vicknair N, Sadler R, Leurgans S. Calcium channel blockers versus other antihypertensive therapies on progression of NIDDM associated nephropathy. Kidney Int 1996;50:1641-1650.

Viberti G, Mogensen CE, Groop LC, Pauls JF. Effect of captopril on progression to clinical proteinuria in patients with insulin-dependent diabetes mellitus and microalbuminuria. European Microalbuminuria Captopril Study Group. J Am Med Assoc 1994; 271:275-279.

EUCLID Study Group. Randomised placebo-controlled trial of lisinopril in normotensive patients with insulin-dependent diabetes and normoalbuminuria or microalbuminuria. Lancet 1997;349:1787-1792.

Ravid M, Brosh D, Levi Z, Bar-Dayan Y, Ravid D, Rachmani R. Use of enalapril to attenuate decline in renal function in normotensive, normoalbuminuric patients with type 2 diabetes mellitus. A randomised, controlled trial. Ann Intern Med 1998;128:982-988.

Kon V, Fogo A, Ichikava I. Bradykinin causes selective efferent arteriolar dilation during angiotensin I converting enzyme inhibition. Kidney Int 1993;44:545-550.

Price DA, De'Oliveira JM, Fisher ND, Hollenberg NK. Renal hemodynamic response to an angiotensin II antagonist, eprosartan, in healthy men. Hypertension 1997;30:240-246.

Pitt B, Poole-Wilson PA, Segal R, Martinez FA, Dickstein K, Camm AJ, Konstam MA, Riegger G, Klinger GH, Neaton J, Sharma D, Thiyagarajan B. Effect of losartan compared with captopril on mortality in patients with symptomatic heart failure: randomized trial—the Losartan Heart Failure Survival Study ELITE II. Lancet 2000;355:1582-1587.

Muirhead N, Feagan BF, Mahon J, Lewanczuk RZ, Rodger NW, Botteri F, Oddou-Stock P, Pecher E, Cheung R. The effects of valsartan and captopril on reducing microalbuminuria in patients with type 2 diabetes mellitus: a placebo-controlled trial. Curr Ther Res 1999;60:650-660.

Lacourciere Y, Belanger A, Godin C, Halle JP, Ross S, Wright N, Marion J. Long-term comparison of losartan and enalapril on kidney function in hypertensive type 2 diabetics with early nephropathy. Kidney Int 2000;58:762-769.

Parving HH, Lehnert H, Brochner-Mortensen J, Gomis R, Andersen S, Arner P. The effect of irbesartan on the development of diabetic nephropathy in patients with type 2 diabetes. N Engl J Med 2001;345:870-878.

Lewis EJ, Hunsicker LG, Clarke WR, Berl T, Pohl MA, Lewis JB, Ritz E, Atkins RC, Rohde R, Raz I. Renoprotective effect of the angiotensin-receptor antagonist irbesartan in patients with nephropathy due to type 2 diabetes. N Engl J Med 2001;345:851-860.

Selection of Therapy Based on Subsets of Hypertension

Selection of antihypertensive therapy based on the subsets of hypertension approach allows for the categorization of drugs into three groups: drugs of choice, alternatives, and contraindicated drugs. Diseases in the left-hand column are often associated with hypertension. A drug should be selected considering all disease factors. Drugs are listed in *alphabetical order,* not by preference, in each column.

Key Code

AB = Alpha Blocker	CAA = Central Alpha Agonist
ABB = Alpha Beta Blocker	CCB = Calcium Channel Blocker
ACEI = Angiotensin Converting Enzyme Inhibitor	D = Diuretic
	DHP = Dihydropyridine
ARB = Angiotensin Receptor Blocker	DV = Direct Vasodilator
BB = Beta-Blocker	SARA = Serum Aldosterone Receptor Antagonist

Concomitant Condition	Drug(s) of Choice	Alternatives	Relative or Absolute Contraindication
Abnormal Vascular Compliance	ACEI ARB CCB	D	Selective BB Non-selective BB
Addictive Syndromes: withdrawal from tobacco, alcohol, opiates	CAA (clonidine)		Non-selective BB
Angina: mixed	BB without ISA CCB, (especially non-DHP)	ARB ACEI AB CAA D ABB	BB with ISA DV
Angina: obstructive	BB without ISA CCB, (especially non-DHP)	ARB ACEI AB CAA D ABB	BB with ISA DV
Angina: vasospastic	CCB (especially DHP)	ARB ACEI AB CAA D	BB without ISA BB with ISA DV ABB

260

Concomitant Condition	Drug(s) of Choice	Alternatives	Relative or Absolute Contraindication
Anxiety/Stress	CAA BB without ISA		
Cerebrovas-cular disease Post CVA (Progress Trial)	ACEI ARB CCB Indapamide Thiazide D	AB CAA DV ABB	BB without ISA BB with ISA
Chronic Liver Disease	AB BB CCB CAA	ACEI DV D ABB	Methyldopa
CHF Systolic Failure	ARB ACEI BB without ISA Carvedilol D-(caution in CRI) Spironolactone Epleronone	CAA DHP-CCB	AB BB with ISA Verapamil Diltiazem DV
Cognitive Dysfunction and Prevention of Vascular Dementia	ACEI CCB (DHP) Indapamide	ARB D	BB
Coronary Heart Disease High-Risk	ACEI ARB CCB	AB BB CAA D	DV
Cyclosporine-induced hypertension	CCB		
Depression	ARB ACEI AB CCB	D DV	BB ABB CAA Reserpine

Concomitant Condition	Drug(s) of Choice	Alternatives	Relative or Absolute Contraindication
Diabetes mellitus	ARB** ACEI CCB	AB BB with ISA CAA DV Indapamide ABB	BB without ISA Thiazide D Methyldopa
Diabetic diarrhea and gustatory sweating	CAA clonidine		
Diastolic dysfunction or failure	BB with ISA CCB ARB ACEI	BB without ISA CAA ABB D (caution with volume status)	AB DV
Dyslipidemia	AB CAA ACEI ARB CCB	ABB BB with ISA DV Indapamide	BB without ISA D (Thiazides) Methyldopa
Essential tremor	B$_{1,2}$-blocker without ISA CAA		
Exercise	ARB* ACEI* AB* CCB CAA	BB with ISA D* DV ABB	BB without ISA

* – Watch out for volume depletion, especially hot weather.
** – These products are not approved for use during pregnancy.

Concomitant Condition	Drug(s) of Choice	Alternatives	Relative or Absolute Contraindication
GERD	ACEI ARB	AB D BB CAA	CCB (decreases LES tone)
Glaucoma	BB CAA D	BB without ISA	
Homo-systeinemia	ACEI ARB CCB	ABB BB CAA DV	D
Hyperuricemia	ARB-(Losartan)	DV ABB ACEI AB CCB CAA	BB without ISA D
Hyper-thyroidism	BB	CAA	
LVH	ARB ACEI CCB CAA Indapamide ABB	AB BB without ISA D (Thiazide)	BB with ISA DV
Menopausal symptoms	CAA	BB without ISA	DV

Concomitant Condition	Drug(s) of Choice	Alternatives	Relative or Absolute Contraindication
Metabolic Syndrome	ACEI ARB CCB	AB SARA Indapamide	BB* Thiazide/Thiazide-like D** DV

* – BB if compelling indications
* – D as required for BP control or compelling indications.

Microvascular angina	CCB	ARB ACEI AB CAA	BB without ISA BB with ISA DV D ABB
Migraine headache (prophylactic)	Non-selective BB without ISA CCB	ARB ACEI AB BB with ISA	DV
Mitral valve prolapse	BB without ISA CCB (Non-DHP) CAA	ARB ACEI AB ABB	BB with ISA DV D
Obesity	ACEI ARB AB CCB CAA	DV D ABB	BB without ISA* BB with ISA

* – Unless compelling indicators.

Concomitant Condition	Drug(s) of Choice	Alternatives	Relative or Absolute Contraindication
Obstructive Airway	AB CCB CAA	ARB ACEI DV D	$B_{1,2}$-blocker B_1-blocker especially high dose BB without ISA BB with ISA ABB
Peptic ulcer disease	CCB CAA	ARB ACEI AB BB DV D ABB	Reserpine
Peripheral vascular disease	CCB (Especially DHP)	ARB ACEI AB CAA DV D	Non-selective BB Selective BB BB without ISA BB with ISA ABB
Post-MI: non–Q-wave Normal left-ventricular function	Diltiazem* Verapamil* ACEI ARB? BB without ISA	AB CAA CCB (DHP) ABB	BB with ISA DV D

* – These products are not approved for use during pregnancy.

Concomitant Condition	Drug(s) of Choice	Alternatives	Relative or Absolute Contraindication
LV systolic dysfunction	ARB ACEI BB SARA	CCB (DHP)	AB Non-DHP CCB
Post-MI: Q-wave Normal left ventricular function	ACEI SARA ARB-? BB without ISA	CCA ABB CCB - Non-DHP	BB with ISA D DV CCB (DHP)
Pregnancy (first and second trimester)	Hydralazine Methyldopa CAA	Possibly AB CCB*	ARB ACEI BB without ISA BB with ISA D
Premature ventricular contractions	BB without ISA Verapamil	ARB ACEI AB CAA ABB Diltiazem Nifedipine	BB with ISA DV D
Prostatism	AB		
Proteinuria	ACEI SARA ARB	D BB	
Pulmonary hypertension	CCB (DHP) DV	ARB ACEI AB CAA D ABB	BB

* – These products are not approved for use during pregnancy.

Concomitant Condition	Drug(s) of Choice	Alternatives	Relative or Absolute Contraindication
Raynaud's phenomenon	CCB (DHP)	ARB ACEI AB CAA DV	BB without ISA BB with ISA ABB
Renal insufficiency	ACEI AB ARB CCB CAA	DV BB (if compelling indications) BB with ISA Loop D Metolozone ABB Indapamide	Thiazide D
Renin Status*	*PRA > 0.65 = HRH PRA < 0.65 = LRH		
High Renin (HRH)	ACEI ARB BB		
Low Renin (LRH)	SARA D CCB AB		
Renovascular Disease (renal artery disease) Bilateral	CCB CAA AB	BB D	ACEI* ARB**

* – Drugs of choice for unilateral RAS
** – Use with caution, but can be highly effective. Need to monitor K+, creatinine, especially initially.

Concomitant Condition	Drug(s) of Choice	Alternatives	Relative or Absolute Contraindication
Sexual Dysfunction	ARB ACEI AB CCB	DV	CAA ABB BB with ISA BB without ISA D Methyldopa Reserpine
Sick Sinus Syndrome or Atrio-ventricular (AV) Block	ARB ACEI AB CCB (DHP)	DV D	ABB BB without ISA BB with ISA CAA Diltiazem Verapamil Reserpine
Sinusitis/ Rhinitis	CAA	ARB ACEI AB CCB DV D	BB ABB Reserpine

Concomitant Condition	Drug(s) of Choice	Alternatives	Relative or Absolute Contraindication
Supraventricular Tachycardia	BB (No ISA) CAA Non-DHP CCB	Other agents as required to control BP	DV
Toxemia of Pregnancy (eclampsia)	CAA CCB* Hydralazine Methyldopa	AB* ABB	ACEI BB without ISA BB with ISA D

* – These products are not approved for use during pregnancy.

Use of NSAIDs	CCB	AB CAA D (may need ↑ dose) ARB (may need ↑ dose) ACEI (may need ↑ dose) BB with or without ISA (may need ↑ dose) ABB (may need ↑ dose)	DV
Volume Overload	D ARB ACEI	AB CCB CAA ABB	BB (systolic HF after volume control) DV

* – Use with caution, but can be highly effective. Need to monitor K+, creatinine, especially initially.

Demographics and Antihypertensive Drugs

Key Code

AB = Alpha Blocker	CAA = Central Alpha Agonist
ABB = Alpha Beta Blocker	CCB = Calcium Channel Blocker
ACEI = Angiotensin Converting Enzyme Inhibitor	D = Diuretic
	DHP = Dihydropyrhidine
ARB = Angiotensin Receptor Blocker	DV = Direct Vasodilator
BB = Beta-Blocker	NI = Neuronal Inhibitor

Demographic Profile	Drug(s) of Choice	Alternatives	Relative or Absolute Contra-indication
*Young patient	ARB ACEI CCB	AB BB with ISA DV AB BB CAA	BB without ISA D NI Reserpine

*If pregnant, avoid ACEI, ARB, BB, and diuretic.

Demographic Profile	Drug(s) of Choice	Alternatives	Relative or Absolute Contra-indication
Elderly patient	ARB ACEI CCB CAA D	BB without ISA BB with ISA AB BB	AB DV NI Reserpine
African-American patient	ARB ACEI CCB CAA D ARB	DV AB BB	AB BB with ISA BB without ISA NI Reserpine
White patient	ARB ACEI CCB CAA	DV AB BB D	AB BB with ISA BB without ISA NI Reserpine

Resistant Hypertension

Definition

The patient's DBP remains above 90 mm Hg despite full doses of three appropriate antihypertensive medications and has been documented on at least two separate visits in the office under proper conditions *and* out of the office with home BP monitoring or 24-hour ambulatory blood pressure monitoring (ABPM).

Causes

An inadequate drug regimen and patient noncompliance account for 70% of total causes.

1. Patient noncompliance to therapy
2. Inadequate drug regimen
   a. Drug doses too low
   b. Drug interactions—antihypertensive agents (two central alpha-agonists, two ACEI or beta-blockers and central alpha-agonist with beta-blocker) or alpha blocker with central alpha agonist.
   c. Rapid metabolism or inactivation (hydralazine)
   d. Other drug interactions and interfering agents
      (1) Corticosteroids and anabolic steroids
      (2) Aldosterone (florinef)
      (3) Sympathomimetics and phenylpropanolamine
      (4) NSAIDs (ACEIs, beta-blockers, diuretics, ARBs)
      (5) Antidepressants—tricyclics and central alpha-agonist
      (6) Decongestants—pseudoephedrine, nasal sprays
      (7) Excess alcohol ingestion (over 30 mL/day) for 7-10 weeks
      (8) Excess caffeine ingestion (variable)
      (9) Excess tobacco use (variable)
      (10) Oral contraceptives
      (11) Erythropoietin
      (12) Cyclosporine
      (13) MAO inhibitors and phenothiazines
      (14) Cocaine and amphetamines
      (15) Appetite suppressants

(16) Omeprazole (Prilosec)
(17) See other drugs listed in
Secondary Causes of Hypertension section

3. Volume overload states
   a. Inadequate diuretic therapy
   b. High sodium intake (10 to 15 g/day)
   c. Secondary to BP reduction with some agents (direct vasodilators) and some beta-blockers pseudotolerance caused by reflex volume overload, tachycardia, or vasoconstriction)
   d. Nephrosclerosis and CRF

4. Obesity and rapid weight gain

5. Secondary hypertension (10%)
   (See other drugs listed in *Secondary Causes of Hypertension* section)
   a. Renovascular hypertension (most common)
   b. Renal insufficiency and failure
   c. Pheochromocytoma
   d. Primary aldosteronism
   e. Cushing's syndrome
   f. Coarctation of aorta
   g. Sleep apnea
   h. Thyroid disease
   i. Hypercalcemia
   j. Licorice intoxication (in chewing tobacco)

6. Pseudo resistance
   a. Using regular adult cuff on obese arm
   b. White coat hypertension
   c. Pseudohypertension in elderly

7. Miscellaneous
   a. Chronic anxiety, panic attacks
   b. Chronic pain
   c. Diffuse vasoconstriction (arteritis)
   d. Insulin resistance
   e. Inappropriate diuretic in patients with renal insufficiency and creatinine clearance below 30 cc/min (i.e., thiazide)

Isolated Systolic Hypertension (ISH) in the Elderly

- All randomized placebo-controlled trials of antihypertensive therapy have demonstrated dramatic reductions in cardiovascular and cerebrovascular morbidity and mortality in the treatment of ISH in the elderly with a wide variety of drugs. The DHP-CCB and diuretics (+ beta- blockers) and ACEIs are efficacious as initial and in combination along with ARBs.
- ISH is defined as SBP > 160 mm Hg with a DBP < 95 mm Hg (Except in SHEP where DBP < 90 mm HG).

Randomized Placebo-controlled Trials of Antihypertensive Drug Therapy in Isolated Systemic Hypertension in the Elderly					
Trial	No. of Patients	Entry BP mm Hg	Mean Age (yr)	Duration (yr)	Primary Drug
EWPHE	172	178/92	73	4.3	Diuretic
MRC-I	428	174/92	62	5.2	β-B/diuretic
Coope and Warrender	349	191/85	70	3.6	β-B
SHEP Coop	4,736	170/77	72	4.4	Diuretic
STOP-H	268	194/91	76	1.9	β-B/diuretic
MRC-II	2,651	182/83	70	6.1	β-B/diuretic
Syst-Eur	4,695	174/85	70	2.0	CCB
Syst-China	2,394	170/86	67	3.0	CCB

ISH in the Elderly: Drug Treatment Categories
Incidence of Cardiovascular Events
per 1000 Patient-Years

Study	Age (Years)	Cardiovascular Events Placebo	Treatment	Cerebrovascular Events Placebo	Treatment	Cardiac Events Placebo	Treatment
EWPHE	60-96	114.8	74.2†	36.3	20.7‡	22.0	18.5
SHEP	≥60	68.3	49.3†	14.9	9.7§	20.2	14.8‡
STOP-Hypertension	70-84	55.5	33.5†	31.3	16.8†	16.5	14.4
MRC-II	65-74	25.2	21.0‡	10.8	8.1*	12.7	10.3
		Placebo	Calcium Antagonist	Placebo	Calcium Antagonist	Placebo	Calcium Antagonist
Syst-Eur	68-98	33.9	23.3§	13.7	7.9	20.5	15.1‡
Syst-China	≥60	33.3	21.4†	20.8	13.0†	10.8	6.9
		ACE-I	Calcium Antagonist	ACE-I	Calcium Antagonist	ACE-I	Calcium Antagonist
GLANT	60±10	12.7	22.7	4.9‡	14.7	4.9	2.9
PATE-Hypertension	70±7	22.5	19.7	9.3	9.1	13.3	10.7

* Diuretics or ß-blockers; † P < .01; ‡ P < .05; § P < .001.

ISH in the Elderly: Drug Treatment Categories
Incidence of Cardiovascular Events
per 1000 Patient-Years

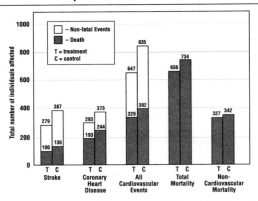

Entry BP average 174/83 mm Hg. Mean difference in treated and control: 10.4/4.1 mmHg. Median follow-up 3.8 years. Summary results of 15,693 patients with ISH (8 trials).

Reprinted from Staessen JA, Gasowski J, Wang JG, et al. Risks of untreated and treated isolated systolic hypertension in the elderly. Lancet 2000;355:865-872, (with permission).

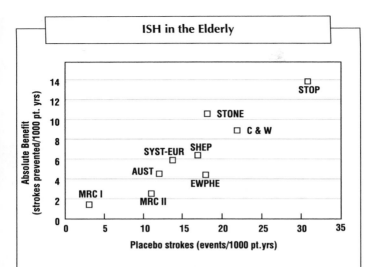

Stroke reduction: absolute benefit. Absolute benefit of antihypertensive treatment in terms of stroke reduction is related to the stroke risk (stroke events in the placebo group) of the patient population. Each point represents data from a major placebo-controlled outcome trial.

Meredith, P. Do Pharmacologic Differences Among Antihypertensive Agents point to Clinical Benefits. AM J. Cardiol. 1999; 84:22S-27S.

Beta-blocker monotherapy is not effective in reducing CHD mortality, total CV mortality or total mortality in elderly patients with hypertension. Beta-blockers as initial treatment or as a monotherapy are effective in reducing CVA morbidity and mortality but are inferior to other antihypertensive drugs..[198]

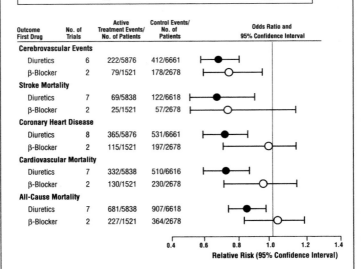

Meta-analysis of Prospective Clinical Trials in Elderly Patients with Hypertension According to First-line Treatment Strategy

Outcome First Drug	No. of Trials	Active Treatment Events/ No. of Patients	Control Events/ No. of Patients	Odds Ratio and 95% Confidence Interval
Cerebrovascular Events				
Diuretics	6	222/5876	412/6661	
β-Blocker	2	79/1521	178/2678	
Stroke Mortality				
Diuretics	7	69/5838	122/6618	
β-Blocker	2	25/1521	57/2678	
Coronary Heart Disease				
Diuretics	8	365/5876	531/6661	
β-Blocker	2	115/1521	197/2678	
Cardiovascular Mortality				
Diuretics	7	332/5838	510/6616	
β-Blocker	2	130/1521	230/2678	
All-Cause Mortality				
Diuretics	7	681/5838	907/6618	
β-Blocker	2	227/1521	364/2678	

Relative Risk (95% Confidence Interval)

Stroke reduction: absolute benefit of antihypertension. Absolute benefit of antihypertensive treatment in terms of stroke reduction is related to the stroke risk (stroke events in the placebo group) of the patient population. Each point represents data from a major placebo-controlled outcome trial.

Meredith, P. Do Pharmacologic Differences Among Antihypertensive Agents point to Clinical Benefits? AM J. Cardiol. 1999; 84:22S-27S.

Hypertensive Urgencies and Emergencies

Definitions

1. *Hypertensive urgency:* DBP≥ 120 mm Hg in the absence of significant end-organ damage.
   a. Grade I or II Keith-Wagener fundoscopic changes
   b. Postoperative hypertension
   c. Preoperative hypertension
   d. Pain-induced or stress-induced hypertension
2. *Hypertensive emergency:* DBP >120 mm Hg with one of following:
   a. Intracranial hemorrhage or thrombotic CVA
   b. Subarachnoid bleed
   c. Hypertensive encephalopathy
   d. Acute aortic dissection
   e. Acute pulmonary edema, acute CHF, and acute left ventricular failure
   f. Eclampsia (toxemia of pregnancy)
   g. Pheochromocytoma hypertensive crisis
   h. Grade III or IV Keith-Wagener fundoscopic changes
   i. Acute renal insufficiency or failure
   j. Myocardial insufficiency syndromes (unstable angina pectoris, acute MI)
   k. Hematuria

Precipitating Factors in Hypertensive Crisis

1. Accelerated sudden rise in blood pressure in a patient with preexisting essential hypertension
2. Renovascular hypertension
3. Glomerulonephritis—acute
4. Eclampsia
5. Pheochromocytoma
6. Antihypertensive withdrawal syndromes

7. Head injuries
8. Renin secreting tumors
9. Ingestion of catecholamine precursors in patients taking MAO inhibitors

Malignant Hypertension

1. Fundoscopic changes of necrotizing arteriolitis (hemorrhages, exudates), disc edema, and papilledema (visual changes, nausea, vomiting, headache, confusion, somnolence, stupor, neurologic deficits, seizures, coma)
2. Hypertensive encephalopathy
3. Diastolic blood pressure > 120 mm Hg with target organ damage
4. Decreasing renal function, proteinuria, hematuria, casts, oliguria, azotemia
5. Microangiopathic hemolytic anemia
6. Left ventricular failure and CHF and pulmonary edema

Factors That Constitute Malignant Hypertension

1. Absolute level of blood pressure
2. Rate of development of blood pressure
3. Type and level of vasoactive substances
4. Presence of end-organ damage

Pathophysiology

High blood pressure level

+

Increased vascular reactivity

+

Critical circulating levels of vasoactive and "vasculotoxic"
agents (angiotensin II, NE, vasopressin)

Relative narrowing efferent arteriole

Sodium "pressure" diuresis (differential effect on
afferent and efferent renal arteriole)

Hypovolemia

Increased
angiotensin II
± norepinephrine
± vasopressin

Narrowing in
interlobular arteries

Proliferation of
myointimal cells

Migration of myointimal
cells to lumen

Platelet and fibrin
migration and mitogenic factors

Platelet and fibrin deposition

"Sausage-string"
change in arteries

Endothelial damage
and platelet aggregation

Release of platelet
factors and thromboxane

Microangiopathic
hemolytic anemia and
intravascular coagulation

Treatment: General Principles

Balance the benefit of immediate reduction in BP to prevent irreversible organ damage against the risk of marked decrease in perfusion and blood flow to vital organs, particularly to the brain, myocardium, and kidney or regional blood flow changes within each organ.

1. Reduce DBP to no less than 100 mm Hg, the SBP to no less than 160 mm Hg, or the MAP to no less than 120 mm Hg the first 24 to 48 hours except in hypertensive emergencies as indicated. Attempt an average reduction of 25% below baseline BP or to the minimum BP indicated above.

2. Acute lowering of blood pressure may decrease blood flow to the brain, myocardium, and kidneys.

3. Attempt to establish normotension within a few days.

4. Avoid hypotension or normotension during first 24 hours except in hypertensive emergencies as indicated.

5. Parenteral or oral antihypertensives are appropriate depending on the clinical setting.

6. Begin concomitant long-term therapy soon after the initial emergency treatment.

7. Assess volume status of patient. Do not overuse diuretics, and avoid sodium restriction in the early phases of malignant hypertension. Volume expansion is often indicated.

8. Reflex volume retention may occur after a few days on some nondiuretic antihypertensive drugs, such as betablockers and direct vasodilators—concept of pseudotolerance.

Treatment: Rapidity of Onset

1. Aortic dissection.

2. Pulmonary edema (caution in acute MI).

3. Malignant hypertension in certain clinical settings with encephalopathy, papilledema—controlled reduction.

4. Subarachnoid bleed or intracerebral bleed—controversial. Non-treatment of BP may be appropriate.

Treatment: Choice of Drug

1. Rapidity of blood pressure drop desired and level of blood pressure.
2. Duration of action of antihypertensive agent.
3. Hemodynamic effect of drug (i.e., use in presence of pulmonary edema, CHF, angina, MI, CVA, aortic dissection, renal insufficiency).
4. Effect on RBF, GRF, and function.
5. Potential and known adverse effects.

Acute Nonparenteral Therapy

Drugs	Route	Onset	Maximum Effect	Duration	Dosage
Clonidine (Catapres)	Oral	30 min	1–2 hr	8–12 hr	0.1–0.2 mg initial then 0.05–0.1 mg q hr to maximum 0.8 mg
Nitroglycerin (Nitrostat)	Sublingual	1 min	15 min	1 hr	0.4 mg

• *Use of sublingual short-acting nifedipine is never medically appropriate.*

Acute Parenteral Therapy

Drugs	Route	Onset	Maximum Effect	Duration	Dosage
*Sodium nitroprusside (Nipride, Nitropress)	IV	seconds	1–2 min	3–5 min	16 μg/min to 1–6 μg/kg/min
*Fenoldopam mesylate (Corlopam)	IV	< 5 min	5–10 min	30 min	0.1–0.3 μg/kg per min
Trimethaphan (Arfonad)	IV	1–5 min	2–5 min	10 min	0.5–5 mg/min (limited availability)
Diazoxide (Hyperstat)	IV	1–5 min	2–3 min	4–24 hr	7.5–30 mg/min 1 propranolol load
					Bolus infusion 50 mg IV q 5–10 min
					Infusion method
					7.5–30 mg/min 1 propranolol load
Hydralazine (Apresoline)	IV	10–20 min	20–40 min	3–8 hr	10 to 20 mg
Methyldopa (Aldomet)	IV	2–3 hr	3–5 hr	6–12 hr	250–500 mg q 6 hr
Phentolamine (Regitine)	IV	(for catechol-amine excess)			load 5–10 mg IV q 5 min, infuse 0.2–0.5 mg/min
*Labetalol (Trandate, Normodyne)	IV	5 min	5–10 min	3–6 hr	2 mg/min IV infusion or 20 mg q 10 min to a maximum 80 mg q 10 min Maximum cumulative dose 300 mg may not be effective in severely hypertensive patients already receiving other antihypertensive agents (propranolol, prazosin)
Nicardipine (Cardene)	IV	10 min	30 min	3–6 hr	5 mg/hr increased 1–2.5 mg/hr every 15 min up to 15 mg/hr
Nitroglycerin	IV	1–2 min	—	2–3 min	5–100 μg/min
Dilevalol	IV	1–5 min	—	3–6 hr	10 mg followed by 25–100 mg every 15 min
Enalapril AT*	IV	10 min	1–4 hr	2–6 hr	1.25 mg then 2.5 to 10 mg every 30–60 min
Esmolol hydrochloride	IV	1–2 min	5 min	10–20 min	250–500 μg/kg/min for 1 min then 50–100 μg/kg/min for 4 min; may repeat sequence

*Preferred drugs

Treatment of Specific Hypertensive Disorders

1.	Hypertension + Congestive heart failure	Nitroglycerin IV Sodium nitroprusside and loop diuretics Fenoldapam DHP-CCB, amlodipine Clonidine ACEI ARB
2.	Hypertension + Coronary insufficiency	Non DHP-CCB Nitroglycerin Beta-blockers Clonidine
3.	Aortic dissection aneurysm	Trimethaphan + propranolol or Nitroprusside + propranolol Labetalol or esmolol
4.	Catecholamine excess (pheochromocytoma)	Phentolamine
5.	Hypertension alone	Fenoldapam Sodium nitroprusside Labetalol-parenteral alternate Nicardipine Nitroglycerin Clonidine (urgency)

Hypertension in Pregnancy

Classification

1. Pregnancy–induced hypertension (PIH) or gestational hypertension.
2. Chronic hypertension: Preexisting, before 20 weeks of gestation.
3. Preeclampsia: Hypertension with proteinuria and edema. Occurs after 20th week of gestation (usually after 36th week).
4. Eclampsia: Preeclampsia + convulsions, coma.

Definition

1. BP usually falls during the first and second trimester.
2. PIH occurs if BP rises more than 30/15 mm Hg or MAP >25 mm Hg or to a level above 140/90 in the last trimester, MAP >95.
3. Most PIH occurs after the 35th week.
4. Preeclampsia develops after 20th week.
5. About 10% of pregnancies are complicated by hypertension.

Pathogenesis: Preeclampsia

1. Increased sensitivity to pressure effects of angiotensin II
2. Reduced intravascular volume
3. Decreased PRA
4. Decreased prostacyclin/thromboxane ratio
5. Increased atrial natriuretic peptide
6. Increased endothelin
7. Decreased endothelin relaxing factor (nitrous oxide)
8. Activation of coagulation
9. Increased fibrin degradation products
10. Thrombocytopenia
11. Increased factor XII
12. Decreased factor X and XI
13. Increased fibrinogen
14. High fibronectin
15. Low antithrombin III
16. Low alpha$_1$, anti-plasmin
17. Increased plasminogen activator inhibitor activity
18. Vasospasm
19. Reduced cardiac output
20. Increased peripheral vascular resistance
21. Decreased sodium exchange
22. Decreased renal blood flow
23. Decreased glomerular filtration
24. Hyperuricemia
25. Hypomagnesimia

Generalized reduced organ perfusion occurs with widespread hemorrhage and necrosis in brain, liver, heart, and kidney with vascular endothelial damage and marked vasoconstriction of small arterioles. Preeclampsia may be a result of abnormal trophoblastic implantation and immunologic disorder.

Disease Spectrum: Preeclampsia

Clinical spectrum of coagulation disorders varies from thrombocytopenia to HELLP syndrome (hemolysis, elevated liver enzymes, low platelet count).

Predisposing Factors

PIH

a. Young primigravida c. Diabetes mellitus
b. Primary hypertension d. Renal disease

Preeclampsia and eclampsia

a. Extremes of reproductive age f. Chronic hypertension
b. Nulliparas   g. Renal disease
c. Multi-fetal pregnancy h. Thalassemia and Rh
d. Fetal hydrops   incompatibility
e. Diabetes mellitus   i. Family history of preeclampsia

Management

1. PIH
   a. Do *not* restrict sodium
   b. Bed rest and mild sedation, hospitalization
   c. Avoid thiazide diuretics, beta-blockers except labetalol, ACE inhibitors, and ARBs
   d. Use hydralazine, methyldopa, clonidine, calcium channel blockers, labetalol.
2. Preeclampsia and eclampsia
   a. Calcium supplement, 1–2 gm/day
   b. Aspirin, 60–100 mg/day
   c. Dipyridamole
   d. Dipyridamole + heparin
   e. Bed rest and sedation
   f. Liberal sodium intake
   g. $MgSO_4$ in eclampsia for convulsions and lower BP
   h. Volume expansion: controversial (?)
   i. Medications to control BP: calcium channel blockers, clonidine, methyldopa, hydralazine, labetalol
   j. Avoid diuretics, beta-blockers except labetalol, ACE inhibitors, and ARBs.

Quality of Life and Antihypertensive Therapy (Selected Trials)*

Study	Beta-Blocker	Diuretic	Central Alpha-Agonist	Calcium Channel Blocker	ACE† Inhibitor	ARB
MRC[39]	↓ (Propranolol)	→				
Croog[95]	↓ (Propranolol)	→	↓ (Methyldopa)		↑ (Captopril)	
Jachuck[96]	↓ (Propranolol)	→	↓ (Methyldopa)			
Curb[97]		→	↓ (Methyldopa)			
Avorn[98]	↓ (Propranolol)					
Testa[99]	↓ (Atenolol)					
Os[100]				↑ (Nifedipine)		
Croog[101]	→/↑ (Atenolol)			→ (Nifedipine)	→ (Lisinopril)	
Fletcher[102]	→ (Atenolol)			→/↑ (Verapamil)	→/↑ (Captopril)	
Life[190]	↓ (Atenolol)				→ (Captopril)	Losartan

*Quality of life is decreased with beta-blockers and diuretics but is unchanged or improved with calcium channel blockers and ACE inhibitors.
†Quality of life with Ang-II receptor antagonists appears to be similar to ACE inhibitor.

Antihypertensive Drug Compliance[193, 194, 195]

- Diuretics and beta-blockers (BB) have the lowest compliance rate and refill rate with chronic use.
- ARBs, ACEIs and CCBs have the highest compliance rate and refill rate with chronic use. These differences are *significant* compared to BBs and diuretics (p< 0.0001).

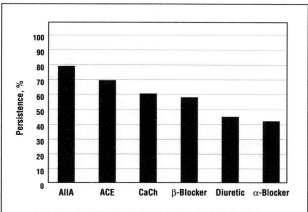

Persistence with antihypertensive therapy by drug class in the Saskatechewan Health Database. ACE—angiotensin converting enzyme inhibitor; AIIa—angiotensin antagonist; CaCh—calcium channel antagonist.

Patient Status at 12 Months in the Merck-Medco Study

Drug (number of patients)	No. of Patients	Patients remaining on initial therapy %	Patients switching to new therapy %
AT1 receptor blocker (5567)	64	7	29
Angiotensin converting enzyme inhibitor (5842)	58	9	33
Calcium channel blocker (5094)	50	9	41
β-Blocker (4994)	43	7	50
Diuretic (5226)	38	6	56

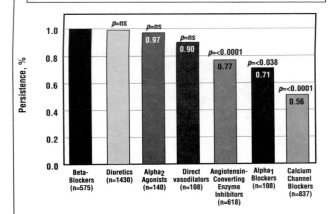

Relative Likelihood of Discontinuing Antihypertensive Therapy Over 7 Years According to Drug Class

p values vs. beta-blockers. N= 2829 patients; 1196 patients dropped out over 7 years.

Adapted from Elliot WJ. Am J Hypertens. 1994;7:26A.

Total Cost of Antihypertensive Therapy[5],[117]

1. Acquisition cost.
2. Coprescription of secondary drugs.
3. Office visits.
4. Ancillary laboratory costs (electrolytes, glucose, lipids, ECG).
5. Costs to patient's lifestyle: quality of life and adverse effects.
6. Cost of increasing end-organ damage.
7. Mean costs per drug cost category—1-year use.[117]

	Acquisition Cost	Supplemental Drug Cost	Laboratory Cost	Clinic Visit Cost	Side Effect Cost	Total Cost
Diuretics	$133	$232	$117	$298	$263	$1043
β-Blockers	$334	$115	$56	$187	$203	$895
α-Blockers	$401	$290	$114	$227	$256	$1288
Centrally acting α-agonists	$285	$295	$125	$267	$193	$1165
ACE inhibitors+ Ang-II receptor antagonists	$444	$291	$95	$218	$195	$1243
Calcium entry blockers	$540	$278	$87	$214	$306	$1425

Characteristics of the Ideal Antihypertensive Drug

1. Efficacious as monotherapy in more than 50% of all patients.
2. BP control during all activities for 24 hours. Avoid excessive nocturnal dipping.
3. Once-a-day dosing with high trough to peak ratio.
4. Hemodynamically logical and effective: Reduces SVR, improves arterial compliance, preserves CO, and maintains perfusion to all vital organs.
5. Lack of tolerance or pseudotolerance: No reflex volume retention or stimulation of neurohumoral mechanisms.
6. Favorable biochemical effects, metabolic effects, and risk factor profile.
7. Reverses structural, vascular smooth muscle, and cardiac hypertrophy; improves systolic and diastolic compliance and left ventricular contractility and function; reduces ventricular ectopy, if present.
8. Reduces all end-organ damage: cardiac, cerebrovascular, renal, retinal, and large artery.
9. Maintains normal hemodynamic response to aerobic and anaerobic exercise.
10. Low incidence of side effects, good quality of life.
11. Good compliance with drug regimen.
12. Good profile for concomitant diseases or problems.
13. Reasonable cost (cost/benefit ratio).
14. No withdrawal symptoms and prolongation of BP control with missed dose due to long biological half-life and efficacy of drug.

Combination Antihypertensive Therapy: Selected Drugs[125]

1. Calcium channel blocker plus:
   a. Alpha-blocker *or*
   b. ACE inhibitor, Ang-II receptor blocker or
   c. CCB of different class: Non DHP with DHP
   d. Central alpha-agonist
   e. Diuretic
   f. Beta-blocker (see comment with 6 a.)
2. Alpha-blocker plus:
   a. Calcium channel blocker *or*
   b. ACE inhibitor, Ang-II receptor blocker
   c. Diuretic
   d. Do not generally use with central alpha-agonist (reduced response rate).
3. Central alpha-agonist plus:
   a. Calcium channel blocker *or*
   b. ACE inhibitor, Ang-II receptor blocker
   c. Diuretic
   d. Do not generally use with alpha-blocker (reduced response rate).
4. ACE inhibitor plus:
   a. Calcium channel blocker *or*
   b. Alpha-blocker
   c. ARB
   d. Central alpha-agonist
   e. Diuretic
5. Diuretic plus:
   a. Any other antihypertensive class
6. Beta-blocker plus:
   a. Calcium channel blocker—use caution in the presence of systolic dysfunction or conducting problems, particularly with verapamil or diltiazem.
   b. ACE inhibitor, Ang-II receptor blocker
   c. Diuretic
   d. Alpha-blocker
   e. Do not use with central alpha-agonist because of possible central antagonism and potential for severe withdrawal syndrome

7. Ang-II receptor blocker plus:
    a. ACE Inhibitor
    b. Calcium channel blocker
    c. Central alpha-agonist
    d. Alpha-blocker
    e. Diuretic

Combination Antihypertensive Therapy: Selected Drugs–*Summary*

	Calcium Channel Blocker	Alpha-Blocker	Alpha-Agonist	ACE Inhibitor	ARB	Diuretic
Calcium channel blocker	√	√	√	√	√	√
Alpha-blocker	√	Ø	Ø	√	√	√
Central alpha-agonist	√	Ø	Ø	√	√	√
Ang-II blocker/	√	√	√	√	Ø	√
ACE inhibitor	√	√	√	Ø	√	√

√, Appropriate combination; Ø, avoid.

Combinations of these *classes* of antihypertensive drugs in low doses can achieve:

1. Additive or synergistic reduction in blood pressure
2. Reduced adverse effects
3. Improvement of the structural and metabolic components of the hypertension syndrome
4. Most patients need 3 to 4 drugs to reach goal BP of ≤ 130/85 mm Hg or better.

Antihypertensive Therapy: Efficacy of Monotherapy

Drug Class	White (%)	African-American (%)	Elderly (%) (both races)
Diuretic	50	60	50
Beta-blocker	50	30–40	20–30
Calcium channel blocker	75	75–80	75–80
ACE inhibitor	60	60	60
Alpha-blocker	60	60	60
Central alpha-agonist	60	60	60
Ang-II blocker	60	60	60
Alpha-beta-blocker	50	50	50

Selected Drug Interactions with Antihypertensive Therapy*116

Class of Agent	Increase Efficacy	Decrease Efficacy	Effect on Other Drugs
Diuretics	• Diuretics that act at different sites in the nephron (e.g., furosemide + thiazides)	• Resin-binding agents • NSAIDs • Steroids	• Diuretics raise serum lithium levels. • Potassium-sparing agents may exacerbate hyperkalemia due to ACE inhibitors.
Beta-blockers	• Cimetidine (hepatically metabolized beta-blockers) • Quinidine (hepatically metabolized beta-blockers) • Food (hepatically metabolized beta-blockers)	• NSAIDs • Withdrawal of clonidine • Agents that induce rifampin and phenobarbital	• Propranolol hydrochloride induces hepatic enzymes to increase clearance of drugs with similar metabolic pathways. • Beta-blockers may mask and prolong insulin-induced hypoglycemia. • Heart block may occur with nondihydropyridine calcium antagonists. • Sympathomimetics cause unopposed alpha-adrenoceptor-mediated vasoconstriction. • Beta-blockers increase angina-inducing potential of cocaine.
ACE inhibitors	• Chlorpromazine or clozapine	• NSAIDs • Antacids • Food decreases absorption (moexipril)	• ACE inhibitors may raise serum lithium levels. • ACE inhibitors may exacerbate hyperkalemic effect of potassium-sparing diuretics.

Class of Agent	Increase Efficacy	Decrease Efficacy	Effect on Other Drugs
Calcium antagonists	• Grapefruit juice (some dihydropyridines) • Cimetidine or ranitidine (hepatically metabolized calcium antagonists)	• Agents that induce hepatic enzymes, including rifampin and phenobarbital	• Cyclosporine levels increase† with diltiazem hydrochloride, verapamil hydrochloride, mibefradil dihydrochloride, or nicardipine hydrochloride (but not felodipine, isradipine, or nifedipine). • Nondihydropyridines increase levels of other drugs metabolized by the same hepatic enzyme system, including digoxin, quinidine, sulfonylureas, and theophylline. • Verapamil hydrochloride may lower serum lithium levels.
Alpha-blockers		N/A	• Prazosin may decrease clearance of verapamil hydrochloride.
Central alpha₂-agonists and peripheral neuronal blockers		• Tricyclic antidepressants (and probably phenothiazines) • Monoamine oxidase inhibitors • Sympathomimetics or phenothiazines antagonize guanethidine monosulfate or guanadrel sulfate • Iron salts may reduce methyldopa absorption	• Methyldopa may increase serum lithium levels. • Severity of clonidine hydrochloride withdrawal may be increased by beta-blockers. • Many agents used in anesthesia are potentiated by clonidine hydrochloride.

*Reproduced with permission from Joint National Committee on Prevention, Detection, Evaluation, and Treatment of High Blood Pressure. The Sixth Report of the Joint National Committee on Prevention, Detection, Evaluation, and Treatment of High Blood Pressure. Arch Intern Med. 1997;157:2413–2446.

Maximum Recommended Doses* of Antihypertensive Drugs with Best Treatment Characteristics

	Dose/Day (mg)
Calcium channel blockers	
Amlodipine (Norvasc)	10
Diltiazem (Cardizem SR and CD, Dilacor XR, Tiazac)	540
Felodipine (Plendil)	10
Isradipine (DynaCirc)	10
Nicardipine (Cardene and Cardene SR)	120
Nifedipine (Adalat Oros and CC, Procardia XL)	90
Nisoldipine (Sular)	60
Verapamil (Calan SR, Isoptin SR, Verelan)	540
ACE inhibitors	
Benazepril (Lotensin)	40
Captopril (Capoten)	50
Enalapril (Vasotec)	40
Fosinopril (Monopril)	80
Lisinopril (Prinivil, Zestril)	40
Moexipril (Univasc)	30
Quinapril (Accupril)	80
Ramipril (Altace)	20
Trandolapril (Mavik)	8
Perindopril (Aceon)	16
Central alpha-agonists	
Clonidine (Catapres and Catapres-TTS)	0.4/TTS-3
Guanabenz (Wytensin)	16
Guanfacine (Tenex)	2
Alpha-blockers	
Doxazosin (Cardura)	10
Prazosin (Minipress)	10
Terazosin (Hytrin)	10
Diuretics	
Indapamide (Lozol)	2.5
Chlorthalidone	25
HCTZ	25

Angiotensin II blockers

Losartan (Cozaar)	100
Valsartan (Diovan)	320
Irbesartan (Avapro)	300
Telmisartan (Micardis)	80
Candesartan cilexetil (Atacand)	32
Eprosartan (Teveten)	1200
Olmesartan (Benicar)	1200

*Approximately 80% to 90% of total antihypertensive effect achieved in most patients.

Diuretics[103–105]

The mechanism of action of diuretics is inhibition of NaCl resorption in the renal tubules. There is an initial reduction in CO secondary to reduction in plasma volume and extracellular fluid volume, but SVR is reduced with long-term therapy (after 4 to 8 weeks), and volume reduction reverses over the same time frame.

Diuretics are used as monotherapy to treat mild to moderate hypertension or as an adjunct to other antihypertensives. The major differences among the diuretics are related to duration and site of action as well as potency of diuretic action. The adverse effects are similar, particularly among the thiazide diuretics. *Lower doses* of diuretics (i.e., HCTZ 12.5 to 25 mg/day or its equivalent) are now recommended by JNC-7 for treatment of essential hypertension during the initial treatment period; the dose is then adjusted as necessary. The maximum antihypertensive dose should not exceed 25 mg of HCTZ or its equivalent. Approximately 80% of the antihypertensive effect of HCTZ is achieved with a 12.5 mg/day dose; 95% is achieved with a 25 mg/day dose.[105] Thiazide-type diuretics (except indapamide) generally lose their effectiveness in patients with serum creatinine levels in excess of 1.7 mg/dl. Indapamide remains effective in patients with moderate to severe chronic kidney disease. Therefore, there is a relatively flat dose-response curve for the *antihypertensive efficacy* of thiazide diuretics, whereas the *diuretic effect may* continue up to doses of 100 mg/day of HCTZ.

Indapamide offers many advantages over other diuretics, is more potent than other diuretics in reducing BP, has mild CCB and AB effects which may make it the diuretic of choice in treating hypertension.[106,107] Indapamide has a better metabolic profile (lipid neutral, no glucose intolerance, and less effect on potassium and magnesium) and may be less nephrotoxic compared to thiazide and thiazide-like diuretics. It reduces LVH and platelet aggregation. There is no effect on insulin resistance. Indapamide is also effective in the presence of renal insufficiency. Indapamide was used in the PROGESS trial. Electrolyte abnormalities ($\downarrow$Na+, $\uparrow$K+) are still seen with this agent.

1. *Classification:* Diuretic inhibition of NaCl resorption in renal tubules.

2. *Mechanism:*
   a. Initial reduction in CO secondary to reduction in plasma volume and extracellular fluid volume
   b. Long-term reduction in SVR
   c. Direct vasodilator action.

3. *Pharmacology:* See individual diuretics listings.

4. *Hemodynamics:*
   a. MAP reduced
   b. CO slightly reduced (1%–5%)
   c. SVR reduced
   d. HR increased
   e. RBF, RPF, and GFR slightly reduced
   f. Renin, aldosterone, and angiotensin II increased
   g. Postural hypotension (mild) decreased IVV
   h. Glomerular pressure increased.

5. *Clinical use:*
   a. Adjunctive with other antihypertensives
   b. Monotherapy, initial therapy in mild to moderate hypertension in absence of compelling indications for other agents
   c. Relatively inexpensive acquisition cost
   d. Reduces supine and upright BP
   e. Fairly well tolerated
   f. No tachyphylaxis.

6. *Major differences in diuretics:*
   a. Duration and site of action
   b. Potency of diuretic action (loop diuretics > thiazides)
   c. Efficacy with renal insufficiency (loop > metolazone > indapamide > thiazides)
   d. Efficacy on BP control (thiazides > loop) - indapamide> thiazides> loops
   e. Hemodynamic regulatory mechanisms
   f. Hormonal regulatory mechanisms.

7. *Most common adverse effects:*
   a. Hypokalemia

   b. Hypomagnesemia

   c. Hyperuricemia

   d. Hyperglycemia (less with loop diuretics), insulin resistance and new onset type 2 DM (except indapamide)

   e. Hyponatremia

   f. Hypochloremia

   g. Hyperlipidemia (mostly thiazides) including hypertriglyceridemia, hypercholesterolemia, increased LDL cholesterol, decreased HDL cholesterol

   h. Azotemia and renal insufficiency, ↓ GFR. Renal vascular fibrosis, proteinuria, and MAU

   i. Hypercalcemia (usually only thiazide-like diuretics)

   j. Impotence—20%–25% of male patients

   k. Dermatologic reactions, rash, purpura

   l. Blood dyscrasias

   m. Cardiac arrhythmias

   n. Volume depletion and postural hypotension

   o. Metabolic alkalosis

   p. Hyperreninemia

   q. Hyperaldosteronism (secondary)

   r. Pancreatitis

   s. Allergic disorders

   t. Vasculitis

   u. Homocysteinemia

   v. Renal cell carcinoma (increased by 55%) and colon carcinoma

   w. Increased PAI-I and PAI-I/TPA ratio

   x. Increased fibrinogen and thrombotic risk.

8. *Contraindications:*

   a. Anuria

   b. Known allergy (some sulfa-allergic patients)

9. *Dose and tablet strength:*
   a. Start with a low dose (12.5 mg of chlorthalidone, HCTZ or equivalent) to control BP, and titrate dose up to a maximum of 25 mg/day. These doses are more effective in volume-dependent, low-renin hypertension; 95% of patients respond to 25 mg/day. For indapamide start with 1.25 mg/day up to a maximum of 2.5 mg/day
   b. For treatment of hypertension, but not for the diuretic effect, there is a *flat dose response* over 25 mg/day of HCTZ or its equivalent
   c. HCTZ and other thiazides are not effective if the creatinine clearance is less than 30 ml/min
   d. Indapamide offers many advantages over other diuretics.

Diuretics Highlights*

Preparation		Mechanism of Action	Pharmacodynamics
Thiazides (benzothiadiazine derivatives)			
Chlorothiazide (Diuril)—Merck	250 mg 500 mg	See HCTZ	Duration: 6–12 hr
Cyclothiazide (Anhydron)—Lilly	2 mg	See HCTZ	Duration: 12 hr
HCTZ (Oretic)—Abbott (Esidrix)—Novartis (Hydro-DIURIL)— Merck	25–50 mg 25–50 mg 25–100 mg	Inhibits resorption of NaCl and thereby increases the quantity of Na^1 traversing the distal tubule and volume of water excreted. Initial antihypertensive effect is due to volume contraction and lower CO. Long-term antihypertensive effect due to lower SVR.	Duration: 6–12 hr
Mircozide (Watson)	12.5		

302

Hemodynamics	Adverse Effects	Contra-indications	Daily Dosage	Drug Interactions
See HCTZ	See HCTZ	See HCTZ	250–500 mg	See HCTZ
See HCTZ	See HCTZ	See HCTZ	1–2 mg on alternate days	See HCTZ
MAP reduced	Hyponatremia	Anuria	6.25–50 mg	Cholestyramine:
CO slightly	Hypokalemia	Hypersensitivity		decreased
reduced initially	Hyperuricemia	to sulfonamilde		thiazide effect
Plasma volume	Hypercalcemia	derivatives		Corticosteroids:
reduced	Hyperglycemia			increased
SVR decreased	Hypomagnesemia			potassium loss
HR increased	Hypochloremia			Diazoxide:
NE increased	Metabolic			increased hyper-
Aldosterone	alkalosis			glycemic effect
increased	Volume			Digitalis glycosides
PRA increased	depletion			increased
Angiotensin II	Postural			digitalis toxicity
increased	hypotension			(hypokalemia
PGC Increased	Hyperlipidemia			and hypomagnesemia)
	Increased total			Indomethacin:
	cholesterol			decreased
	triglycerides			antihypertensive
	Decreased HDL			and natriuretic
	Increased LDL			effects
	Not renoprotective			NSAIDs:
				decreased
				diuretic and
				antihypertensive
				effects

Preparation		Mechanism of Action	Pharmacodynamics
Methyclothiazide (Enduron)—Abbott	2.5 mg 5 mg	See HCTZ	Duration: 24 hr Peak: 2 hr
Polythiazide (Renese)—Pfizer Chlorthalidone (Hygroton)— Adventis (Thalitone)—BI	1 mg 2 mg 4 mg 25 mg 50 mg 100 mg 25 mg	See HCTZ Increases excretion of Na^+ and H_2O Site of action is at the cortical diluting segment of the distal tubule	Duration: 24–48 hr Duration: 24–72 hr Onset: 2 hr
Loop diuretics Bumetanide (Bumex)—Roche	Oral: 0.5 mg, 1 mg, 2 mg IV: 0.25 mg/mL	Decreases chloride and secondary sodium resorption in ascending limb of the loop of Henle	Onset: ½ hr Peak: 1–1½ hr Half-life: 4–6 hr Metabolism: liver Excretion: renal
Ethacrynic acid (Edecrin)—Merck	25 mg 50 mg IV powder: 50 mg diluted to 100 mL	See Furosemide	Duration: 1–4 hr Onset: 1 hr
Torsemide (Demadex)— Roche	5 mg 10 mg 20 mg 100 mg IV: 2 mL (20 mg) vial IV: 5 mL (10 mg/mL) vial	See Furosemide	Onset: ½ hr— simultaneous food intake delays absorption Peak: 1 hr Half-life: 3.5 hr Metabolism: liver Excretion: renal Less protein bound

Hemodynamics	Adverse Effects	Contra-indications	Daily Dosage	Drug Interactions
e HCTZ	See HCTZ	Renal decompensation Hypersensitivity	2.5–5 mg	See HCTZ
e HCTZ	See HCTZ	See HCTZ	1–4 mg	See HCTZ
e Thiazides	Hypomagnesemia Increases cholesterol, triglycerides, and LDL Decreases HDL	See HCTZ	12.5–50 mg	See Thiazides
FR, RPF, RBF eserved eduction in ee water earance	Hypokalemia Hypochloremic alkalosis Hyperuricemia Ototoxicity Muscle pain and tenderness Dizziness Hypotension Weakness	See HCTZ	Average dose: 1–2 mg Range: 0.5–10 mg Maximum: 10 mg	Probenecid: reduces bumetanide effectiveness Indomethacin: blunts sodium excretion associated with bumetanide Lithium: reduces renal clearance of bumetanide, high risk of lithium toxicity
e Furosemide	Gastrointestinal symptoms common with larger doses Hyperuricemia	Anuria	50–100 mg Should not exceed 400 mg	Oral anticoagulants: increased anticoagulant effect Aminoglycoside antibiotics, digitalis: see Furosemide
FR, RPF, RBF id base balance eserved creased urinary .cretion of sodium Ioride + H$_2$O	Dizziness Headache Nausea Weakness Vomiting Hyperglycemia Excessive urination Hyperuricemia Hypokalemia Excessive thirst	Anuria Hypersensitivity	Intial: 5 mg qd Range: 5–10 mg qd Maximum: 10 mg qd	Salicylates: salicylate toxicity NSAIDs: possible renal dysfunction Indomethacin: blunts sodium excretion associated with torsemide Probenecid: reduces torsemide effectiveness Lithium: reduces renal clearance of torsemide, high risk of torsemide toxicity

Preparation		Mechanism of Action	Pharmacodynamic
Furosemide (Lasix)— Adventis	20 mg 40 mg 80 mg	Primarily inhibits the resorption of Cl^-, Na^+, and H_2O in the ascending loop of Henle and exerts a weak diuretic effect in the proximal and distal tubules	Duration: 1–4 hr Onset: 1 hr Peak: 1–2 hr Metabolism: liver Excretion: renal
Diuretic of the pyridine-sulfonylurea class (Demadex)— Boehringer Mannheim	5 mg 10 mg 20 mg 100 mg	Acts within the lumen of the thick ascending portion of the loop of Henle where it inhibits the $Na^+/K^+/Cl^-$ carrier system	Duration: oral 6–8 hr IV 6–8 hr Onset: oral 1 hr IV 10 min Peak: oral 1–2 hr IV 1 hr Excretions: hepatic 80% renal 20% Bioavailability: 80%

emodynamics	Adverse Effects	Contra-indications	Daily Dosage	Drug Interactions
ecreased ulmonary edge pressure ▸WP) ecreases CO ▸ecreases SVR	Fluid and electrolyte imbalance Hypomagnesemia Hypokalemia Mild diarrhea Nerve deafness Decreases HDL	Anuria Azotemia	20–150 mg	Digitalis glycosides: increased digitalis toxicity (hypokalemia and hypomag-nesemia) Indomethacin: decreased antihypertensive and natriuretic effect Probenecid: decreased diuretic effect NSAIDs: decreased diuretic and antihypertensive effects Aminoglycoside antibiotics: increased ototoxicity and nephrotoxicity
▸FR, RPF ▸eserved ▸O decreased VR decreased	Fluid and electrolyte imbalance Dizziness Headache Excessive urination Rhinitis Nausea	Known sensitivity to Demadex or to sulfonylurea Use with caution: Hepatic disease with cirrhosis and ascites Ototoxicity Volume and electrolyte depletion	Hypertension: Initial dose 5 mg qd Increase to 10 mg qd if inadequate BP response after 4–6 weeks Maximum rec-ommended: 10 mg qd	Indomethacin: natriuretic effects partially inhibited Lithium: may decrease renal clearance Salicylates: salicylate toxicity Cholestyramine: decreases the absorption of oral Demadex

Preparation		Mechanism of Action	Pharmacodynamic
Potassium-sparing diuretics			
Amiloride (Midamor)—Merck	5 mg	Inhibits K^+/Na^+ exchange in the distal tubule—a weak diuretic antihypertensive	Duration: 24 hr Onset: 2 hr Peak: 6–10 hr Excretion: kidney
Spironolactone (Aldactone) Pharmacia	25 mg 50 mg 100 mg	Antagonist of aldosterone through competitive binding of receptors at the aldosterone-dependent Na^+/K^+ exchange site in the distal convoluted renal tubule; causes an increase in Na^+ and water excreted	Duration: 12–48 hr
Triamterene (Dyrenium)— Wellspring	50 mg 100 mg	Not a diuretic but has a diuretic effect on the distal renal tubules, inhibiting the resorption of Na^+ in exchange for K^+	Duration: 7–9 hr Onset: 2–4 hr
Epleronone (Pfizer) (INSPRA)	25 mg 50 mg 100 mg 200 mg 400 mg	High selectivity for Aldosterone receptor	

emodynamics	Adverse Effects	Contra-indications	Daily Dosage	Drug Interactions
	See Triamterene	Hyperkalemia Should not be used with other potassium-conserving drugs in patients with impaired renal function	5–10 mg Should not exceed 20 mg	NSAIDs: renal failure, hyperkalemia ACE inhibitors: hyperkalemia
	Gynecomastia Menstrual irregularity or amenorrhea Postmenopausal bleeding Hyperkalemia Hyponatremia Gastrointestinal symptoms Impotence Fever Rash	Anuria Acute renal insufficiency Significant impairment of renal function Hyperkalemia	100–400 mg to treat hyper-aldosteronism 50–100 mg to treat essential hypertension	Salicylates: decreased diuretic effect Anticoagulations decreased anticoagulant effect Captopril: hyperkalemia Ether, nitrous oxide: hypotension
	Blood dyscrasias Photosensitivity Skin rash Hyperkalemia Hyperglycemia Metabolic acidosis Triamterene Kidney Stones	Anuria Renal insufficiency Severe hepatic disease	100 mg bid after meals Should not exceed 300 mg	Indomethacin and NSAIDs: renal failure Captopril and ACE inhibitors: hyperkalemia (additive) Ether, nitrous oxide: hypotension (additive)
	Minimal Rare Hyperkalemia (2.7%)		25 to 400 mg per day Effective in reducing BP LVH. CHF and proteinuria	Other K^+ sparing agents

Preparation	Mechanism of Action	Pharmacodynamic
Combination diuretics		
HCTZ 50 mg + amiloride 5 mg (Moduretic)—Merck	Combination tablet only	Amiloride is a K^+-conserving diuretic with weak, natriuretic antihypertensive activity. HCTZ blocks the resorption of Na^+ and K^+, thereby increasing the quantity of Na^+ traversing the distal tubule and the volume of water excreted	Duration: 24 hr Onset: 1–2 hr
HCTZ 25 mg + spironolactone 25 mg (Aldactazide)— Pharmacia/Pfizer	Combination tablet only	Combination of diuretic agents with different but complementary mechanisms and sites of action, providing additive diuretic and anti-hypertensive effects and preserving K^+	Duration: 24 hr Onset: 1–2 hr
HCTZ 25 mg + Triamterene 50 mg (Dyazide)— SmithKline Glaxo	Combination capsule only	HCTZ blocks resorption of Na^+ and Cl^- and thereby increases the quantity of Na^+ traversing the distal tubule and volume of water excreted. Triamterene has a weak diuretic effect on the distal renal tubules, inhibiting the resorption of Na^+ in exchange for K^+	Duration: 7–9 hr

emodynamics	Adverse Effects	Contra-indications	Daily Dosage	Drug Interactions
ee Thiazides	Electrolye imbalance Elevates BUN Hyperkalemia Mild skin rash	Renal impairment Patients receiving K$^+$-conserving agents Hyperkalemia	1–2 tablets	See HCTZ and Amiloride
ee Thiazides	Gynecomastia Gastrointestinal symptoms Hyperkalemia Rash	Anuria Acute renal insufficiency Acute, severe hepatic failure Hyperkalemia	Optimal dosage established by individual titration of the components	See HCTZ and Spironolactone
educes SVR lild reduction CO lild reduction plasma olume (See hiazides)	Electrolye imbalance Muscle cramps Rash Weakness Photosensitivity Gastrointestinal disturbances	Renal dysfunction Azotemia Hyperkalemia Anuria	1–2 capsules Not to exceed 4 capsules†	See HCTZ and Triamterene

Preparation		Mechanism of Action	Pharmacodynamic
HCTZ 50 mg + Triameterene 75 mg (Maxzide)— Bertek	Tablet (scored) 25 mg HCTZ + 37.5 mg Triameterene	HCTZ blocks NaCl resorption and later reduces SVR. Triameterene has a weak diuretic effect on distal renal rubule, preserves K$^+$	Duration: 6–12 hrs Onset: 2 hrs Peak: 4 hrs Excretion: kidney Improved bioavailab over Dyazide (Thiazides)
Quinazoline diuretic derivative Metolazone (Zaroxolyn)—Celltech (Diulo) Mykrox	2.5 mg 5 mg 10 mg .5 mg	Acts primarily to inhibit Na$^+$ resorption at the cortical diluting site and in the proximal convo- luted tubule	Duration: 12–24 hrs Onset: 1 hr Peak: 24 hrs Excretion: renal
Indoline diuretic derivative Indapamide (Lozol) Aventis	1.25 mg 2.5 mg 5 mg	Similar to thiazides— acts on the cortical diluting segment; may be effective in mild renal insufficiency	Duration: 24 hr Onset: 1 hr Peak: 2 hr Metabolism: liver Excretion: renal 70% bile 23%

*Consult the *Physicians' Desk Reference* for full prescribing information.
†Bioequivalence is low, with only 30% absorption.
‡Bioequivalence is improved compared with Dyazide; 60% absorption.

emodynamics	Adverse Effects	Contra-indications	Daily Dosage	Drug Interactions
educes SVR	Electrolyte	Renal dysfunction	½ to 1 tablet‡	See HCTZ and
ild reduction	imbalance	Azotemia		Triamterene
CO	Muscle cramps	Hyperkalemia		
ild reduction	Rash	Anuria		
plasma	Weakness			
lume (See	Photosentivity			
astrointestinal				
sturbances				
ee Thiazides	Azotemia	Renal insufficiency	2.5–5 mg	See Thiazides
	Hyperglycemia		Higher doses	
	Hyperuricemia		may be	
	Hypercalcemia		indicated with	
	Hyponatremia		other disorders	
	Hypokalemia			
	Hypomagnesemia			
AP reduced	Hypokalemia	See Thiazides	Average:	See Thiazides
O reduced	Hypomagnesemia		1.25–2.5 mg	
VR reduced	Hyperuricemia		Maximum:	
inimal change	Hyponatremia		2.5 mg	
RBF, RPF,	Hypochloremia			
FR				

Central Alpha-Agonists[103,104]

The central alpha-agonists all stimulate the central postsynaptic $alpha_2$ receptor in the brain stem, which reduces sympathetic nervous system activity to the periphery. These CNS effects result in a reduction in SVR, plasma and urine NE levels, and PRA, CO, RBF, and GFR. The CO is preserved at rest and with exercise.

Common side effects are sedation and dry mouth, which are minimized with low-dose long-term therapy. Concern about withdrawal syndrome has been overemphasized with all these drugs, particularly clonidine. When low doses are used, the frequency of withdrawal syndrome is minimal and probably less than that with beta-blockers.

Antihypertensive efficacy is excellent and similar with all of the central alpha-agonists. Selection of therapy depends more on some of the unique side effects, duration of action, and cost.

Clonidine, guanabenz, and guanfacine all have a neutral or favorable effect on serum lipids and glucose compared with methyldopa, which has an unfavorable effect. Methyldopa reduces HDL cholesterol and increases triglycerides. There is little reason to use methyldopa now because the side effects are greater than and efficacy is inferior to those of the other central alpha-agonists:[108–110]

1. Clonidine (Catapres): oral and transdermal patch
2. Guanabenz (Wytensin)
3. Guanfacine (Tenex)
4. Methyldopa (Aldomet)

Alpha Receptors

Alpha receptors are primarily of two types:

1. *Presynaptic (prejunctional):* located at the membranes of the neurons that contain the neurotransmitter NE. Stimulation inhibits the release of NE from the postganglionic sympathetic nerve ending. NE in the synaptic cleft inhibits its own release.
2. *Postsynaptic:* located on the target organ. Activation results in an agonist effect (vasoconstriction in the periphery) but reduced sympathetic activity centrally.

314

Central Alpha-Agonists: Similarities

1. Stimulation of central postsynaptic alpha$_2$ receptors in the nucleus tractus solitarii of the medulla oblongata results in:
   a. Reduced sympathetic nervous system activity.
   b. Reduced NE levels in serum and urine.
   c. Reduced PRA owing to reduced NE levels.
   d. Increased vagal stimulation (bradycardia):
      (1) Clonidine: direct.
      (2) Guanabenz: direct.
      (3) Guanfacine: direct.
      (4) Methyldopa: indirect (alpha-methylnorepinephrine).
2. Peripheral alpha-agonist pressor response is overwhelmed by central alpha-agonist effect except rarely with:
   a. Intravenous doses (transient pressor effects).
   b. High oral doses.
3. Peripheral sympathetic reflexes remain intact, so fewer problems occur with:
   a. Postural hypotension: methyldopa effect greater than that of clonidine, guanabenz, guanfacine.
   b. Exercise: preserved with all four drugs.
   c. Sexual dysfunction: methyldopa effect greater than that of clonidine, guanabenz, or guanfacine.
4. Lowering of BP is not associated with reduction of systemic or regional blood flow.
5. Minimal to no sodium or water retention or weight gain occurs except with methyldopa. Natriuresis occurs in some patients with clonidine, guanabenz, and guanfacine.
6. Hemodynamic effects are similar.
7. Drugs are effective as monotherapy.
8. Adjunctive therapy with other antihypertensive drugs allows for additive or synergistic effects at lower doses of each drug. The recommended average maximum is:
   a. Clonidine: 0.4 mg (oral); TTS-3 mg once/week.
   b. Guanabenz: 16 to 24 mg/day.
   c. Guanfacine: 2 mg/day.
   d. Methyldopa: 2000 mg/day.
9. Dose equivalency: Clonidine 0.1 mg = guanabenz 4 mg = guanfacine 0.5 mg = methyldopa 500 mg.

Central Alpha-Agonists Highlights*

Preparation		Mechanism of Action	Pharmacodynamics
Clonidine (Catapres)— Boehringer Ingelheim	0.1 mg (oral) 0.2 mg (oral) 0.3 mg (oral) TTS 1–3	Selective stimulation of postsynaptic alpha$_2$ adrenergic receptors in depressor site of vasomotor center of medulla, nucleus tractus solitarii, and hypothalamus. Reduces efferent sympathetic tone and increases vagal tone to heart, peripheral vasculature, and kidney. Reduces SVR, causing vasodilation and lowering blood pressure. Spares peripheral reflexes. Reduces PRA	Onset: ½–1 hr Peak: 3–5 hr Plasma half-life: 12–16 hr Metabolism: liver (minimal) Excretion: renal TTS—duration of antihypertensive effect: 1 week

Hemodynamics	Adverse Effects	Contra-indications	Daily Dosage	Drug Interactions
MAP reduced	Sedation and	Sick sinus	Initial:	Tricyclic anti-
CO unchanged	drowsiness	syndrome	0.1 mg hs	depressants
HR reduced	Dry mouth	Second-or third-	and increase	and beta-
(10%)	Dizziness	degree AV	by 0.1 mg q	adrenergic
SVR reduced	Withdrawal	block	3–4 days,	blockers:
RBF, RPF, GFR: no	syndrome and	Depression	giving larger	loss of
change or increase	rebound hyper-		bid doses	antihypertensive
RVR reduced	tension (uncom-		at bedtime.	effect in some
Plasma and urinary	mon with doses		Some qd,	patients
NE and EPI reduced	<1.2 mg qd)		usually bid	
Angiotensin II	Weakness		Average:	
reduced	Headache		0.4–0.6 mg	
PRA reduced	Bradycardia		Maximum:	
Aldosterone	Constipation		1.2 mg	
reduced	Impotence (un-		Range:	
Exercise response	common—4%)		0.2–1.2 mg	
preserved	Depression		TTS: once	
PWP reduced	Nightmares		per week	
Fluid retention:			TTS—1, 2,	
minimal to			or 3	
none				
Diuresis in some				
patients				

Preparation		Mechanism of Action	Pharmacodynamics
Guanabenz (Wytensin)— Wyeth-Ayerst	4 mg 8 mg	Stimulation of post-synaptic alpha$_2$ receptors in medulla reduces sympathetic activity. SVR and PRA	Onset: 1 hr Peak: 4 hrs Plasma and half-life: 6 hrs Metabolism: 75% (site undetermined) Excretion: renal: 80%
Guanfacine (Tenex)— Wyeth	1 mg 2 mg	Reduces sympathetic tone, SVR, and HR	Onset: 1 hr Peak: 4 hrs Plasma half-life: 12 hrs Excretion: renal

Hemodynamics	Adverse Effects	Contra-indications	Daily Dosage	Drug Interactions
MAP reduced CO unchanged HR reduced (minimal) SVR reduced RBF, RPF, GFR: no change RVR reduced Plasma and urinary NE and EPI reduced Aldosterone reduced PRA reduced Angiotensin II reduced Exercise response preserved Plasma volume: unchanged Diuresis in some patients	Dry mouth Sedation and drowsiness Fatigue Impotence Withdrawal syndrome Rebound and overshoot hypertension Dizziness Weakness Headache Constipation	Pregnancy	Average dose: 16 mg Range: 8–48 mg Maximum: 48 mg	Potentiates central nervous system depressant depressant drugs
MAP reduced CO unchanged HR reduced (10%) SVR reduced RBF, RPF, GFR: no change or increase RVR reduced Plasma and urinary NE and EPI reduced Angiotensin II reduced PRA reduced Aldosterone reduced Exercise response preserved PWP reduced Fluid retention: minimal to none Diuresis in some	See Clonidine	Allergy to guanfacine	1 mg hs Maximum: 3 mg hs	See Clonidine

	Preparation	Mechanism of Action	Pharmacodynamics
Methyldopa (Aldomet)— Merck	125 mg 250 mg 500 mg Also available in elixir, 250 mg/mL	Alpha-methylnorepi-nephrine stimulates a postsynaptic alpha$_2$ adrenergic receptor in the medulla and decreases sympathetic outflow, which reduces SVR and PRA. Also has some peripheral action	Onset: 2–3 hr Peak: 5 hr Plasma half-life: 12 hr Metabolism: hepatic Excretion: renal

*Consult the *Physicians' Desk Reference* for full prescribing information.
†Variable oral absorption, 50%–80%.

Hemodynamics	Adverse Effects	Contra-indications	Daily Dosage	Drug Interactions
MAP reduced	Lassitude	Active hepatic disease	Average: 250–3000 mg bid schedule Maximum: 3000 mg†	Beta-adrenergic blockers: loss of antihypertensive action in some patients Oral contraceptives: decreased antihypertensive effect
CO unchanged or some decrease	Drowsiness and sedation			
HR slightly decreased	Dry mouth			
SVR decreased	Mild orthostasis			
RBF, RPR, GRF: no change	Positive Coombs' test and anemia			
RVR reduced	Positive rheumatoid factor and lupus erythematosus preparation			
Angiotensin II reduced	Impotence			
PRA reduced	Hepatitis			
Aldosterone reduced	Withdrawal syndrome			
Exercise response preserved	Rebound and overshoot hypertension			
Plasma volume increased	Altered mental acuity			
	Depression			

Comparison of Commonly Used Oral Central Alpha-Agonists

Drug	Initial Dose (mg)	Range of Usual Total Daily Dose (mg)	Orthostasis	Effect on RBF and GFR	Fluid Retention	CO	HR	Effect on Plasma Renin	Insufficiency States Needing Dose Change	Available Tablet/ Capsule Sizes (mg)
Clonidine	0.1 bid	0.2–1.2	Rare	→/↑	Minimal or none	↑	→	→	Renal insufficiency	0.1, 0.2, 0.3, and TTS 1, 2, 3
Guanabenz	4 bid	8–48	Rare	↑	Minimal or none	↑	→/↓	→	Renal insufficiency	4, 8
Guanfacine	1 hs	1–3	Rare	→/↑	Minimal or none	↑	→/↓	→	Renal insufficiency	1, 2
Methyldopa	250 bid	250–3000	Yes (mild)	↑	Yes	→/↓	→/↓	→	Renal and hepatic insufficiency	125, 250, 500

↑ Increased; ↓ decreased; → no change.

322

Postganglionic Neuron Inhibitors[103,104]

The postganglionic neuron inhibitors act by depleting catecholamine stores or inhibiting the release of catecholamines in peripheral sympathetic nerve endings. The onset of action is slow except for guanadrel, and the drugs have a long half-life. This class of antihypertensive drugs is best *avoided* unless it is necessary to treat severe refractory hypertension unresponsive to all other medications. The adverse effects are similar, and they are poorly tolerated by most patients.

Postganglionic Neuron Inhibitors Highlights*

	Preparation (mg)	Mechanism of Action	Pharmaco-dynamics	Hemo-dynamics
Guanadrel (Hylorel)— Fisons	10 25	Decreases adrenergic neuronal activity by inhibiting NE release and depleting NE stores in the peripheral nerve endings. Does not cross into central nervous system	Duration: 10–14 hr Onset: 2 hr Peak: 4–6 hr Excretion: renal Metabolism: hepatic	CO reduced Venous capacitance increased SVR reduced Marked Na$^+$ an H$_2$O retention
Guanethidine (Ismelin)— Novartis	10 25	Interferes with release of NE from sympathetic nerve terminals	Onset: 5–7 days Half-life: 7–14 days Excretion: renal	CO reduced Venous capacitance increase SVR reduced GFR, RBF, R reduced Severe NA$^+$ a H$_2$O retention

Adverse Effects	Contraindications	Daily Dosage (mg)	Drug Interactions
Faintness Orthostatic hypotension Diarrhea Severe volume retention	Avoid use in CHF, angina, cerebro-vascular disease	5–50 mg in divided doses	Tricyclic antidepressants: decreased antihy-pertensive effect Sympathomimetic amines: de-creased antihy-pertensive effect Antihistamines: hypertensive response
False-negative urine vanillylmandelic acid (VMA) and catecholamines Orthostatic and postexertional hypotension Severe Na$^+$ and H$_2$O retention Impotence Retrograde ejacu-lation Bradycardia CHF Exacerbates angina Diarrhea	Pheochromocytoma Simultaneous use of EPI	10–25 Maximum: 100	Tricyclic anti-depressants: decreased antihy-pertensive effect Oral contraceptives: decreased guanethidine effect Minoxidil: severe orthostatic hypotension Phenothiazines: decreased antihy-pertensive effect Sympathomimetic amines: decreased anti-hypertensive effect Hypoglycemia drugs: enhanced hypoglycemic effect

	Preparation (mg)	Mechanism of Action	Pharmaco-dynamics	Hemo-dynamics
Reserpine	0.1 0.25 1	Depletes catecholamine stores in both peripheral sympathetic nervous system and central nervous system	Onset: 4–6 weeks Half-life: 7 days or more	Bradycardia CO reduced SVR reduced

*Consult the *Physicians' Desk Reference* for full prescribing information.

Adverse Effects	Contraindications	Daily Dosage (mg)	Drug Interactions
False-negative VMA and urine catecholamines Bradycardia Premature ventricular contractions Nasal congestion Depression Na$^+$ and H$_2$O retention Postural hypotension Weight gain Nightmares Extrapyramidal reactions Lowers HDL cholesterol	History of or current depression Active peptic ulcer Hypotension	0.1–0.25 Maximum: 0.25	May prolong or inhibit effects of Sympathomimetic amines

Beta-Blockers—General[103,104]

1. Proposed mechanisms of action in hypertension:
   a. Slowing of heart rate with reduction of CO.
   b. Reduction of cardiac contractility and CO.
   c. Block of renal renin release.
   d. Sympathetic outflow reduced because of central beta effect.
   e. Blockade of postsynaptic peripheral beta receptors.
   f. Competitive antagonism of catecholamines at receptor site.
   g. Increased prostaglandin levels in vascular tissue (indomethacin blocks).
   h. Increased baroreflex sensitivity.
2. At equipotent doses, there is little or no difference in *antihypertensive* effect among the various beta-blockers, and side effects are similar.
3. Antihypertensive efficacy depends on patient profile:
   a. Age: not as effective in the elderly (reduced beta receptors).
   b. Race: not as effective in African-Americans (low renin, volume dependent).
   c. Renin status: best in high-renin and normal-renin patients; not as effective in low-renin patients.
   d. Duration of hypertension:
      (1) Recent onset, younger patient—hyperdynamic with relatively increased CO and relatively increased SVR: possibly effective.
      (2) Established—hypodynamic with reduced CO and elevated SVR: less effective.
4. Antihypertensive effect correlates poorly with plasma levels.
5. All beta-blockers without ISA increase SVR and decrease CO, which is the *opposite* hemodynamic effect desired to reduce BP.

Beta-Blockers and Beta Receptors

Beta$_1$ stimulation:

1. Cardiac stimulation: increased myocardial contractility, stroke volume, and CO; tachycardia; increased AV conduction and automaticity
2. Renin release from kidneys
3. Lipolysis of free fatty acids

Beta$_2$ stimulation:

1. Bronchodilation
2. Vasodilation
3. Glycogenolysis (liver, skeletal muscle) and lactate production
4. Pancreatic insulin release
5. Smooth muscle relaxation (uterus)
6. Skeletal muscle stimulation: tremor

Beta$_1$ blockade:

1. Reduction in myocardial contractility and CO
2. Bradycardia and heart block, depressed automaticity
3. Decreased renin release
4. Reduced release of free fatty acids

Beta$_2$ blockade:

1. Bronchoconstriction
2. Vasoconstriction
3. Abnormal glucose metabolism (liver, skeletal muscle glycogenolysis reduced)
4. Hyperglycemia (inhibited pancreatic insulin release)
5. Smooth muscle contraction (uterus)
6. Skeletal muscle: reduced tremor

Beta-blockers differ mainly in seven properties:

1. Cardioselectivity
2. ISA
3. Membrane-stabilizing activity (MSA)
4. Lipid solubility versus water solubility
5. Pharmacokinetics
6. Potency
7. Platelet aggregation effect

Beta-Blockers: Selectivity

1. *Nonselective:* blockade of both beta$_1$ and beta$_2$ receptors.
   Nadolol
   Penbutolol
   Pindolol
   Propranolol
   Timolol

2. *Cardioselective:* blockade of beta$_1$ receptor with *relative* sparing of blockade of beta$_2$ receptor (susceptible to stimulation by EPI). Cardioselectivity *diminishes* with *increasing doses.*
   Acebutolol
   Atenolol
   Metoprolol
   Betaxolol
   Bisoprolol

3. *ISA:*
   Acebutolol
   Pindolol
   Penbutolol
   Carteolol

4. *Alpha and beta blockade:*
   Labetalol
   Carvedilol

Side Effects and Contraindications of Beta-Blockers[103,104]

Contraindications

1. Sinus bradycardia
2. Heart block greater than first degree
3. Cardiogenic shock
4. Overt cardiac failure
5. Bronchial asthma/chronic obstructive pulmonary disease
6. Known hypertensitivity to product.

Side Effects

1. Myocardial depression: CHF, reduced CO (less with drugs with ISA), dyspnea
2. Bradycardia and heart block (electrical depression) (less with drugs with ISA)
3. Central nervous system (due to penetration of blood-brain barrier): fatigue, lethargy, poor memory, weakness, drowsiness, emotional lability, mental depression, paresthesias, disorientation, hallucinations, psychosis, delirium, catatonia, insomnia, nightmares, dreams, headache, dizziness, vertigo
4. Gastrointestinal: nausea, diarrhea, constipation, pain, flatulence, ischemic colitis
5. Respiratory: bronchospasm, wheezing, exacerbation of asthma and chronic obstructive pulmonary disease
6. Perpheral vascular constriction: Raynaud's phenomenon, claudication, cold extremities (less with pindolol and acebutolol)
7. Inhibition of glycogenolysis
8. Withdrawal syndrome: severe hypertension, unstable angina, arrhythmias, MI, death
9. Drug interactions: indomethacin blocks antihypertensive action

10. Hyperglycemia: exacerbated diabetes mellitus, inhibited insulin release, and insulin resistance
11. Hypertriglyceridemia HDL cholesterol decreased LDL cholesterol increased, HDL/LDL ratio decreased (except for drugs with ISA) and dense small–atherogenic LDL is increased
12. Hypertriglyceridemia: additive with thiazides
13. Muscle fatigue and exercise-induced fatigue
14. Impotence and decreased libido
15. Postural hypotension
16. Hyperuricemia: additive with thiazides
17. Hyperkalemia (blocks intracellular transport of K^+)
18. Hyperthyroidism symptoms after sudden withdrawal
19. Hypoglycemia in:
    a. Diabetes mellitus: masked and prolonged symptoms
    b. Postanesthesia
    c. Dialysis
    d. Fasting (children)
    e. Prolonged exercise
20. Severe hypertensive response in hypoglycemic patients on beta blockade
21. Crosses placenta (fetal bradycardia, hypotension, and hypoglycemia)
22. Precipitates labor by increasing uterine contractions in eclampsia
23. Paradoxic hypertension in presence of catecholamine excess owing to EPI, pheochromocytoma, hypoglycemia, withdrawal of central alpha-agonist during combined therapy, or volume-dependent hypertension
24. Reduction in GFR, RBF, RPF, which may persist for 6 months to 1 year or longer after discontinuing therapy
25. Reduced birth weight (atenolol).

Drug Interactions with Beta-Blockers

Interacting Drugs	Adverse Effect
Alcohol	Signs of delirium tremens may be blocked
Barbiturates	Decreased beta-blocker effect
Chlorpromazine	Increased effects of both drugs
Cimetidine	Increased beta-blocker effect
Clonidine	Paradoxic hypertension
Contraceptives, oral	Increased metoprolol and possibly propranolol effect
Diazoxide	Hypotension (additive)
Diltiazem	Cardiac failure
	AV conduction disturbances and sinus bradycardia
Disopyramide	Cardiac failure
Hydralazine	Increased propranolol and metoprolol effects
Hypoglycemics, sulfonylurea	Decreased effect of hypoglycemic agent
	After overdose, prolonged hypoglycemia and decreased glycogenolysis (blocked beta effects of EPI); beta receptor blockade masks tachycardia and tremor during hypoglycemia
Indomethacin	Decreased antihypertensive effect
Insulin	With overdose, prolonged hypoglycemia and decreased glycogenolysis (blocked beta effects of EPI); beta receptor blockade masks tachycardia and tremor during hypoglycemia
Lidocaine	Increased lidocaine toxicity with propranolol
Methyldopa	Hypertensive episode
Nicotine	Decreased propranolol effects; vasoconstriction and hypertension
Nifedipine	Cardiac failure—rare
Prazosin	Increased hypotensive effect of first dose of prazosin
Rifampin	Decreased beta-blocker effects
Sympathomimetic amines	Decreased antihypertensive effect; hypertensive reactions
Sympathomimetic bronchodilators	Decreased bronchodilator effects
Theophyllines	Increased theophylline toxicity; reported only with propranolol
Verapamil	Cardiac failure; AV conduction disturbances and sinus bradycardia

Beta-Blockers Highlights*

	Preparation (mg)	Mechanism of Action	Pharmaco-dynamics	Hemo-dynamics
Acebutolol (Sectral)— Wyeth-Ayerst	200 400	Cardioselective beta-adrenergic receptor block with weak ISA and MSA	Onset: ½–1 hr Peak: 2½ hrs Half-life: 3–4 hrs ISA: 1+ MSA: 1+ Lipid solubility: low (1+) Metabolism: hepatic Excretion: renal	HR, CO, PRA, RPF, RBF, GFR, aldo-sterone reduced SVR and RVR unchanged MAP reduced Plasma volume increased or no change
Atenolol (Tenormin)— Astra-Zeneca	25 mg 50 100	$Beta_1$ selective blocking agent without MSA or ISA. Prefer-ential effect not absolute. Higher doses inhibit beta adrenorecep-tors located in the bronchial and vascular musculature	Onset: 1 hr Peak: 2–4 hrs Half-life: 6–9 hrs ISA: none MSA: none Lipid solubility: low (1+), more water soluble Metabolism: minimal, hepatic (10%) Excretion: renal, unchanged	HR, CO, PRA, GFR, RBF, RPF, aldo-sterone reduced SVR and RVR increased MAP reduced Plasma volume increased

Adverse Effects	Contraindications	Daily Dosage (mg)	Drug Interactions
See separate list of side effects	See separate list of contraindications	Initial: 400 Average: 600 Range: 200–1200 Maximum: 1200	See separate list of drug interactions
See separate list of side effects	See separate list of contraindications	Initial: 25–50 Average: 50 Maximum: 100	See separate list of drug interactions

	Preparation (mg)	Mechanism of Action	Pharmaco-dynamics	Hemo-dynamics
Betaxolol (Kerlone)— Pharmacia	10 20	Cardioselective	Onset: 1 hr Peak: 3 hr Half-life: 14–22 hr ISA: none MSA: 1+ Lipid solubility: none Metabolism: hepatic Excretion: renal	HR, CO, PRA, GFR, RBF, RPF, aldo-sterone reduced SVR and RVR increased MAP reduced Plasma volume increased or no change
Metoprolol (Lopressor)— Novartis	50 100	Selective beta-adrenergic blocking agent with relative selectivity for beta adrenore-ceptors located primarily in cardiac muscle.	Onset: 1 hr Peak: 1½–2 hr Half-life: 3–4 hr ISA: none MSA: minimal (1+) to none	HR, CO, PRA, RPF, RBF, GFR, and aldo-sterone reduced SVR and RVR increased MAP reduced Plasma volume increased
(Toprol XL)— Astra-Zeneca	25 mg 50 100 200	Specificity is lost with large doses	Lipid solubility: moderate (3+) Metabolism: hepatic Excretion: hepatic to renal	
Nadolol (Corgard)— Monarch	20 40 80 120 160	Nonselective beta-adrenergic re-ceptor antagonist	Onset: 1–2 hr Peak: 3–4 hr Half-life: 20–24 hr ISA: none MSA: none Lipid solubility: low (1+), more water soluble Metabolism: minimal, hepatic (27%) Excretion: renal, unchanged	HR, CO, PRA, aldosterone reduced May not alter RPF and GFR RVR unchanged SVR increased MAP reduced Plasma volume increased

Adverse Effects	Contraindications	Daily Dosage (mg)	Drug Interactions
See separate list of side effects	See separate list of contraindications	Initial: 10 Average dose: 10 Maximum dose: 20	See separate list of drug interactions
See separate list of side effects	See separate list of contraindications	Initial: 50 (qd or bid) Average: 200 (lose beta selectivity at 150) Range: 50–450 Maximum: 450 Initial: 50–100 qd Maximum: 400	See separate list of drug interactions
See separate list of side effects	See separate list of contraindications	Initial: 40 Average: 160 Range: 40–340 Maximum: 340	See separate list of drug interactions

	Preparation (mg)	Mechanism of Action	(73%) Pharmaco-dynamics	Hemo-dynamics
Carteolol (Cartrol)- Abbott Laboratories	2.5 5	Nonselective beta-adrenergic receptor antagonist with ISA	Onset: ½–1 hr Peak: 1–3 hr Half-life: 6 hr ISA: yes MSA: none Lipid solubility: low Metabolism: 30–50% hepatic Excretion: renal, unchanged (50–70%)	HR reduced < with other beta blockers (2–5 beats/min) CO reduced < with other beta blockers or not at all MAP reduced Plasma volume increased SVR unchange or reduced GFR, RBF, RI preserved or slightly reduce
Penbutolol (Levatol)— Schwarz Pharma	20	Nonselective beta-adrenergic antagonist with mild ISA, mild partial agonist activity	Onset: ½–1 hr Peak: 1½–3 hrs Half-life: 5 hr ISA: 0–1⁺ MSA: none Lipid solubility: low (1⁺) Metabolism: hepatic Excretion: renal	HR, CO, PRA, aldosterone reduced GFR, RBF, RPF unchange MAP reduced Plasma volume unchanged or increased
Pindolol (Visken)— Novartis	5 10	Nonselective beta-adrenergic antagonist with ISA	Onset: ½–1 hr Peak: 1–2 hrs Half-life: 3–4 hrs ISA: yes (3⁺) MSA: minimal (1⁺) to none Lipid solubility: moderate (3⁺) Metabolism: hepatic (60%) Excretion: renal (40%)	HR reduced le than with othe beta-blockers (4–8 beats/mir CO reduced le than with othe beta-blockers or not at all SVR unchange or reduced MAP reduced GFR, RBF, RI preserved or slightly reduce RVR unchang or reduced Plasma volum increased

Adverse Effects	Contraindications	Daily Dosage (mg)	Drug Interactions
See separate list of side effects	See separate list of contraindications	Initial: 2.5 Range: 5–10 Maximum: 10	See separate list of drug interactions
See separate list of side effects	See separate list of contraindications	Initial: 10 Average: 20–40 Maximum: 50	See separate list of drug interactions
Neutral effects on lipids See separate list of side effects	See separate list of contraindications	Initial: 10 bid Average: 20 Range: 10–50 Maximum: 60	See separate list of drug interactions

	Preparation (mg)	Mechanism of Action	Pharmaco-dynamics	Hemo-dynamics
Propranolol (Inderal)— Wyeth-Ayerst	10 20 40 60 80	Nonselective beta-adrenergic receptor blocker	Onset: 1–2 hrs Peak: 2–4 hrs Half-life: 2½–6 hrs ISA: none MSA: 3+	HR, CO, PRA, RPF, RBF, GFF aldosterone reduced SVR and RVR increased MAP reduced
(Inderal LA)— Wyeth-Ayerst	60 80 120 160		Lipid solubility: high (4+) Metabolism: hepatic Excretion: hepatic to renal	Plasma volume increased
Timolol (Blocadren)— Merck	5 10 20	Nonselective beta-adrenergic receptor blocking agent	Onset: ½–1 hr Peak: 1–2 hrs Half-life: 3–4 hrs ISA: none to minimal (1+) MSA: none Lipid solubility: low (2+) Metabolism: hepatic (80%) Excretion: renal (20%)	HR, CO, PRA, RPF, RBF, GFF aldosterone reduced SVR, RVR increased MAP reduced Plasma volume increased
Alpha-beta–blocker Labetalol (Trandate)— Promethus (Normodyne) Schering Plough-	100 200 300 Also intra venous (5 mg/mL) —	Competitive antagonist at both alpha and beta receptors Oral: Alpha/beta ratio is 1:3 IV: Alpha/beta ratio is 1:7 Beta₂ agonist: Beta₁ and beta₂ antagonist; alpha₁ blocker; nonselective	Onset: 1 hr Peak: 2–4 hrs Half-life: 6–8 hrs ISA: none to 1+ MSA: 1+ Lipid solubility: low (1+) Metabolism: hepatic (40%) Excretion: renal (60%)	HR, CO, PRA reduced RPF, RBF, GFF unchanged to reduced SVR and RVR unchanged to slightly reduced MAP reduced Plasma volume increased or unchanged
Carvedilol (Coreg)— SmithKline Glaxo	3.125 6.25 12.5 25	Nonselective beta-adrenergic blocker with alpha₁ blocking activity	Onset: ½ hr Absorption:80%, first pass in liver 23% Peak: 1–2 hrs Half-life: 7–10 hrs	Similar to label also mild calci channel blocke antioxidant and antiproliferativ actions

Adverse Effects	Contraindications	Daily Dosage (mg)	Drug Interactions
See separate list of side effects	See separate list of contraindications	Initial: 40 Average: 80 bid Range: 10–640 Maximum: 640	See separate list of drug interactions
See separate list of adverse effects	See separate list of contraindications	Initial: 10 Average: 20 Range: 10–60 Maximum: 60	See separate list of drug interactions
See separate list of adverse effects	See separate list of contraindications	Initial: 100 bid Average: 200–400 bid Range: 400–800 Maximum: 2400	See separate list of drug interactions
Dizziness (6.2%) Fatigue (4.3%)	NYHA Class IV Asthma 2° or 3 ° AVB Bradycardia Cardiogenic shock Hepatic disease	Initial: 6.25 bid Average: 12.5 bid Maximum: 25 bid Take with food	Catecholamine-depleting agents Clonidine Digoxin Rifampin Diltiazem

Preparation	Mechanism of Action (mg)	Pharmaco-Action	Hemo-dynamics	dynamics
Carvedilol (continued)			ISA: none MSA: ? Lipid solubility: high Metabolism: hepatic (98%), P-450 enzymes Excretion: renal (2%)	
Bisoprolol (Zebeta)-Lederle	5 10	Beta, cardio-selective adreno-receptor blocking agent. Specificity lost with higher doses	Onset: 1 hr Peak: 2–4 hrs ISA: none MSA: minimal to none Lipid solubility: low Metabolism: 50% hepatic 50% renal Excretions: 50% renal 50% nonrenal	HR, CO, PRA, RBF reduced MAP reduced SVR, RVP increased

*Consult the *Physicians' Desk Reference* for full prescribing information.

Adverse Effects	Daily Contraindications	Dosage (mg)	Drug Interactions
	Hypersensitivity to drug		Verapamil Insulin Oral hypoglycemics Cimetidine
See separate list of side effects	See separate list of contraindications	Initial: 5 Average: 10 Maximum: 20	See separate list of drug interactions

Direct Vasodilators

The direct vasodilators have a potent relaxation effect on the vascular smooth muscle of arteries, reducing SVR. The hemodynamics of the vasodilators are similar, but adverse effects differ. Because of increased PRA, CO, plasma volume, and reflex tachycardia, direct vasodilators require the concomitant use of either beta-blockers or central alpha-agonists and diuretics. The direct vasodilators hydralazine and minoxidil therefore should *not* be used alone (as monotherapy) to treat chronic hypertension. Minoxidil is much more potent than hydralazine. See Highlights next page.

Direct Vasodilators Highlights*

	Preparation	Mechanism of Action	Pharmacodynamics	Hemo-dynamics	Adverse Effects	Contra-indications	Daily Dosage	Drug Interactions
Hydralazine (Apresoline)— Novartis	10 mg 25 mg 50 mg 100 mg 20 mg/mL IV	Peripheral vasodilator that acts by direct relaxation on the vascular smooth muscles	Rapid absorption Duration: 6 hr Onset: 20–30 min (IV), 1 hr (oral) Peak: 2–4 hr Excretion: renal Metabolism: liver	Peripheral vasodilation SVR, PVR reduced HR, CO increased PRA increased GFR increased RBF, RPF increased	Postural hypo-tension Headaches Reflex tachy-cardia Nausea Palpitations Fatigue Fluid retention Lupus syndrome Nasal congestion	Aortic aneurysm Coronary artery disease Mitral valve or rheumatic heart disease	Initial: 10 mg qid Range: 40–400 mg Usual dose: 100–200 mg bid schedule	Diazoxide: severe hypotension Digoxin: decreased digoxin effect with IV hydra-lazine Beta-adrenergic blockers: en-hanced hydra-lazine effect
Minoxidil (Loniten)— Pharmacia & Upjohn	2.5 mg 5 mg 10 mg	Direct relaxation of arterial smooth muscle. Reduces SVR and PVR (little effect on venous smooth muscle)	Duration: 12 hr Onset: 1 hr Peak: 4–8 hr Excretion: renal Metabolism: liver	SVR, PVR reduced Reflex tachy-cardia HR, CO increased PRA, NE, Ang-II, aldos-terone increased RPF, RBF, GFR increased	Hypertrichosis Fluid retention and weight gain Precipitation of angina Cardiac tamponade ECG changes Reflex tachy-cardia ↓ T-cell Function ↑ RVH ↑ LVH	CHF Pheochromo-cytoma	Initial: 5 mg single dose Range: 10–40 mg bid schedule	Guanethidine: severe ortho-static hypo-tension

*Consult the *Physicians' Desk Reference* for full prescribing information.

Alpha$_1$-Blockers[103]

The alpha$_1$-blockers (indirect vasodilators) prazosin, doxazosin, and terazosin block the peripheral postsynaptic alpha$_1$-adrenergic receptor and reduce SVR but usually do not cause reflex tachycardia. CO is preserved or increased, and plasma volume is usually unchanged. These favorable hemodynamic changes reverse the abnormalities in essential hypertension and preserve organ perfusion.

Monotherapy with modest sodium restriction is effective in 50% to 60% of patients with mild hypertension but is generally not recommended since ALLHAT. Concomitant use of diuretics is *not* necessarily required.

The alpha$_1$-blockers have favorable effects on serum lipids and no adverse effects other than CHD risk factors.

Side effects are infrequent and minor. First-dose syncope and hypotension are rare (less than 1%) and have been overemphasized. They are more likely to occur in patients who are volume depleted, are on diuretics, or are elderly.

Initiation at a low dose (1 mg hs) and slow titration to 10 mg/day improve compliance and minimize adverse effects while maximizing efficacy as initial monotherapy.

They are useful in BPH, and may prevent or reduce progression of prostate carcinoma.

Alpha₁-Blockers Highlights*

	Preparation (mg)	Mechanism of Action	Pharmacodynamics
Doxazosin (Cardura)— Pfizer	1 2 4 8	Selective blockade of alpha₁ receptor. Antagonizes pressor effects of phenylephrine and NE	Duration: 24 hrs Onset: 1 hr Peak: 2–6 hrs Metabolism: liver Excretion: urinary and fecal
Prazosin (Minipress)— Pfizer	1 2 5 10	Vasodilator effect is related to blockade of peripheral post-synaptic alpha adrenoreceptors	Duration: 8–12 hrs Onset: 1 hr Peak: 2–3 hrs Metabolism: liver Excretion: biliary, feces
Terazosin (Hytrin)—Abbott	1 2 5 10	Postsynaptic alpha₁ blockade	Duration: 18–24 hrs Onset: 1 hr Peak: 1–2 hrs Metabolism: liver Excretion: biliary, feces

*Consult the *Physicians' Desk Reference* for full prescribing information.

Hemo-dynamics	Adverse Effects	Contra-indications	Daily Dosage (mg)	Drug Interactions
HR unchanged or increased CO unchanged SVR reduced Venous capacitance increased PRA unchanged RBF, RPF, GFR increased or unchanged PWP reduced or unchanged	Syncope (rare) Dizziness Increased sweating Fatigue Palpitations Edema	Hypersensitivity to quinazolines	Initial: 1 hs Maximum: 16 Average: 4–6	Vardenafil (Levitra) and Tadalafil Cialis): Hypotension
HR and CO unchanged or increased SVR reduced Venous capacitance increased PRA unchanged RPF, RBF, GFR unchanged or slightly increased PWP reduced or unchanged	Syncope with first dose (rare, <1%) Postural hypotension (uncommon) Palpitations Dizziness Weakness Headache	None	Initial: 1 bid with first dose at bedtime Maintenance: 5–15 in divided doses (bid) Maximum: 40	Beta-adrenergic blockers: increased hypotensive effect of the first dose Indomethacin: decreased hypotensive effect Vardenafil Tadalafil
See Prazosin	Syncope Postural hypotension Headache Tachycardia Asthenia Edema Dry mouth Nasal congestion Dizziness	None	Initial: 1 Average: 1–5 Maximum: 40; may require bid dosing	See Prazosin Vardenfil Tadalafil

Angiotensin-Converting Enzyme Inhibitors (ACEIs) [103,104]

These agents inhibit the conversion of angiotensin I to angiotensin II, thus interrupting the renin-angiotensin-aldosterone system. Plasma renin activity is increased; angiotensin II and aldosterone levels are decreased. The net antihypertensive mechanism appears to be a decrease in fluid volume and vasodilation. ACE inhibitors may be used alone or in combination with other antihypertensive agents that enhance the effect. The agents may also affect the kinin-bradykinin and prostaglandin systems and increase angiotensin 1-7, a potent vasodilator.

ACE inhibitors are effective in all forms of hypertension (HRH, NRH, LRH). Side effects are minor and infrequent, and most patients tolerate these agents well. Cough occurs in 10% to 15% of patients and is more common in women. ACE inhibitors are useful as initial therapy and as monotherapy. They are effective in African-Americans, elderly, whites and young patients if dosed to adequate levels.

ACE inhibitors also have a favorable effect in preserving renal function in both nondiabetic and diabetic hypertensives and in diabetics with proteinuria to reduce proteinuria and IGCP.

A triphasic BP response may occur with high renin levels:
1. Initial abrupt fall (occasionally to hypotensive levels) for several hours.
2. Return of BP but to below pretreatment levels.
3. Chronic gradual reduction of blood pressure over several days, but not as low as with initial therapy. Maximum effect at 2 to 4 weeks is predicted by initial response.

Patients with normal or low renin levels have a more prolonged and gradual decrease in BP. Volume depletion or concurrent antihypertensive therapy exaggerates the response.

ACE is the key enzyme in the RAAS and kinin system. ACE is found primarily in tissues such as the endothelium and blood vessels, where it stems from local synthesis secondary to gene expression. The adverse effects of ACE are related to its conversion of angiotensin I to angiotensin II and its degradation of bradykinin. In addition to causing vasoconstriction, increased angiotensin II levels, and an increase in PAI-1, EDCF and endothelin promote vascular smooth muscle growth and migration, matrix synthesis, platelet aggregation, and thrombosis. Degradation of bradykinin inhibits its vasodepressor, antiproliferative, and fibrinolytic effects due to decreases in endothelium-derived relaxing factor (EDRF)/NO, prostacyclin, and t-PA. The processes mediated by angiotensin II and bradykinin occur primarily at the tissue level and are implicated in a number of cardiovascular conditions, including hypertension, ischemia, atherosclerosis, vascular hypertrophy, and restenosis after vascular injury.

Approach to Initiation of ACE Inhibitor Therapy

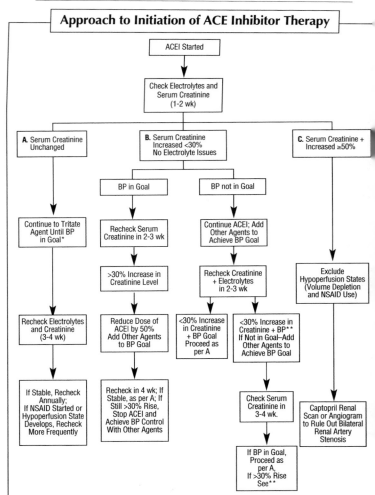

A schematic approach to patient with renal, insufficiency started on therapy with an angiotensin-converting enzyme inhibitor (ACE).

*– blood pressure (BP) less than 130/85 mm Hg for those with renal insufficiency or diabetes;
** – if serum creatinine level increases more than 30%, reduce ACEI dose by 50% and add other BP-lowering agents; + – if serum creatinine rise is greater than 30% and less than 50% within the first month of therapy, causes for hypoperfusion are eliminated, and nonsteroidal anti-inflammatory drugs (NSAIDs) are not given, treat as if bilateral renal arterial disease is present.

ARCH Intern Med/Vol 160, March 13, 2000; 692

Renin-Angiotensin-Aldosterone System (RAAS)

General and Major Points: Two RAAS

1. Classic RAAS: BP regulation. Circulating ACE 10%
2. Tissue RAAS: Regulates vascular and cardiac structure and function (90%)

   Angiotensin-converting enzyme (ACE) is an ectoenzyme that faces lumen of vascular system (i.e., protrudes from cell membranes into extracellular space).

ACE is located on:

1. Vascular endothelial cells: lumen and vasa vasorum
2. Media of VSMC

   Angiotensin-ll (A-ll) is a potent vasoconstrictor, growth promoter, thrombogenic, pro-oxidant, proinflammatory, atherogenic hormone.

   Other types of angiotensins exist with variable cardiovascular effects, both qualitatively and quantitatively.

   Aldosterone produces similar cardiovascular effects as A-II.

   Alternate pathways exist for conversion of A-l → A-ll other than ACE.

   Alternate pathways become quantitatively more important under conditions of disease.

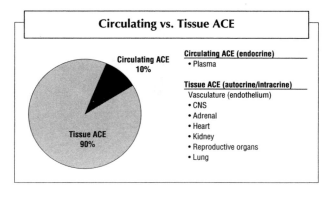

Circulating vs. Tissue ACE

Circulating ACE 10%

Tissue ACE 90%

Circulating ACE (endocrine)
- Plasma

Tissue ACE (autocrine/intracrine)
Vasculature (endothelium)
- CNS
- Adrenal
- Heart
- Kidney
- Reproductive organs
- Lung

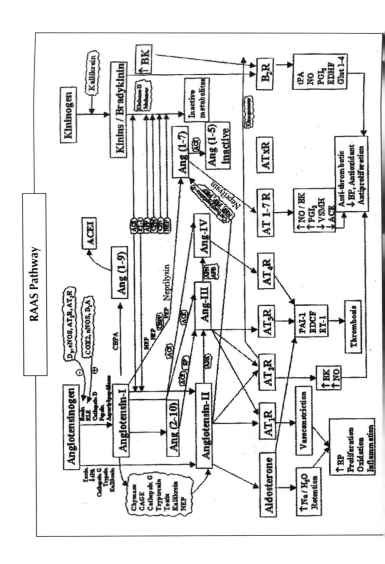

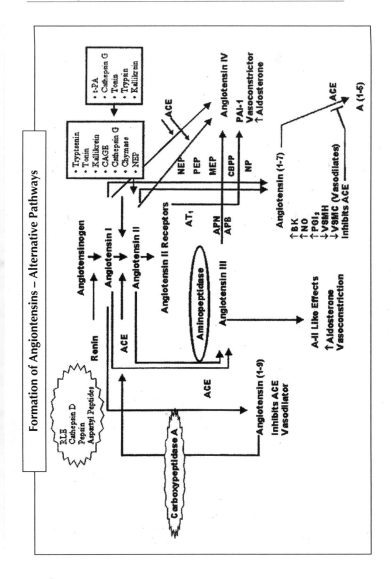

Formation of Angiontensins – Alternative Pathways

ACE and ACEI: Clinical-Basic Science Correlations

Extracellular engagement of ACEI to ACE is a function of:

1. Affinity (tissue selectivity, lipophilicity)
2. Tissue blood flow

ACEIs differ in:

1. Enzyme binding affinities (tissue selectivity)
2. On and off rates
3. Duration of action

Tissue ACE and conversion of A-l to A-ll is an autocrine, and intracrine function.

ACEIs interact differently with ACE active sides, depending on their structural configurations (ACE and other endogenous degradation).

Potency of ACE Inhibitors in Plasma and Tissue

Plasma		Tissue
Quinaprilat (400)	High	Quinaprilat (33)
Cilazaprilat (28)		Benazeprilat (27)
Benazeprilat(17)		Perindoprilat(17)
Fosinoprilat (14)		Ramiprilat (11)
Ramiprilat (12)		Lisinopril (6)
Lisinopril (5)		Enalaprilat (2.3)
Enalaprilat (5)		Fosinoprilat (1.7)
Captopril (1)	Low	

Adapted from Fabris B, et al. Br) Pharmacol. 1990:100:651-655. Fabris B, etal. I Cardiovasc Pharmacol. 1990;15(suppl 21-.56-513. Johnston C1, et al.) Hypertens. 1989;7 (suppl 5):511-516.

Content points:

- Radioligand inhibitor binding (RIB) studies demonstrate a wide range of ACE binding affinity among the available ACE inhibitors.
- Quinaprilat, the active metabolite of quinapril, possesses the highest ACE binding affinity in both tissue and plasma.
- Tissue ACE and the endothelium appear to play important roles in the development of atherosclerosis. It is plausible that differences in ACE binding affinity could translate into differential clinical responses.

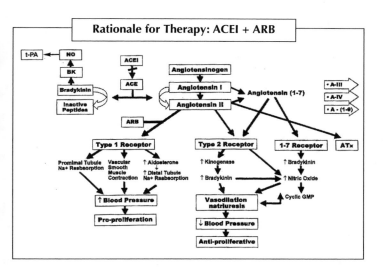

Rationale for Therapy: ACEI + ARB

ACE Inhibitors Highlights*

	Preparation (mg)	Mechanism of Action	Pharmacodynamics
Benazepril (Lotensin)— Novartis	5 10 20 40	ACE Inhibitor	Onset: 1 hr Peak: 2–4 hrs Plasma half-life: 10–11 hr Metabolism: hepatic, renal Excretion: renal Absorption: unaffected by food
Captopril (Capoten)— PAR–	12.5 25 50 100	A specific inhibitor of angiotensin-converting enzyme; interrupts the renin-angiotensin system and formulation of angiotensin II	Onset: 1–2 hrs Peak: 4 hrs Plasma half-life: 8–12 hrs (increases with dose) Metabolism: liver (15%) Excretion: renal (85%—unchanged 50% metabolites 35%) Absorption: reduced by food
Enalapril (Vasotec)— Biovail	5 10 20	ACE Inhibitor	Onset: 1 hr Peak: 3–4 hrs Plasma half-life: 12–24 hr Metabolism: liver Excretion: renal (40%) Absorption: unaffected by food

Hemo-dynamics	Adverse Effects	Contra-indications	Daily Dosage (mg)	Drug Interactions
Exercise response preserved Angiotensin II and aldosterone reduced PRA and angiotensin I increased GFR, RPF, RBF unchanged or increased RVR reduced HR unchanged or rarely increased SVR reduced MAP reduced	Headache Dizziness Fatigue Cough Nausea Angioedema (rare)	Similar to lisinopril	Initial: 10 Average: 10–40 Maximum: 80 Interval: qd	Lithium K+ supplements K+- sparing diuretics: risk of hyperkalemia
See Benazepril	Taste disturbances Cutaneous rash Proteinuria Leukopenia Renal insufficiency Cough Angioedema (rare)	Renal impairment Renal artery stenosis (caution) Connective tissue disease (caution)	Initial: 25 bid or tid Average: 100–150 Range: 75–450 Maximum: 450 Intervals: bid or tid Lower doses now recommended	Cimetidine: severe neuropathies in patients with renal impairment Indomethacin: decreases hypotensive effect Spironolactone and triamterene: hyperkalemia (monitor K+ concentration) Lithium: Increased lithium levels K+ supplements, K+-sparing diuretics (combination, i.e., Dyazide, Maxzide): risk of hyperkalemia
See Benazepril	Less rash and loss of taste than with captopril Other side effects are similar	Renal impairment Renal artery stenosis (caution) Connective tissue disease (caution)	Initial: 5 Average: 20 Range: 10–140 Maximum: 40 Intervals: qid or bid	See Captopril

	Preparation (mg)	Mechanism of Action	Pharmacodynamics
Fosinopril (Monopril)— Bristol-Myers Squibb	10 20 40	ACE inhibitor	Onset: 1 hr Peak: 2–6 hrs Plasma half-life: 12 hrs Metabolism: hepatic, renal Excretion: renal, feces Absorption: unaffected by food
Quinapril (Accupril)— Pfizer	5 10 20 40	ACE inhibitor	Onset: 1 hr Peak: 1–2 hrs Plasma half-life: 25 hrs Metabolism: hepatic Excretion: renal (96%) Absorption: 60% decreased by food
Lisinopril (Prinivil)—Merck (Zestril)— Astra-Zeneca	2.5 5 10 20 30 40	ACE inhibitor	Onset: 1 hr Peak 6 hrs Plasma half-life: 12–24 hrs Metabolism: none Excretion: renal (100%) Absorption: unaffected by food
Ramipril (Altace)— Monarch	1.25 2.5 5 10	ACE inhibitor	Onset: 1 hr Peak: 3–6 hrs Plasma half-life: 13–17 hrs Metabolism: liver Excretion: renal (60%), hepatic (feces) (40%) Absorption: reduced by food
Moexipril (Univasc)— Schwarz Pharma	7.5 15	ACE inhibitor	Onset: 1 hr Peak: 1 ½ hrs Plasma half-life: 12–14 hrs Metabolism: liver Excretion: bile and urine Absorption: reduced by food
Trandolapril (Mavik)— Abbott	1 2 4	ACE inhibitor	Onset: 1 hr Peak: 4–10 hrs Plasma half-life: 6–10 hrs Metabolism: hepatic Excretion: urine, feces, bile
Perindopril (Aceon)— Solvay Metabolism: Liver	2 mg 4 mg 8 mg	ACE inhibitor Rhinitis	Onset: 1 hour Peak: 3–7 hourss Plasma half-life:3–10 hr ACE inhibitor Excretion: Renal Absorption: Unaffected by food

Hemo-dynamics	Adverse Effects	Contra-indications	Daily Dosage (mg)	Drug Interactions
See Benazepril	Headache Dizziness Fatigue Cough Nausea Diarrhea Angioedema[†]	Similar to lisinopril	Initial: 10 Average: 20–40 Maximum: 80 Interval: qd	See above Digoxin: may cause false low digoxin levels
See Benazepril	Headache Fatigue Nausea Dizziness Cough Angioedema[†]	Hypersensitivity to drug	Initial: 10 Average: 20–40 Maximum: 80 Interval: bid	See Captopril
See Benazepril	Dizziness Headache Fatigue Diarrhea Cough Interval: qd Angioedema[†] Hypotension[†] Neutropenia[†]	Hypersensitivity to drug Renal impairment Renal artery stenosis (caution) Connective tissue disease (caution)	Initial: 5–10 monother-apy Average: 20–40 Maximum: 80 Interval: qd	Diuretics: hypotension Indomethacin renal insuffi-ciency K+-sparing agents and K+ supple-ments: increased risk of hyper-kalemia
See Benazepril	Headache Dizziness Fatigue Cough Nausea Angioedema[†]	Hypersensitivity to drug	Initial: 2.5 Average: 2.5–20 Maximum: 20 Interval: qd	Benazepril
	As above	As above	Initial: 7.5 Maximum: 30 Interval:qd	As above
See Benazepril	Cough Dizziness Diarrhea Headache Fatigue	As above	Initial: 1–2 Average: 2–4 Maximum: 4 Interval: qd or bid	As above
See Benazepril	Dizziness Headache Asthenia Dyspepsia Proteinuria Palpitations	History of angio-edema related to previous 4–8 mg Pregnancy Renal impairment (caution) Renal artery stenosis (caution)	Initial: 4 mg qd Average: and K+supple- Maximum: 16 mg Intervals: qd or bid	Diuretic: hypo-tension K+sparing agents and K+ supple-ments may increase risk of hyperkalemia Gentamicin use with caution

Non Hypertensive Treatment Effects of ACEIs

- ↑ BK
- ↑ NO
- ↑ EDHF
- ↓ Vasopressin
- ↓ ET-1
- ↑ PGI-2
- ↑ Enkephalins
- ↑ EDV
- ↓ CAMS
- ↓ PAI-1 and ↑ t-PA (↑ Fibrinolysis)
- ↓ Growth Factors and VSMH
- ↓ ROS/O_2

- ↑ AC_1, ↑ C_1AC, ↑ C_2AC, ↓ PWV, ↑ AGI, ↓ ASI, ↓ PP, ↓ AD, ↓ ASI
- ↓ Plaque Rupture
- Angiogenesis (myocardial)
- ↓ Atherosclerosis
- ↓ Platelets effects
- ↑ Ang 1-7
- ↓ Ang II – transient
- ↓ Microalbuminuria (MAU) and proteinuria
- ↓ MLR
- ↓ Fibrinogen

Calcium Channel Blockers[149]

Calcium channel blockers inhibit the influx of calcium ions through slow channels in vascular smooth muscle tissue and cause relaxation of the arterioles of the body. These agents are useful in the treatment of all degrees of hypertension (mild, moderate, or severe).

1. The higher the BP, the greater the therapeutic reduction in BP.
2. Low-renin hypertensive patients (volume-dependent patients) have the best response (75% to 80% response rate as monotherapy), but most patients respond well.
3. African-Americans and elderly patients also respond well (75% to 80% with monotherapy).
4. Mild edema in the absence of weight gain may be seen with long-term use. Diuretic and natriuretic effects occur. ACEI and ARB will counteract this edema. The edema is due to an increase in interstitial fluid related to dilation of the afferent arteriole of the capillary bed. *Diuretics* are *not* effective treatment for CCB-induced edema; ARBs may be effective and similar to ACEIs.

5. Antihypertensive effect is enhanced by most other antihypertensive agents.
6. The effect on lipids is neutral or favorable. No adverse effect is seen on K^+, Mg^{2+}, glucose, uric acid, etc.
7. There is a low adverse effect profile.
8. Calcium channel blockers preserve renal function, and actually reduce microalbuminuria and proteinuria if the initial values are below about 400 mg/day.
9. LVH is reduced.
10. Calcium channel blockers are very effective as monotherapy.
11. Calcium channel blockers have been shown to reduce incidence of dementia (cognitive function improves with reduction in blood pressure). (Forette F, Seux ML, Staessen JA, et al. Prevention of dementia in randomized double-blind placebo-controlled Systolic Hypertension in Europe (Syst-Eur) trial. Lancet 1998;352:1347–1351.)
12. Amlodipine (ALLHAT) and other CCB in meta-analysis studies may reduce CVA better than any other antihypertensive drug classes (NS). Amlodipine was equal to chlorthalidone in reduction of fatal CHD and non fatal MI, as well as, all cause mortality (ALLHAT), and equal to Valsartan in reducing combined cardiac morbidity and mortality (VALUE).

Calcium Channel Blockers Highlights

	Preparation	Mechanism of Action	Pharmacodynamics
Amlodipine (Norvasc)—Pfizer	2.5 mg 5 mg 10 mg	Coronary and vascular smooth muscle vasodilation	Absorption: 100% unchanged unaltered by food Bioavailability: 64%–90% Onset: 6 hrs Peak: 6–12 hrs Half-life: 30–50 hrs Protein binding: 93% Metabolism: hepatic: 90% Excretion: urine (60%): metabolites No alteration with renal insufficiency
Diltiazem SR (Cardizem SR, Cardizem CD)—Biovail (Cardizem LA)	60 mg 90 mg 120 mg 120 mg 180 mg 240 mg 300 mg 360 mg 420 mg	Selective relaxation of smooth muscle prevents protienuria	Absorption: well absorbed > 90% Bioavailability: 45%–67% (first pass-hepatic) Onset: 1 hr Peak: 3 hrs Half-life: 4 hrs Protein binding: 80%
(Tiazac)—Forest/UAD	120 mg 180 mg 240 mg 300 mg 360 mg 420 mg	Relaxation of smooth muscle Reduces proteinuria	Metabolism: hepatic (60% fecal excretion) Excretion: renal (35%) Plasma levels: 40–200 ng/mL
(Dilacor XR)—Watson	180 mg 240 mg 360 mg	Relaxation of smooth muscle	
(Tiamate)—	120 mg 240 mg	Relaxation of smooth muscle Reduces proteinuria	
Isradipine (DynaCirc, DynaCirc SR†)—Novartis Reliant	2.5 mg 5 mg 10 mg	Selective relaxation of smooth muscle in systemic vasculature. Mild diuretic activity	Absorption: 90%–95% Bioavailability: 15%–24% Onset of action: 20 min Peak: 2–3 hrs Food increases time to peak by 1 hr

*Consult the *Physicians' Desk Reference* for full prescribing information.

Hemo-dynamics	Adverse Effects	Contra-indications	Daily Dosage (mg)	Drug Interactions
SVR reduced HR Palpitations CO unchanged or increased RBF, RPF, GFR preserved, increased No effect on sinotrial (SA) or AV node Coronary vasodilation Afterload reduction Dilates coronary and peripheral arteries	Dizziness Flushing Edema	Hypersensitivity to	Initial: 5 Average: 5 Maximum: 10 Interval: qd Long T 1/2 - intrinsic High trough to peak ratio	None yet established
Depresses SA and AV nodal function Negative inotropic effect Reduces HR Reduces SVR Increases MVO^2 CO unchanged	Headache AV block disorders and sinus arrest Dizziness Pedal edema Bradycardia Electrocardiographic abnormalities Asthenia Constipation Dyspepsia Nausea Palpitations	Sick sinus syndrome, AV block (2nd-degree, 3rd-degree), severe CHF, digitalis toxicity Acute MI and pulmonary congestion Additive effects with beta blockers and digoxin	Average: 240–360 Range: 120–360 Maximum: 360 Interval: bid or tid Initial: 120–240 Average: 180–360 Maximum: 540 Interval: once daily	Beta-adrenergic blockers: cardiac failure (additive effects on contractility and blockade of compensating reflexes) AV conduction disturbances and sinus brady-cardia (additive)
Vasodilation with increased coronary, cerebral, and skeletal muscle blood flow SVR reduced HR increased CO increased	Headache Dizziness Edema Palpitations Fatigue Flushing	Hypersensitivity to drug	Initial: 2.5 bid Average: 5–10 in divided doses Maximum: 20	

	Preparation	Mechanism of Action	Pharmacodynamics
Isradipine (continued)			Half-life: biphasic; early: 1½–2 hrs terminal: 8 hrs Protein binding: 95% Excretion: urine 60%–65%, feces 25%–30%
Nicardipine (Cardene)— Roche	20 mg 30 mg	Selective relaxation of vascular smooth muscle. More selective on smooth muscle than myocardium. Greater effect on cerebral and coronary vessels than peripheral vessels	Absorption: >95% Bioavailability: 35% Onset: 30 min Peak: 1 hr
(Cardene SR)— Roche	30 mg 45 mg 60 mg		Half-life: 8.6 hrs Protein binding: 95% Metabolism: liver Excretion: urine 60%, feces 35% Plasma levels: 10–100 ng/mL

*Absorption of Adalat is altered with food, whereas Procardia XL is not.

Hemo-dynamics	Adverse Effects	Contra-indications	Daily Dosage (mg)	Drug Interactions
SVR reduced Reflex increase in HR MAP reduced RBF, RPF, GFR preserved CO unchanged or increased No effect on sinoatrial or AV nodal conduction Coronary artery vasodilation	Flushing Headache Pedal edema Asthenia Palpitations Dizziness Tachycardia	Advanced aortic stenosis Hypersensitivity to drug	Initial: 20 tid Average: 30 tid Maximum: 40 tid	Food: increases time to peak by 1 hr Cimetidine: increases nicardipine levels Cyclosporine: increases cyclosporine plasma levels Beta-blockers: CHF

	Preparation	Mechanism of Action	Pharmacodynamics
Nifedipine (Adalat CC)— Bayer (Procardia XL)— Pfizer	30 mg 60 mg 90 mg extended-release tablets	Selective relaxation of vascular smooth muscle by reducing intracellular calcium concentration	Absorption: 90% Bioavailability: 75% Onset: immediate First peak: 2.5–5 hrs Second peak: 6–12 hrs Half-life: 2 hrs Protein binding: 92%–98% Metabolism: liver— complete Excretion: renal (60%–80%) Plasma levels: C_{max} is 36% greater avg concentration 70% greater in subjects age >60 yr 6–120 ng/mL
Nisoldipine (Sular)— Astra-Zeneca	10 mg 20 mg 30 mg 40 mg	Inhibits calcium influx into vascular smooth muscle and cardiac muscle	Absorption: 87% Bioavailability: 5% Onset: 2 hrs Peak: 6–12 hrs Half-life: 7–12 hrs Protein binding: 99% Metabolism: liver Excretion: urine (60–80%

Hemo-dynamics	Adverse Effects	Contra-indications	Daily Dosage (mg)	Drug Interactions
SVR reduced	Headache	Hypersensi-tivity to drug	Initial: 30	Beta-adrenergic blockers: cardiac failure (additive effects on contractility and blockade of compensating-reflexes)
PRA decreased	Dizziness		Average: 30	
MAP reduced	Lightheadedness		Range: 30–90	
RBF, RPF, GFR preserved	Tachycardia		Maximum: 90	
CO increased or unchanged by reflex sympa-thetic activity and decreased SVR	Tremor		Interval: qd on empty stomach	
	Nervousness			Digoxin: increased digoxin effect (rare)
	Palpitations			
	Leg cramps			
	Fatigue			Hypoglycemics, sulfonylurea: in-creased hypogly-cemic effect with oral nifedipine (decreased glu-cose metabolism)
No effect on sino-atrial or AV nodal function	Weakness			
	Nausea			
	Diarrhea			
Smooth muscle relaxation (generalized)	Edema			
	Flushing			Cimetidine: in-creased nifedi-pine plasma levels
	Orthostatic hypotension			
	Tinnitus			
Similar to nifedipine	Similar to nifedipine	Allergy	Average: 20 Range: 10–60 qd Maximum: 60	Cimetidine: in-creased plasma levels
				Quinidine: de-creased bioavail-ability

	Preparation	Mechanism of Action	Pharmacodynamics
Verapamil (Calan SR)— Pharmacia (Isoptin SR)— Abbott (Verelan)— Wyeth-Ayerst Verelan PM— (Schwarz) Pharma	Oral: 120 mg 180 mg , 240 mg SR tab 40 mg, 80 mg 120 mg, 180 mg 240 mg 180 mg 200 mg 300 mg	Selective relaxation of smooth muscle by reducing intra-cellular calcium concentration in coronary and peri-pheral vasculature and inhibiting slow-channel Ca^{2+} transport Reduces proteinuria	Absorption: 95% Bioavailability: 10%–20% (extensive hepatic first pass) Onset: 1 hr Peak: 2 hrs Half-life: 3–6 hrs (up to 9 hr with long-term therapy) Protein binding: 90% Metabolism: hepatic (85% fecal (15%); accumu- lates in liver disease Excretion: renal (70%), biexponential elimina- tion (fast/slow) Plasma levels: 80–300 ng/mL
(Covera HS)— Pharmacia	180 mg 240 mg	See above. Unique delivery system designed for 4–5 hr delay to be taken hs for max. concentration in the A.M.	Absorption: 65% Bioavailability: 33%–65% Onset: 4–5 hrs Peak: 11 hrs Half-life: 14–16 hrs Protein binding: 94% Metabolism: hepatic Excretion: renal (70%), fecal (16%)
Felodipine (Plendil) Astra-Zeneca	2.5 mg 5 mg 10 mg	Selective relaxation of vascular smooth muscle, more than on myocardium	Absorption: 95% Bioavailability: 20% Onset: 1/2-1 hrs Peak: 2.5-5 hrs Half-life: 11-16 hrs Protein binding: 99% Metabolism: liver Excretion: urine 70% feces 10%

*Consult the *Physicians' Desk Reference* for full prescribing information.   †Not found in

Hemo-dynamics	Adverse Effects	Contra-indications	Daily Dosage (mg)	Drug Interactions
Sinoatrial and AV nodal function depressed reentrant pathways, ventricular response slowed SVR arterial reduced (no venous effect) MAP reduced—less pronounced CO reduced, negative inotropic action Mild bradycardia Myocardial oxygen supply increased by increasing coronary blood flow Myocardial oxygen demand reduced by decreasing HR and reducing afterload No adverse effect on pulmonary function Smooth muscle relaxation—generalized (vascular, gut, bronchial)	Constipation: most common Headache Vertigo, dizziness, lightheadedness Weakness Nervousness Pruritus, flushing Gastric disturbances Hepatitis SGOT Alkaline phosphatase Orthostatic hypotension AV block AV dissociation Asystole Sinus arrest Pedal edema Pulmonary edema and CHF Paresthesias (cold, numbness) Hyperprolactinemia and galactorrhea	Sick sinus syndrome, second-degree or third-degree AV block, digitalis toxicity, cardiogenic shock	Average: 240 Range: 120–480 Maximum: 540 Interval: qd, bid

Average: 240 Range: 180–540 Maximum: 540 Interval: qhs (swallow whole) | Beta-adrenergic blockers: cardiac failure (additive effects on contractility and blockade of compensating reflexes) Digoxin: increased digoxin toxicity (possibly decreased renal excretion) Hypoglycemics, sulfonylurea: increased hypoglycemic effect (increased glucose metabolism) Lithium: increased lithium levels Rifampin: reduced bioavailability of Calan Carbamazepine: increased carbamazepine concentrations Neuromuscular blocking agents: Calan may potentiate their effects |
| SRV reduced HR increased RBF, RPF, GFR preserved CO unchanged or increased No effect on SA or AV conduction Coronary artery vasodilation | Edema Headache Flushing Dizziness Asthenia Tachycardia Fatigue Extrasystoles Nausea Palpitations | Hypersensitivity to drug | Initial: 5 mg Average 5-10 mg Maximum: 20 mg Adjust every 2 weeks if necessary Take tablet whole | Cimetidine: increased felodipine levels Digoxin: increased digoxin levels Phenytoin, carbamazepine, phenobarbital: decreased felodipine levels |

Treatment: Non-Hypertensive Effects of Some CCBs: 155A

- Counteracts A-II via ↑ in NO bioavailability
- Counteracts ET-1
- Increases eNOS and NO
- Antioxidant (membrane lipid) (↓ROS, ↓O2)
- Enhances EDHF
- Interferes with cyclooxygenase-derived contracting factors
- ↑ EDV
- Endothelial cell cytoprotection (↓cytokines, ↓CAMs)
- Modifies of VCMC membrane defect
- Inhibits VSMC proliferation and migration
- Inhibits ACAT in macrophages » Inhibits cholesterol esterification and oxidation of LDL via lipid peroxide
- Decreases insulin resistance
- ↑ AC, ↑ C_1AC, ↑ C_2AC, ↓ PP, ↑ AD, ↓ASI, ↓ PVW, ↓AGI
- ↓ Atherosclerosis
- Anti-platelet effect
- Inhibits tissue necrosis factor
- Inhibits platelet-derived growth factor
- Decrease media/lumen ratio (MLR)
- Decrease xanthine oxidase and catalase
- Decrease βFGF
- Decrease leukotrienes
- Decrease thromboxane B_2
- Decrease fibrinogen

AGI = augmentation index

AD = aortic distensibility

ASI = aortic stiffness index

βFGF = beta fibroblastic growth factor

Angiotensin II Receptor Blockers (ARBs)

Ang-II receptor blockers are the newest class of antihypertensives. Like ACE inhibitors, these agents interfere with the renin-angiotensin-aldosterone system. ACE inhibitors block the conversion of A-I to Ang-II, whereas ARBs block the binding of Ang-II to one of its receptor sites, AT_1. It is thought that the actions of Ang-II are more effectively blocked by direct AT_1 receptor antagonism.

Ang-II receptor blockers have a more favorable safety and tolerability profile than ACE inhibitors. They do not cause the adverse effects, such as cough and angioedema, that are attributed to ACE inhibitor interactions with the bradykinin system.

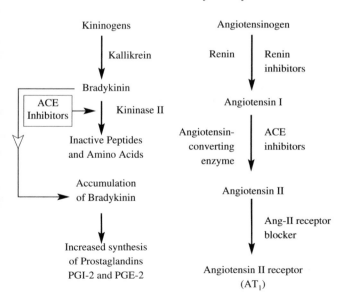

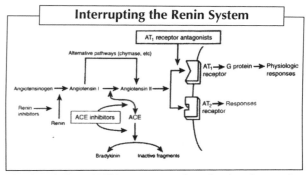

Site of angiotensin II type 1 (AT_1) receptor antagonists and angiotensin-converting enzyme (ACE) inhibitors in the renin-angiotensin-aldosterone system. (Adapted from Johnston CI: Angiotensin receptor antagonists: focus on losartan. Lancet 1995;346:1403-1407).

Angiotensin II Receptors and the Effects of Blockade

Vascular AT_1 receptors
      Constantly expressed
      Mediate vasoconstriction
      Mediate angiotensin II arterial wall growth effects
Vascular AT_2 receptors
      Expressed only after injury (sustained hypertension
      might provoke expression)
      Mediate vasodilation
      Mediate antiproliferative actions
      Activate other factors (e.g., nitric oxide)
Potential double action of selective AT_1 blockers
      Directly block vasoconstrictor and growth actions of
      angiotensin II at AT_1 receptors
      Increase circulating angiotensin II levels
      Unblocked AT_2 receptors (if expressed), stimulated by
      increased angiotensin II activity, mediate vasodilation
      and growth inhibition
      Net effects: AT_1, blockade + AT_2 stimulation
      Unknown effect on other AT receptors

AT1, angiotensin II type 1; AT2, angiotensin II type 2.

From Weber MA: Interrupting the renin-angiotensin system: The role of angiotensin-converting enzyme inhibitors and angiotensin II receptor antagonists in the treatment of hypertension. Am J Hypertens 1999;12:189S-194S.

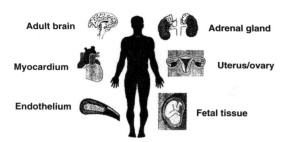

Distribution of the AT2 receptor, which is ubiquitous in fetal tissue, and is present in high concentrations in adults only in the adrenal medulla, uterus, ovary, vascular endothelium, and distinct brain areas. (From Chung O, Unger T: Angiotensin II receptor blockade and end-organ protection. Am J Hypertens 1999;12:150S-156S, with permission).

Examples of Genes That Can Be Regulated by Angiotensin II

Early genes/proto-oncogenes	*fos, myc, myb, jun, jun-B, egr-1*
Growth factor genes	Transforming growth factor β_1, platelet-derived growth factor-A chain, fibroblast growth factor-2, insulin-like growth factor-1 receptor
Cell matrix factor genes	Fibronectin, collagen type 1-α_1, collagen type III-α_1, laminin-β_1, laminin-β_2,
Hypertrophic marker	Atrial natriuretic peptide, brain natriuretic peptide, skeletal muscle action-α_1
Fibrinolytic system genes	Plasminogen activator inhibitor, types 1 and 2
Miscellaneous genes	Aldosterone synthase (CYP11B2), endothelial nitric oxide synthase

From Kurtz TW, Gardner DG: Transcription-modulating drugs: a new frontier in the treatment of essential hypertension. Hypertension 1998;32:380-386. December 1999-Vol. 12, No. 12, Part 3, with permission.

Pharmacologic Properties of Available ARB

Compound	Solubility in Water/Alcohol	Bioavailability (%)	Food Effect	Active Metabolite	Half-life (h)	Protein Binding (%)	Dosing (mg)
Irbesartan[8]	–/*	60-80	No	No	11-15	90	150-300 daily
Losartan[9]	+/+	33	Minimal	Yes	2 (6-9)	98.7 (99.8)	50-100 daily, twice daily
Valsartan[10]	*/+	25	40%-50% decrease	No	6	95	80-320 daily
Candesartan[11]	–/*	15	No	Yes	9	>99	8-32 daily, twice daily
Telmisartan[12]	–/NR	42-58	6%-20% decrease	No	24	99.5	40-80 daily
Eprosartan	-	13	Yes Minimal < 25%	No	20	98	400-1200 daily
Olmesartan	-	25%	No	No	13	99	20-40 daily

*Low solubility; NR, not reported.

From Zusman RM: Are there differences among angiotensin receptor blockers? Am J Hypertens 1999;12:231S–235S, (with permission).

Ang-II Receptor Blockers (ARBs) Highlights*

	Preparation	Mechanism of Action	Pharmaco-dynamics	Hemo-dynamics	Adverse Effects	Contra-indications	Daily Dosage	Drug Interactions
Candesartan cilexetil (Atacand)— Astra-Zeneca	4 mg 8 mg 16 mg 32 mg	Selective AT_1 angiotension II receptor antagonist (see Irbesartan)	Onset: 0.5 hr Peak: 3–4 hrs Plasma half-life: 9 hrs Metabolism: hepatic and renal Excretion: urine and feces	(see Irbesartan)	Headache Dizziness Upper respiratory infections Pharyngitis Rhinitis	Pregnancy Hypersensitivity to drug	Initial: 16 mg qd Range: 8–32 mg Maximum: 32 mg qd	No significant interactions reported
Eprosartan (Teveten)— Unimed	400 mg 600 mg	Vascular and pre-synpetic AT_1 blockade	Peak 1-2 hrs T 1/2 20 hrs Metabolism: none Excretion: bile Absorption: 13%	Similar to other ARBs	Rare facial edema Similar to other ARBs	Pregnancy Hypersensitivity	400-1200 mg	None
Irbesartan (Avapro)— Bristol Myers Squibb	75 mg 150 mg 300 mg	Blocks vasoconstrictor and aldosterone-secreting effects of angiotensin II by selectively binding to the AT_1, angiotensin II receptor.	Peak: 1.5–2 hrs Plasma half-life: 11–15 hrs Metabolism: biliary and renal Excretion: urine: 20% feces: 80% Absorption: (not affected by food) 60–80%	Exercise response preserved All and PRA increased Aldosterone reduced No effect on bradykinin GFR, RPF, RBF unchanged MAP reduced HR unchanged	Diarrhea Dyspepsia/heartburn Musculo-skeletal trauma Fatigue Upper respiratory infection	Hypersensitivity to drug Pregnancy	Initial: 150 mg qd Range: 150–300 mg qd Maximum: 300 mg qd	May be administered with other hypertensives. Hydrochlorothiazide has shown additive effect

*Consult the *Physicians' Desk Reference* for full prescribing information.

Ang-II Receptor Blockers (ARBs) Highlights (*Continued*)*

	Preparation	Mechanism of Action	Pharmaco-dynamics	Hemo-dynamics	Adverse Effects	Contra-indications	Daily Dosage	Drug Interactions
Losartan (Cozaar)— Merck	25 and 50 mg 1000 mg	Blocks vasoconstrictor-and aldosterone-secreting effects of Ang-11	Onset: 1 hr Peak: 3–4 hrs (active metabolite) Plasma half-life: 6–9 hrs (active metabolite) Metabolism: hepatic and renal Excretion: renal and biliary Absorption: food slows absorption	Exercise response preserved Ang-II and PRA increased Aldosterone reduced No effect on bradykinin GFR, RPF, RBF unchanged MAP reduced HR unchanged	Dizziness Asthenia/ fatigue Headache Cough	Pregnancy Hypersensitivity Caution with decreased liver function	Initial: 25–50 mg Range: 25–100 mg qd or bid Maximum: 100 mg qd or bid	May be administered with other hypertensives
Telmisartan (Micardis)— Boehringer Ingelheim	40 mg 80 mg	(see Irbesartan)	Peak: 0.5–1 hr Plasma half-life: 24 hrs Metabolism: gut wall Excretion: feces (> 97%) Absorption: slightly affected by food	(see Irbesartan)	Upper respiratory infection Back pain Sinusitis Diarrhea Pharyngitis	Pregnancy Nursing mothers Hypersensitivity to drug Caution with biliary obstruction and hepatic insufficiency	Initial: 40 mg qd Range: 20–80 mg qd Maximum: 80 mg qd	Digoxin: ↑ peak plasma concentration

Ang-II Receptor Blockers (ARBs) Highlights (*Continued*)*

	Preparation	Mechanism of Action	Pharmaco-dynamics	Hemo-dynamics	Adverse Effects	Contra-indications	Daily Dosage	Drug Interactions
Valsartan (Diovan) Novartis	80 mg caps 160 mg caps 320 mg	Blocks the vasocon-strictor and aldosterone secreting effects of AII by selectively blocking binding of AII to AT_1 receptor tissues.	Onset: 2 hrs Peak: 2–4 hrs Half-life: 6 hrs Metabolism: liver and renal Absorption: 30–50% Excretion: urine 13%, feces 83%	Exercise response preserved AII and PRA increased Aldosterone reduced No effect on bradykinin GFR, RPF, RBF unchanged MAP reduced HR unchanged	Headache Dizziness Viral infections Fatigue Abdominal pain	Hypersensitive to drug Pregnancy Caution with liver function tests	Initial: 80 mg qd Average: 80–160 mg qd 320 mg qd Maximal BP reduction seen in 4 weeks	No significant interactions reported
Olmesartan (Benicar) Sanyko	50 mg 20 mg 40 mg	High affinity and specific binding at AT_1R Insurmountable inhibition of A-II	Onset: 2 hrs Peak: 2–4 hrs T 1/2 13 hrs Bioavailability 25% Albumin bound 99% Not metabolized by CYP450 Renal: 35-50% Hepatic: 50-65% 24 hr duration	Similar to other ARBs	Similar to placebo dizzyness in 3% withdrawl rate less than placebo	Hypersensitive to drug Pregnancy No dose adjustment for: – elderly – Hepatic disease – Renal disease – Food	Initial: 20 mg qd Average: 20 mg qd Maximum: 40 mg qd	None No dose adjustments needed for – digoxin – warfarin – antacids

*Consult the *Physicians' Desk Reference* for full prescribing information.

Arterial Compliance: Structure/Function: Treatment [199,200,201]

Human trials with gluteal artery biopsies to assess vascular wall structure and function.

  • Correct both structure and function and reduce BP Increase small artery diameter, increase arterial compliance, decrease media/lumen ratio, decrease SVR and BP remodeling or arterioles

  - ACEI
  - ARB
  - CCB

  • Correct BP but no functional or structure change (No change on ED, AC M/L ratio, arterial diameter)

  - Diuretic
  - Beta-blocker

  • Nitroglycerin

  - ↑ AC (C-1)
  - ↓ PWV
  - No change SVR, ditensibility, EM
  - ↓ SBP, ↓ PP (10%), no change DBP

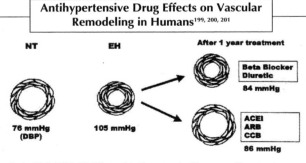

Antihypertensive Drug Effects on Vascular Remodeling in Humans[199, 200, 201]

NT

EH

After 1 year treatment

Beta Blocker
Diuretic
84 mmHg

ACEI
ARB
CCB
86 mmHg

76 mmHg (DBP)

105 mmHg

Park, JB, Schiffrin El. Effects of Antihypertensive Therapy on Hypertensive Vascular Disease. Curr Hypertens Reports. 2000;2: 280-288.

Selected Combination Antihypertensive Drugs

Beta-Adrenergic Blockers and Diuretics

    Atenolol, 50 or 100 mg/chlorthalidone, 25 mg   Tenoretic

    Bisoprolol fumarate, 2.5, 5, or 10 mg/hydrochlorothiazide,   Ziac
    6.25 mg

    Metoprolol tartrate, 50 or 100 mg/Lopressor HCT
    hydrochlorothiazide, 25 or 50 mg

    Nadolol, 40 or 80 mg/bendroflumethiazide, 5 mg   Corzide

    Propranolol hydrochloride, 40 or 80 mg/hydro-
    chlorothiazide, 25 mg   Inderide

    Propranolol hydrochloride (extended release), 80,   Inderide LA
    120, or 160 mg/hydrochlorothiazide, 50 mg

    Timolol maleate, 10 mg/hydrochlorothiazide, 25 mg   Timolide

ACE Inhibitors and Diuretics

    Benazepril hydrochloride, 5, 10, or 20 mg/
    hydrochlorothiazide, 6.25, 12.5, or 25 mg   Lotensin HCT

    Captopril, 25 or 50 mg/hydrochlorothiazide, 15 or 25 mg   Capozide

    Enalapril maleate, 5 or 10 mg/hydrochlorothiazide, 12.5   Vaseretic
    or 25 mg

    Lisinopril, 10 or 20 mg/hydrochlorothiazide, 12.5 or 25 mg   Prinzide, Zestoretic

Moexipril

    7.5 mg or 115 mg + HCTZ: Miretic 12.5 mg or 25 mg

Quinapril

    10 mg or 20 mg + HCTZ: Accuretic 12.5 mg or 25 mg

Angiotensin II Receptor Blockers
and Diuretics

    Valsartan, 80 or 160 mg/hydrochlorothiazide, 12.5 mg   Diovan HCT

    Losartan potassium. 50 mg/hydrochlorothiazide, 12.5 mg   Hyzaar
    and 100 mg/HCTZ 25 mg

Candesartan

    16 mg or 332 mg + Atacand-HCT HCTZ 12.5 mg

Irbesartan

    150 mg or 300 mg: Avalide + HCTZ 12.5 mg

Telmisartan

    40 mg + :Micardis HCT: HCTZ 12.5 mg

Eprosartan

    600 mg + HCTZ 12.5 mg   Teveten HCT

Calcium Antagonists and ACE Inhibitors

    Amlodipine besylate, 2.5 or 5 mg/benazepril   Lotrel
    hydrochloride, 10 or 20 mg

    Diltiazem hydrochloride, 180 mg/enalapril maleate, 5 mg   Teczem

    Verapamil hydrochloride (extended release),   Tarka
    180 or 240 mg/trandolapril, 1, 2, or 4 mg

    Felodipine, 5 mg/enalapril maleate, 5 mg   Lexxel

Other Combinations

Triamterene, 37.5, 50, or 75 mg/hydrochlorothiazide, 25 or 50 mg	Dyazide, Maxide
Spironolactone, 25 or 50 mg/hydrochlorothiazide, 25 or 50 mg	Aldactazide
Amiloride hydrochloride, 5 mg/hydrochlorothiazide, 50 mg	Moduretic
Guanethidine monosulfate, 10 mg/hydrochlorothiazide, 25 mg	Esimil
Hydralazine hydrochloride, 25, 50, or 100 mg/hydrochlorothiazide, 25 or 50 mg	Apresazide
Methyldopa, 250 or 500 mg/hydrochlorothiazide, 15, 25, 30, or 50 mg	Aldoril
Reserpine, 0.125 mg/hydrochlorothiazide, 25 or 50 mg	Hydropres
Reserpine, 0.10 mg/hydralazine hydrochloride, 25 mg/hydrochlorothiazide, 15 mg	Ser-Ap-Es
Clonidine hydrochloride, 0.1, 0.2, or 0.3 mg/chlorthalidone, 15 mg	Combipres
Methyldopa, 250 mg/chlorothiazide, 150 or 250 mg	Aldochlor
Reserpine, 0.125 or 0.25 mg/chlorthalidone, 25 or 50 mg	Demi-Regroton
Reserpine, 0.125 or 0.25 mg/chlorothiazide, 250 or 500 mg	Diupres
Prazosin hydrochloride, 1, 2, or 5 mg/polythiazide, 0.5 mg	Minizide

Hypertension Drug Selection: *Summary*

- Calcium channel blockers (CCBs), angiotensin receptor blockers (ARBs), and angiotensin-converting enzyme inhibitors (ACEIs) have the best overall profile based on the eight parameters in the subsets of approach to hypertension.

- Combination therapy (low dose) with CCBs, ACEIs, ARBs, diuretics (± Beta-blockers) may provide synergistic antihypertensive effects, reduce side effects, and improve surrogate endpoints as well as target organ damage.

- Clinical trials in hypertension with CCBs (especially amlodipine) reduce CHD, MI, and CVA equal to diuretics and better than beta-blockers, and ACEI. See VALUE trial comparing ARB to CCB.

- ACEIs are equal to diuretics and beta-blockers in reducing cardiovascular and cerebrovascular morbidity and mortality in recent clinical trials, with the exception of Lisinopril in ALLHAT (see controversies) related to CHF and CVA (in non-black patients). However CHD and MI morbidity and mortality are equally reduced.

- Clinical trials in hypertension with ARBs proved superior to βB in CV reduction at equal BP levels in the LIFE trial. Valsartan was similiar to Amlodipine in reducing primary endpoints of combined cardiac morbidity and mortality (VALUE). Clinical trials in CHF show benefit with ACEIs and ARBs, and clinical trials in MI show benefit with ACEIs.

- Diuretics may be used as initial or add-on therapy but should never exceed 25 mg/day of HCTZ or its equivalent. Their impact on CHD and MI is suboptimal in all clinical trials except ALLHAT whereas CVA is reduced, as is CHF. HCTZ and chlorthalidone may be nephrotoxic long-term which may limit its usefulness. Indapamide, on the other hand appears to stablize or improve renal function, is more potent in reducing BP and LVH. It is the preferred diuretic. HCTZ and chlorthalidone reduce insulin sensitivity and increase the incidence of new onset type 2 DM.

- Beta-blockers as monotherapy do not reduce CHD or MI in the elderly population, and their efficacy in younger populations is questionable. Beta-blockers do reduce CVA but are less effective than ARBs, and are effective in reducing morbidity after an acute MI. They increase insulin resistance and new onset type 2 DM.

- Central alpha-agonists and alpha-blockers are effective as monotherapy or as add-on therapy with favorable metabolic profiles but may be limited due to side effects unless kept at very low doses.
- In patients with diabetes mellitus and hypertension, recent clinical trials indicate that CCBs, ACEIs and ARBs are superior to diuretics and beta-blockers in reducing cardiovascular, cerebrovascular and renal morbidity and mortality.
- In ISH a CCB/ACEI prevents CVA better than D/BB combination (STOP - 2 Trial).

Effects on Structural and Functional Changes in Compliance Appear to Vary Among Antihypertensive Drug Classes*

Drug Class	No. of Agents Tested	No. of Studies	No. of Patients	Increase in Arterial Compliance Yielded
ACE inhibitors	8	15	~273	With Agents studied (perindopril was most used agent)††
Calcium Channel Blockers	8	11	~150	With agents studied
β-blockers	7	10	~326	With none, except "vasodilating" β-blockers
Diuretics	4	5	~75	Little effect beyond that associated with ↓ BP (an attempt was made methodologically to separate pressure-dependent from direct effects)

* – studies are primarily cross-sectional and short term. Thus, these studies can only be used for information regarding directional effects and by and large cannot distinguish functional from structural changes. The number of published studies using nitrovasodilators, α-blockers, and clonidine are too few for inclusion.

† Certain studies of ACE inhibitors included evaluation of biopsy-demonstrated improvement in vascular remodeling. †† Of the ACE-inhibition studies cited, perindopril was the agent tested in greatest total number of patients. Perindopril is the only ACE inhibitor with FDA-approved labeling that cites an increase in the compliance of large arteries.

Modified from Glasser SP et al. J Clin Pharmacol. 1998;38:202-212.

New Antihypertensive Drug Classes

1. Renin inhibitors
2. Vasopressin antagonists
3. Neuropeptidase inhibitors
4. Serotonin receptor antagonists (ketanserin)
5. Dopamine receptor antagonists (fenoldopam)
6. Prostaglandin analogs (PGI_2-iloprost)
7. Lipoxygenase inhibitors (phenidone)
8. Cicletanine
9. Potassium channel activators (BRL-34915)
10. Sodium channel blockers (6-iodoamiloride)
11. Endothelin antagonists (bosentan)
12. Selective aldosterone receptor antagonsists (SARAs)

Subset Selection of Antihypertensive Therapy

1. Pathophysiology and vascular biology
2. Hemodynamics
3. End-organ damage and risk factor reduction
4. Concomitant medical diseases or problems
5. Demographic selection
6. Adverse effects and quality of life with therapy
7. Compliance
8. Total health care cost

Conclusions

1. The treatment of mild hypertension (DBP <110 mm Hg) with certain antihypertensive agents (some diuretics or beta-blockers) may induce metabolic functional or structural changes in the (vascular system or vascular biology and adversely affect other risk factors that *partially or completely* negate the beneficial effects of lowering BP). Optimal reduction in CHD, MI CVA, CHF and CVD is dependent on blood pressure control, but is also dependent on specific non-blood pressure mechanisms. CCB, ACEI and ARBs show superiority over diuretics and beta-blockers in many surrogate as well as clinical CV outcomes.
2. Diuretic agents (except spironolactone, epleronone, amiloride,

methyldopa have adverse effects on the hypertensive-athero-sclerotic syndrome and other risk factors for end-organ damage. These agents also have significant clinical side effects with a corresponding poor quality of life and reduced compliance rate.

3. The only antihypertensive agents available to date that do not adversely affect serum lipids, glucose and insulin sensitivity are calcium channel blockers, alpha$_1$-blockers, central alpha-agonists (except methyldopa), ACE inhibitors, indapamide, and Ang-II receptor blockers. All of these agents are effective as initial monotherapy in about 50% to 60% or more of patients with mild hypertension. All are well tolerated (in >90% of patients) if dosed appropriately (start low, go slow) and have a low side-effect profile. Combination therapy is 90% to 95% effective.

4. Diuretic agents (HCTZ or Chlorthalidone) may induce hypokalemia, hypomagnesemia, or other electrolyte and acid-base abnormalities, insulin resistance, hyperglycemia new-onset type 2 DM or other metabolic abnormalties. There may also be an increase in the incidence of sudden death in predisposed patients secondary to cardiac arrhythmias. Predisposing factors include exercise, the presence of LVH, abnormal ECGs, silent or clinical ischemia, acute stress, or digitalis treatment. Avoid these high doses.

5. The use of lower doses of diuretics (HCTZ 12.5 to 25 mg/day or Chlorthalidone) is effective for the treatment of hypertension and may have fewer adverse effects. A dose of 25 mg/day achieves 95% of the antihypertensive effect and 12.5 mg achieves 80% of the antihypertensive effect.[108] Indapamide is a preferred diuretic, and epleronone shows excellent results as well.

6. The selection of nonpharmacologic therapy or antihypertensive drugs that have a neutral or favorable effect on serum lipids, glucose, electrolytes, and other risk factors and improve endothelial function and arterial compliance (improve vascular biology) may reduce the risk of CHD and other end-organ damage in patients with hypertension. *Optimal* treatment aims to reduce *all* risk factors, thereby reducing *all* end-organ damage.

7. Selection of drug therapy should be individualized and based on the subsets of hypertension approach and reversing the components of the hypertension-atherosclerotic syndrome.

8. An optimal goal BP may be as low as 110/70 mm Hg.

References

1. Levy RI. Lipid regulation. A new era in the prevention of coronary heart disease. Am Heart J. 1985;110:1099–1100.

2. Collins JG. Physician visits. Volume and interval since last visit, United States, 1980. U.S. Department of Health and Human Services (PHS) publication 83–1572, Series 10, No. 144, 1983.

3. Kannel WB. Some lessons in cardiovascular epidemiology from Framingham. Am J Cardiol. 1976;37:269–282.

4. Appel LJ, Moore TJ, Obarzanek E, et al. A clinical trial of the effects of dietary patterns on blood pressure. N Engl J Med. 1997;336:1117-1124.

5. Houston MC. New insights and approaches to reduce end organ damage in the treatment of hypertension: Subsets of hypertension approach. Am Heart J. 1992;123:1337–1367.

6. The Fifth Report of the Joint National Committee on Detection, Evaluation, and Treatment of High Blood Pressure (JNC V). Arch Intern Med. 1993;153:154–183.

7. Kirkendall WM, Feinleib M, Freis ED, Mark AL. Recommendations for human blood pressure determination by sphygmomanometers: Subcommittee of the AHA Postgraduate Education Committee. Circulation. 1980;62:1146A–1155A.

8. Final Report of the Subcommittee on Nonpharmacological Therapy of the 1984 Joint National Committee on Detection, Evaluation, and Treatment of High Blood Pressure: Nonpharmacological approaches to the control of high blood pressure. Hypertension. 1986;8:444–467.

9. Houston MC. New insights and new approaches for the treatment of essential hypertension: Selections of therapy based on coronary heart disease risk factor analysis, hemodynamic profiles, quality of life, and subsets of hypertension. Am Heart J. 1989;117:911–951.

10. Hollifield JW, Slaton P. Demographic approach to initiation of antihypertensive therapy: Treatment strategies in hypertension. Miami: Symposium Specialists, Inc. 1981:51–58.

11. Woods JW, Pittman AW, Pulliam CC, et al. Renin profiling in hypertension and its use in treatment with propranolol and chlorthalidone. N Engl J Med. 1976;294:1137–1143.

12. Buhler FR, Bolli P, Kiowski W, et al. Renin profiling to select antihypertensive baseline drugs: Renin inhibitors for high-renin and calcium entry blockers for low-renin patients. Am J Med. 1984;77:36–42.

13. Letcher RL, Chien S, Laragh JH. Changes in blood viscosity accompanying the response to prazosin in patients with essential hypertension. J Cardiovasc Pharmacol. 1979;1(suppl 6):S8–S20.

385

14. Lund-Johansen P. Hemodynamic changes at rest and during exercise in long-term prazosin therapy for essential hypertension. In: Prazosin Clinical Symposium Proceedings. Special Proceedings by Postgraduate Medicine. New York: Custom Communications, McGraw-Hill Co, 1975:45–52.

15. Okun R. Effectiveness of prazosin as initial antihypertensive therapy. Am J Cardiol. 1983;51:644–650.

16. Itskovitz HD. Hemodynamic effects of antihypertensive drugs. Am Fam Physician. 1983;27:137–142.

17. van Zwieten PA, Thoolen MJ, Timmermans PB. The hypertensive activity and side effects of methyldopa, clonidine and guanfacine. Hypertension. 1984;6:1128–1133.

18. Lund-Johansen P. Hemodynamic changes in long-term diuretic therapy of essential hypertension: a comparative study of chlorthalidone, polythiazide and hydrochlorothiazide. Acta Med Scand. 1970;187:509–518.

19. Ventura HO, Frohlich ED, Messerli FH, et al. Immediate regional blood flow distribution following angiotensin converting enzyme inhibition in patients with essential hypertension. Am J Med. 1984;76:58–61.

20. Frohlich ED. Hemodynamic effects of calcium entry-blocking agents in normal and hypertensive rats and man. Am J Cardiol. 1985;56:21H–27H.

21. Halperin AK, Cubeddu LX. The role of calcium channel blockers in the treatment of hypertension. Am Heart J. 1986;111:363–382.

22. Ekelund LG, Ekelund C, Rossner S. Antihypertensive effects at rest and during exercise of a calcium blocker, nifedipine, alone and in combination with metoprolol. Acta Med Scand. 1982;212:71–75.

23. Lund-Johansen P. Hemodynamic effects of verapamil in essential hypertension at rest and during exercise. Acta Med Scand. 1984;681(Suppl):109–115.

24. Hansson L. Hemodynamics of metoprolol and pindolol in systemic hypertension with particular reference to reversal of structural vascular changes. Am J Cardiol. 1986;57:29C–32C.

25. Lund-Johansen P. Central hemodynamic effects of beta-blockers in hypertension: A comparison between atenolol, metoprolol, timolol, penbutolol, alprenolol, pindolol and bunitrolol. Eur Heart J. 1983;4(suppl D): 1–12.

26. Trap-Jensen J, Clausen JP, Noer I, et al. The effects of beta-adrenoceptor blockers on cardiac output, liver blood flow and skeletal muscle blood flow in hypertensive patients. Acta Physiol Scand. 1976;440(suppl):30.

27. Pedersen EB. Abnormal renal hemodynamics during exercise in young patients with mild essential hypertension without treatment and during long-term propranolol therapy. Scand J Clin Lab Invest. 1978;30:567–571.

28. Hansson L, Pascual A, Julius S. Comparison of guanadrel and guanethidine. Clin Pharmacol Ther. 1973;14:204–208.

29. Woosley RL, Nies AS. Guanethidine. N Engl J Med. 1976;295: 1053–1057.

30. Lund-Johansen P. Exercise and antihypertensive therapy. Am J Cardiol. 1987;59:98A–107A.

31. Kannel WB, Wolf PA, Verter J, McNamara PM. Epidemiologic assessment of the role of blood pressure in stroke: The Framingham Study. JAMA. 1970;214:301–310.

32. Mortality Experience According to Blood Pressure After Treatment: Blood Pressure Study. Chicago: Society of Actuaries and Association of Life Insurance Medical Directors of America, 1979.

33. Hypertension Detection and Follow-up Program Cooperative Group. Five-year findings of the Hypertension Detection and Follow-Up Program: I. Reduction in mortality of persons with high blood pressure including mild hypertension. JAMA. 1979;242:2562–2571.

34. Veterans Administration Cooperative Study Group on Antihypertensive Agents. Effects of treatment on morbidity in hypertension: II. Results in patients with diastolic blood pressure averaging 90 through 114 mmHg. JAMA. 1970;213:1143–1152.

35. Smith WM. Treatment of mild hypertension: Results of a ten-year intervention trial. Circ Res. 1977;40(suppl I):198–205.

36. Perry HM Jr. Treatment of mild hypertension: Preliminary results of a two-year feasibility trial. Circ Res. 1977;40(suppl I):1180–1187.

37. Helgeland A. Treatment of mild hypertension: A five year controlled drug trial: The Oslo Study. Am J Med. 1980;69:725–732.

38. Report by the Management Committee: The Australian Therapeutic Trial in Mild Hypertension. Lancet. 1980;1:1261–1267.

39. Greenberg G, Brennan PJ, Miall WE. Effects of diuretic and beta-blocker therapy in the Medical Research Council Trial. Am J Med. 1984;76:45–51.

40. Multiple Risk Factor Intervention Trial Research Group. Multiple Risk Factor Intervention Trial: Risk factor changes and mortality results. JAMA. 1982;248:1465–1477.

41. Amery A, Birkenhäger W, Brixko P, et al. Mortality and morbidity results from the European Working Party on High Blood Pressure in the Elderly Trial. Lancet. 1985;1:1349–1354.

42. Miettinen TA, Huttunen JK, Naukkarinen V, et al. Multifactorial primary prevention of cardiovascular diseases in middle-aged men: Risk factor changes, incidence, and mortality. JAMA. 1985;254:2097–2102.

43. Wilhelmsen L, Tibblin G, Werkö L. A primary preventive study in Gothenburg, Sweden. Prev Med. 1972;1:153–160.

44. MRC Working Party. Medical Research Council trial of treatment of hypertension in older adults: Principal results. Br Med J. 1992;304:405–412.

45. Sacks FM, Svetkey LP, Vollmer WM, Appel LJ, Bray GA, et al. Effects on blood pressure of reduced dietary sodium and the dietary approaches to stop hypertension (DASH) diet. N Engl J Med. 2001; 344:3-10.

46. Perry HM Jr, Goldman AI, Lavin MA, et al. Evaluation of drug treatment in mild hypertension: VA-NHLBI feasibility trial. Ann NY Acad Sci. 1978;304:267–288.

47. IPPPSH Collaborative Group. Cardiovascular risk and risk factors in a randomized trial of treatment based on the beta-blocker oxprenolol: The International Prospective Primary Prevention Study in Hypertension (IPPPSH). J Hypertens. 1985;3:379–392.

48. Coope J, Warrender TS. Randomised trial of treatment of hypertension in elderly patients in primary care. Br Med J. 1986;293:1145–1151.

49. Wilhelmsen L, Berglund G, Elmfeldt D, et al. Beta-blockers versus diuretics in hypertensive men: Main results from the HAPPHY trial. J Hypertens. 1987;5:561–572.

50. Wikstrand J, Warnold I, Olsson G, et al. Primary prevention with metoprolol in patients with hypertension: Mortality results from the MAPHY study. JAMA. 1988;259:1976–1982.

51. SHEP Cooperative Research Group. Prevention of stroke by antihypertensive drug treatment in older persons with isolated systolic hypertension (SHEP): Final results of the Systolic Hypertension in the Elderly Program. JAMA. 1991;265:3255–3264.

52. Dahlöf B, Lindholm LH, Hansson L, et al. Morbidity and mortality in the Swedish Trial in Old Patients with Hypertension (STOP-Hypertension). Lancet. 1991;338:1281–1285.

53. Castelli WP. Epidemiology of coronary heart disease: The Framingham Study. Am J Med. 1984;76:4–12.

54. Castelli W, Leaf A. Identification and assessment of cardiac risk: An overview. Cardiol Clin. 1985;3:171–178.

55. Kannel WB. Status of risk factors and their consideration in antihypertensive therapy. Am J Cardiol. 1987;59:80A–90A.

56. Kannel WB, Schatzkin A. Risk factor analysis. Prog Cardiovasc Dis. 1983;26:309–332.

57. Bush TL, Barrett-Connor E, Cowan LD, et al. Cardiovascular mortality and noncontraceptive use of estrogen in women: Results from the Lipid Research Clinics Program Follow-Up Study. Circulation. 1987;75:1102–1109.

58. Deutsche RS. The effect of heavy drinking on ischemic heart disease. Primary Cardiol. 1986;12:40–48.

59. Fitzgerald DJ, Roy L, Catella F, Fitzgerald GA. Platelet activation in unstable coronary disease. N Engl J Med 1986;315:983–989.

60. Meade TW, Mellows S, Brozovic M, et al. Haemostatic function and ischaemic heart disease: Principal results of the Northwick Park Heart Study. Lancet. 1986;2:533–537.

61. Spence JD. Hemodynamic effects of antihypertensive drugs: Possible implications for the prevention of atherosclerosis. Hypertension. 1984; 6:163–168.

62. Brunner HR, Laragh JH, Baer L, et al. Essential hypertension: Renin and aldosterone, heart attack and stroke. N Engl J Med. 1972;286:441–449.

63. Giese J. Renin, angiotensin and hypertensive vascular damage: A review. Am J Med. 1973;55:315–332.

64. Chobanian AV. The influence of hypertension and other hemodynamic factors in atherogenesis. Prog Cardiovasc Dis. 1983;26:177–196.

65. Letcher RL, Chien S, Pickering TG, et al. Direct relationship between blood pressure and blood viscosity in normal and hypertensive subjects: Role of fibrinogen and concentration. Am J Med. 1981;70:1195–1202.

66. Reaven GM, Huffman BB. A role for insulin in the aetiology and course of hypertension. Lancet. 1987;2:435–437.

67. Ferrannini E, Buzzigoli G, Bonadonna R, et al. Insulin resistance in essential hypertension. N Engl J Med. 1987;317:435–437.

68. Ames RP, Hill P. Elevation of serum lipid levels during diuretic therapy of hypertension. Am J Med. 1976;61:748–757.

69. Lasser NL, Grandits G, Caggiula AW, et al. Effects of antihypertensive therapy on plasma lipids and lipoproteins in the Multiple Risk Factor Intervention Trial. Am J Med. 1984;76:52–66.

70. Helgeland A, Hjermann L, Leren P, Holme I. Possible metabolic side effects of beta-adrenergic blocking drugs. Br Med J. 1978;1:828.

71. Ames RP. The effects of antihypertensive drugs on serum lipids and lipoproteins: I. Diuretics. Drugs. 1986;32:260–278.

72. Ames RP, Hill P. Increase in serum lipids during treatment of hypertension with chlorthalidone. Lancet. 1976;1:721–723.

73. Glück Z, Weidmann P, Mordasini R, et al. Increased serum low-density lipoprotein cholesterol in men treated short-term with the diuretic chlorthalidone. Metabolism. 1980;29:240–245.

74. Boehringer K, Weidmann P, Mordasini R, et al. Menopause-dependent plasma lipoprotein alterations in diuretic-treated women. Ann Intern Med. 1982;97:206–209.

75. Mauersberger H. Effect of prazosin on blood pressure and plasma lipids in patients receiving a beta-blocker and diuretic regimen. Am J Med. 1984;76:101–104.

76. Goldman AI, Steele BW, Schnaper HW, et al. Serum lipoprotein levels during chlorthalidone therapy: A Veterans Administration–National Heart, Lung, and Blood Institute cooperative study on antihypertensive therapy: mild hypertension. JAMA. 1980;224:1691–1695.

77. Koskinen P, Manninen V, Eisalo A. Quinapril and blood lipids. Br J Clin Pharmacol. 1988;26:478–480.

78. Ames RP. Metabolic disturbances increasing the risk of coronary heart disease during diuretic-based antihypertensive therapy: Lipid alterations and glucose intolerance. Am Heart J. 1983;106:1207–1214.

79. Ames RP. Negative effects of diuretic drugs on metabolic risk factors for coronary heart disease: Possible alternative drug therapies. Am J Cardiol. 1983;51:632–638.

80. Grimm RH Jr, Leon AS, Hunninghake DB, et al. Effects of thiazide diuretics on plasma lipids and lipoproteins in mildly hypertensive patients: A double-blind controlled trial. Ann Intern Med. 1981;94:7–11.

81. Flamenbaum W. Metabolic consequences of antihypertensive therapy. Ann Intern Med. 1983;98:875–880.

82. Weinberger MH. Antihypertensive therapy and lipids: Evidence, mechanisms, and implications. Arch Intern Med. 1985;145:1102–1105.

83. Drayer JI, Gardin JM, Weber MA, Aronow WS. Changes in ventricular septal thickness during diuretic therapy. Clin Pharmacol Ther. 1982; 32:283–288.

84. Lowenthal DT. Hypertension and exercise physiology: Clinical and therapeutic applications. In: Lowenthal DT, Bharadwaja K, Oaks WW, eds. Therapeutics Through Exercise. New York: Grune & Stratton, 1981:133–144.

85. Loaldi A, Polese A, Montorsi P, et al. Comparison of nifedipine, propranolol and isosorbide dinitrate on angiographic progression and regression of coronary arterial narrowings in angina pectoris. Am J Cardiol. 1989;64:433–439.

86. Lichtlen PR, Hugenholtz PG, Rafflenbeul W, et al. Retardation of angiographic progression of coronary artery disease by nifedipine: Results of the International Nifedipine Trial on Antiatherosclerotic Therapy (INTACT). Lancet. 1990;335:1109–1113.

87. Kober G, Schneider W, Kaltenbach M. Can the progression of coronary sclerosis be influenced by calcium antagonists? J Cardiovasc Pharmacol. 1989;13(suppl 4):52–56.

88. The MIDAS Research Group. Multicenter Isradipine Diuretic Atherosclerosis Study (MIDAS). Am J Med. 1989;86(suppl 4A):37–39.

89. Waters D, Lespérance J. Interventions that beneficially influence the evolution of coronary atherosclerosis: The case for calcium channel blockers. Circulation. 1992;86(suppl III):III-116.

90. Rostand SG, Brown G, Kirk KA, et al. Renal insufficiency in treated essential hypertension. N Engl J Med. 1989;320:684–688.

91. Brazy PC, Fitzwilliam JF. Progressive renal disease: Role of race and antihypertensive medications. Kidney Int. 1990;37:1113–1119.

92. Eliahou HE, Cohen D, Hellberg B, et al. Effect of the calcium channel blocker nisoldipine on the progression of chronic renal failure in man. Am J Nephrol. 1988;8:285–290.

93. Alcazar JM, Rodicio JL, Ruilope LM. Long-term diuretic therapy and renal function in essential arterial hypertension. Am J Cardiol. 1990; 65:51H–54H.

94. Warram JH, Laffel LMB, Valsania P, et al. Excess mortality associated with diuretic therapy in diabetes mellitus. Arch Intern Med. 1991; 151:1350–1356.

95. Croog SH, Levine S, Testa MA, et al. The effects of antihypertensive therapy on the quality of life. N Engl J Med. 1986;314:1657–1664.

96. Jachuck SJ, Brierly J, Jachuck S, Willcox PM. The effect of hypotensive drugs on the quality of life. J R Coll Gen Pract. 1982;32:103–105.

97. Curb JD, Borhani NO, Blaszkowski TP, et al. Long-term surveillance for adverse effects of antihypertensive drugs. JAMA. 1985;253:3263–3268.

98. Avorn J, Everitt DE, Weiss S. Increased antidepressant use in patients prescribed β-blockers. JAMA. 1986;255:357–360.

99. Testa MA, Hollenberg HK, Anderson RB, Williams GH. Assessment of quality of life by patient and spouse during antihypertensive therapy with atenolol and nifedipine gastrointestinal therapeutic system. Am J Hypertens. 1991;4:363–373.

100. Os I, Bratland B, Dahlof B, et al. Lisinopril or nifedipine in essential hypertension? A Norwegian multicenter study on efficacy, tolerability and quality of life in 828 patients. J Hypertens. 1991;9:1097–1104.

101. Croog SH, Kong BW, Levine S, et al. Hypertensive black men and women. Quality of life and effects of antihypertensive medications. Arch Intern Med. 1990;150:1733–1741.

102. Fletcher AE, Bulpitt CJ, Hawkins CM, et al. Quality of life on antihypertensive therapy: a randomized double-blind controlled trial of captopril and atenolol. J Hypertens. 1990;8:463–466.

103. Gerber JC, Nies AS. Pharmacology of antihypertensive drugs. In: Genest J, Kuchel O, Hamet P, et al. Hypertension. 2nd ed. New York, NY: McGraw-Hill; 1983:1093–1127.

104. Wollam GL, Gifford RW, Tarazi RC. Antihypertensive drugs. Clin Pharmacol Ther Drugs. 1977;14:420–460.

105. Carney S, Gillies Al, Morgan T. Optimal dose of a thiazide diuretic. Med J Aust. 1976;2:692–693.

106. Campbell DB, Brackman F. Cardiovascular protective properties of indapamide. Am J Cardiol. 1990;65:11H–27H.

107. Clarke RJ. Indapamide: A diuretic of choice for the treatment of hypertension? Am J Med Sci. 1991;301(3):215–220.

108. Oster JR, Epstein M. Use of centrally acting sympatholytic agents in the management of hypertension. Arch Intern Med. 1991;151:1638–1644.

109. Beers MH, Passman LJ. Antihypertensive medications and depression. Drugs. 1990;40(6):792–799.

110. Ames RP. The effects of antihypertensive drugs on serum lipids and lipoproteins. Part II. Non-diuretic drugs. Drugs. 1986;32:335–357.

111. Kaplan NM. Resistant hypertension: What to do after trying "the usual." Geriatrics. 1995;50:24–38.

112. Houston MC. Pathophysiology, clinical aspects diagnosis and treatment of hypertensive crisis. Prog Cardiovasc Dis. 1989;32:99–148.

113. Cunningham FG, Lindheimer H. Hypertension in pregnancy. N Engl J Med. 1992;326:927–932.

114. Sabatini S. Pathophysiology of and therapeutic strategies for hypertension in pregnancy. Curr Opin Nephrol Hypertens. 1993;2:763–774.

115. Kincaid-Smith, P. Hypertension in pregnancy. Blood Pressure. 1994;3:18–23.

116. Joint National Committee on Prevention, Detection, Evaluation, and Treatment of High Blood Pressure. The Sixth Report of the Joint National Committee on Prevention, Detection, Evaluation, and Treatment of High Blood Pressure. Arch Intern Med. 1997;157:2413–2446.

117. Hilleman DE, Mohiuddin SM, Lucas D Jr, et al. Cost-minimization analysis of initial antihypertensive therapy in patients with mild to moderate essential diastolic hypertension (ABST). Circulation 1992;88(Part 2):263.

118. Himmelmann, A, Hansson L, et al. ACE inhibition prescribes renal function better than beta-blockade in the treatment of essential hypertension. Blood Pressure. 1995;4:85–90.

119. Saruta T, Kanns Y, et al. Renal effects of amlodipine. J Hum Hypertens. 1995;9(suppl I):811–816.

120. Reeves RA. Does this patient have hypertension? How to measure blood pressure. JAMA. 1995;273:1211–1218.

121. Drugs for Hypertension. Med Lett. 1995;37:45–50.

122. Eberhardt RT, Kevak RM, Kang PM, Frishman WH. Angiotensin II receptor blockade: An innovative approach to cardiovascular pharmacotherapy. J Clin Pharmacol. 1993;33:1023–1038.

123. Gradman AH, Arcuri KE, Goldberg AI, et al. A randomized, placebo-controlled, double-blind, parallel study of various doses of losartan potassium compared with enalapril maleate in patients with essential hypertension. Hypertension. 1995;25:1345–1350.

124. Bakris, GL, Griffen KA. Combined effects of an angiotensin converting enzyme inhibitor and a calcium antagonist on renal injury. J Hypertens. 1997;15:1181–1185.

125. Bakris GL, Houston MC, Messerli FH. Effective use of combination therapy in hypertension. Patient Care. Fall 1997 suppl., pp 10–21.

126. Gong L, Zhang W. Shanghai Trial of Nifedipine in the Elderly (STONE). J Hypertens. 1996;14:1237–1245.

127. Staessen J. Facard R. et al. Systolic Hypertension in Europe Trial (SYST–EUR). Lancet. 1997;350:757–764.

128. Liu L, Wang JG, Gong L, et al. Comparison of active treatment and placebo in older Chinese patients with isolated systolic hypertension: Systolic Hypertension in China (Syst-China) Collaborative Group. J Hypertens. 1998;16:1823–1829.

129. Hansson L. Zanchetti A, Carruthers SG, et al. Effects of intensive blood pressure lowering and low-dose aspirin in patients with hypertension: Principal results of the Hypertension Optimal Treatment (HOT) randomized trial. Lancet. 1998;351:1755–1762.

130. Messerli FH, Grossman E, Goldbourt U. Are beta-blockers efficacious as first-line therapy for hypertension in the elderly? A systematic review. JAMA. 1998;279:1903–1907.

131. Bakris GL. Progression of diabetic nephropathy: A focus on arterial pressure level and methods of reduction. Diabetes Res Clin Pract. 1998;39(suppl):S35–S42.

132. Epstein M. The benefits of ACE inhibitors and calcium antagonists in slowing progressive renal failure. Focus on fixed-dose combination antihypertensive therapy. Ren Fail. 1996;18:813–832.

133. Hansson L, Lindholm LH, Niskanen L, et al. Effect of angiotensin-converting enzyme inhibition compared with conventional therapy on cardiovascular morbidity and mortality in hypertension: The Captopril Prevention Project (CAPPP). Lancet. 1999;611–616.

134. Tuomilehto J, Rastenyte D, Birkenhäger W, et al. Effects of calcium-channel blockade in older patients with diabetes and systolic hypertension. N Engl J Med. 1999;340:677-684.

135. National Intervention Cooperative Study in Elderly Hypertensives Study Group: Randomized double-blind comparison of a calcium antagnoist and a diuretic in elderly hypertensives. Hypertension 1999;34:1129-1133.

136. Hansson L, Lindholm LH, Ekbom T, et al. For the STOP-Hypertension-2 Study Group: Randomized trial of old and new antihypertensive drugs in elderly patients: Cardiovascular mortality and morbidity the Swedish Trial in Old Patients with Hypertension-2 study. Lancet 1999;354:1751-1756.

137. US Renal Data System. USRDS 1997 Annual Data Report. Bethesda, MD, National Institute of Health, National Institute of Diabetes and Digestive and Kidney Diseases, 1997.

138. Klag MJ, Whelton PK et al. Blood pressure and incidence of end stage renal disease in men. A prospective study. Circulation 1994; 18:941.

139. National High Blood Pressure Education Program Working Group: 1995 update of the working group reports on chronic renal failure and renovascular hypertension. Arch Int. Med 1996;156:1938-1947.

140. Bauer JH, Reams GP, Lai SM. Renal protective effects of strict blood pressure control with enalapril therapy. Arch Intern Med 1987;147:1387-1400.

141. Wee PM, De Mitchell AG, Epstein M. Effects of calcium antagonists on renal hemodynamics and progression of nondiabetic chronic renal disease. Arch Intern Med 1994;154:1185-1202.

142. Hannedouche T, Landais P, et al. Randomised controlled trial of enalapril and beta-blockers in non-diabetic chronic renal failure. BMJ 1994;309:833-837.

143. GISEN Study Group: Randomized placebo controlled trial of the effect of ramipiril on decline in glomerular filtration rate and risk of terminal renal failure in proteinuric nondiabetic nephropathy. Lancet 1997; 349:1857-1863.

144. Maschio G, Alberti D, Hanin G, et al. Effect of the angiotensin-converting enzyme inhibitor benazapril on the progression of renal insufficiency. N Engl J Med 1996;334:939-945.

145. Tarif N, Bakris GL: Angiotensin II receptor blockade and progression of renal disease in non-diabetic patients. Kidney Int 1997;52(suppl 63): S67-S70.

146. Bakris GL (ed). The renin-angiotensin system in diabetic nephropathy: From bench to bedside. Miner Electrolyte Metab 1998; 24(6):361-438.

147. Neutel JM, Smith DHG, Weber MA. Is high blood pressure a late manifestation of the hypertension syndrome? Am J Hypertens 1999; 12:215S-223S.

148. Messerli FH, Grossman E: B-blockers and diuretics: to use or not to use? Am J Hypertens 1999;12:157S-163S.

149. Abernethy, DR, Schwartz JB. Calcium antagonist drugs. N Engl J Med 1999; 341(19):1447-1457.

150. ALLHAT Collaborative Research Group: Major outcomes in high-risk hypertensive patients randomized to angiotensin-converting enzyme inhibitor or calcium channel blocker vs. diuretic. The antihypertensive and lipid-lowering treatment to prevent heart attack trial (ALLHAT). JAMA 220;288:2981-2997.

151. Houston, MC. The role of vascular biology, nutrition and nutraceuticals in prevention of hypertension. Journal of the American Nutraceutical Association April 2002; (suppl.):1-71.

152. Vlachopoulos C, O'Rouke M. Diastolic pressure, systolic pressure or pulse pressure? Curr Hypertens Reports. 2000;2:271-279.

153. Franklin SS. Aging and Hypertension: The assessemnt of blood pressure indices in predicting coronary heart disease. J Hypertens. 1999;17 (suppl 5):S29-S36.

154. Kannel WB. Elevated Blood Pressure as a Cardiovascular Risk Factor. Am J Cardiol. 2000;85:251-255.

155. Blacher J, Staessen JA, Girerd X, et al. Pulse pressure not mean pressure determines cardiovascular risk in older patients. Arch Intern Med. 2000;160:1085-1089.

155A. Houston M. Vascular Biology in Clinical Practice. Philadelphia,PA: Hanley and Belfus; 2002.

156. Staessen JA, Wang JG, Thijs, L. Cardiovascular protection and blood pressure reduction: a meta-analysis. Lancet. 2001;358:1305-1315.

157. Psaty, BM, Smith NL, Siscovick DS, et al. Health Outcomes associated with antihypertensive therapies used as first-line agents. JAMA 1997;277:739-745.

158. Blood Pressure lowering treatment trials. Collaboration effects of ACE inhibitors, calcium antagonists and other blood pressure lowering drugs: results of prospectively designed overview of randomized trials. Lancet. 2000;355:1955-1964.

159. Pahor M, Psaty BM, Alderman MH, et al. Health outcomes associated with calcium antagonists compared with other first line antihypertensive therapies: a meta-analysis of randomized controlled trials. Lancet. 2000: 356: 1949-1954.

160. Neal B, MacMahon S. The world health organization-international society of hypertension. Blood pressure lowering treatment trials collaboration: prospective collaborative overview of major randomized trial of blood pressure–lowering treatments. Current Hypertension Reports. 1999;1:346-356.

161. Carter AB Hypotensive therapy in stroke survivors. Lancet. 1970; I:485-489.

162. Barraclough M. Joy MD, Macgregor GA, et al. Control of moderately raised Blood Pressure. BMJ. 1973;3:434-443.

163. Hypertension-stroke cooperative study group. Effect of antihypertensive treatment on stroke recurrence. JAMA. 1974: 229 :409-418.

164. Kuramoto K. Matsushita S, Kuwajima I etal prospective study on the treatment of mild hypertension in he aged. JPN heart J. 1981;22:75-85.

165. Perry HM, Smith WM, McDonald RH et al. Morbidity and mortality in the systolic hypertension in the elderly program (SHEP) pilot study. Stroke.1989;20: 4-13.

166. Medical research council working party. Medical research council trial of treatment of hypertension in older adults. BMJ. 1992: 304: 405-423.

167. Veterans Administration cooperative study group on antihypertensive agents. Effects of treatment on moribidity in hypertension. JAMA. 1967; 202:1028-1034.

168. Brown MJ, Palmer CR, Castaisne A. Morbidity and mortality in patients randomised to double-blind treatment with a long-acting calcium-channel blocker or diuretic in the international nifedipine GITS study: Intervention as a goal in hypertension treatment (INSIGHT). Lancet. 2000;356;366-372.

169. Hansson L, Hedner T, Lund Johnson P, et al. Randomised trial of effects of calcium antagonists compared with diuretics and beta-blockers on cardiovascular morbidity and mortality in hypertension: The Nordic diliazem (NORDIL) study. Lancet. 2000;356:359-365.

170. Black HR, Elliot WJ, Grandits G, et al. Principal results of the controlled onset verapamil investigation of cardiovascular endpoints (convince trial). JAMA. 2003; 289: 2073-2082.

171. Pitt B, Byington RP, Furberg CD, et al. Effect of Amlodipine on the progression of atherosclerosis and the occurrence of clinical events. Circulaton: 2000;102: 1503-1510.

172. Zanchetti A, Rosei EA, Plau CD. The verapamil in hypertension and atherosclerosis study (VHAS): results of long-term randomized treatment with either verapamil or chlorthalidone on carotid intima-media thickness. J. Hypertens. 1998;16; 1667-1676.

173. Ohihara T. Practitioner's trial on the efficacy of antihypertensive treatment in the elderly on hypertension. (The PATE hypertension study) in Japan. AM J Hypertens. 2000;13:461-467.

174. The GLANT study group: a 12 month comparison of ACE inhibitor and CA antagonist therapy in mild to moderate essential hypertension: the GLANT study. Hypertens Res. 1995;18:235-244.

175. Omae T, Matsuoka H, Arakawa K, Imura O, Ishii M, Ogihara T, Kaneko Y, Kuramochi M, Kokubu T, Takeda R, Hiwada K, Fukiyama K, Fujishima M, Yamada K, Yoshinaga K, Shimuzu U, Nobutomo K: GLANT sudy. Nipppon Iji-shinpo. 1993;3630:26-34 (in Japanese).

176. Hanson L, Lindhol LH, Ekbom T, et al. For the STOP-Hypertension-2 study group: randomized trial of old and new hypertensive drugs in elderly patients: cardiovascular mortality and morbidity The Swedish trial in old patients with hypertension-2 study. Lancet. 1999;354:1751-1756.

177. Lewis, EJ. The role of angiotensin receptor blockers in preventing the progression of renal disease in patients with type 2 diabetes. AM J. Hypertension. 2002;15:1235-1285.

178. Wright JT, Bakris G, Green T. et al. Effect of blood pressure lowering and antihypertensive drug class on progression of hypertensive kidney disease. Results from the AASK trial. JAMA, 2002;288:2421-2431.

179. Estacio RO, Jeffer BW, Giffird N, Schrier RW. Effect of blood pressure control on diabetic microvascular complications in patients with hypertension and type 2 diabetes. Diabetes Care. 2000 Apr;23 (suppl) 2:B54-64.

180. Tatti P. Pahor M, Byington RP, et al. Outcome results of the fosinopril vs. amlodipine cardiovascular events randomized trial (FACET) in patients with hypertension and NIDAM. Diabetics Care. 1998; 21(4);597-603.

181. Zanchetti A, Bond MG, Henniq M, et al. Risk factors associated with alterations in carotid intima-media thickness in hypertension: baseline data from the European lacidipine study on atherosclerosis. J Hypertens. 1998; 16: 949-996.

182. Conti CR, Cooper–Deltoff RM. How will invest and other hypertension trials change clinical practices. Clin Cardiol. 2001;24(II suppl): V24-29.

183. Pepine CJ, Handberg-Thurmond E, Marks RG. Rationale and design of the International Verapamil SR/Trandolapril Study (INVEST): an internet based randomised trial in coronary artery disease patients with hypertension. J Am Coll Cardiol. 1998; 32: 1228-1237.

184. Malacco E, Gnemmi AE, Romagnoli A, et al. Systolic hypertension in the elderly: long-term lacidipine treatment. Objective protocoal and organization. Shell study group. J Cardiovasc, Pharmacol. 1994;23 (suppl 5):562-66.

185. Borhani NO, Mercuri M, Borhani PA, et al. Final outcome results of the multicenter Isradipine diuretic atherosclerosis study (MIDAS). A randomised controlled trial. JAMA. 1996;276:785-791.

186. Devereux RB, Palmier V and Sharpe N, et al. Effects of once-daily angiotensin-converting enzyme inhibition and calcium channel blockade-based antihypertensive treatment regiments on left ventricular hypertrophy and diastolic filling in hypertension: the prospective randomized enalapril study evaluating regression of ventricular enlargement (PRESERVE) trial. Circulation. 2001;104 (11):1248-1254.

187. PROGRESS collaborative group. Randomized trial of a perindopril-based blood-pressure lowering regimens among 6105 individuals with previous stroke or transient ischaemic attack. Lancet 2001;358:1033-1041.

188. Hanson L, Lindholm LH, Niskanew L. Effect of angiotensin-converting enzyme inhibition compared with conventional therapy on cardiovascular morbidity and mortality in hypertension: the captopril prevention project (CAPPP) randomized trial. Lancet. 1999;353:611-616.

189. Kjelosen SE, Dahlof B, Devereux RB. Effects of Losartan on cardiovascular morbidity and mortality in patients with isolated systolic hypertension and left ventricular hypertrophy. JAMA. 2002;288:1491-1498.

190. Dahlof B, Devereux RB, Kjeldsen SE, Julius S, Beevers G, Faire U, Fyhrquist F, Ibsen H, Kristiansson K, Lederballe-Pedersen O, Lindholm LH, Nieminen MS, Omvik P, Oparil S, Wedel H. The Life study group. Cardiovascular morbidity and mortality in the losartan intervention for end-point reduction in hypertension study (LIFE): a randomised trial against atenolol. Lancet. 2002 Mar 23;359(9311):995-1003.

191. Zanchetti A, Rulope LM. Antihypertensive treatment in patients with type-2 diabetes mellitus: guidelines from recent controlled randomized trials. Hypertension. 2002; 20:2099-2110.

192. Nosadini R, Tonolo G. Cardiovascular and renal protection in type 2 diabetes mellitus: the role of calcium channel blockers. J AM Soc Nephrology. 2002;13 (suppl)3:5216-5223.

193. Zarnke KB, Marentette MA, Gert WC. Saskatchewan health and database analysis of antihypertensive persistence. Paper presented at 2nd international forum on angiotensin antagonists. Monte Carlo. January 2001.

194. Bloom BS. Continuation of initial antihypertensive medication after 1 year of therapy. Clin Ther. 1998; 20:671-681.

195. Caro JJ, Speckman JL, Salas M, et al. Effect of initial drug choice on persistence with antihypertensive therapy: the importance of actual practice data. Can Med Assoc J. 1999; 160:41-46.

196. Grossman E, Messerli FH; Goldbourt U: Does diuretic therapy increase the risk of renal cell carcinoma? Am J Cardiol, 1999; 83:1090-1093.

197. Prospective studies collaboration. Age-specific relevance of usual blood pressure to vascular mortality: a meta-analysis of individual data for 1 million adults in 61 prospective studies. Lancet. 2002;360:1903-1913.

198. Messerlu FH, Grossman E. Beta-blockers and diuretics: to use or not to use? AM J Hypertens. 199;12:1573-1635.

199. Cohn JN. ACE-inhibition and vascular remodeling of resistance vessels. Vascular compliance and cardiovascular implications. Heart Disease. 2000;2:S2-S6.

200. Park JB, Schiffrin EL. Effects of Antihypertensive therapy on hypertensive vascular disease. Curr Hypertens Reports. 2000;2:280-288.

201. Oparil S, Weber MA. Hypertension: a Companion to Brenner and Rector's: The Kidney. Philadelphia; WB Saunders, 2000.

202. Collins R, Peto R, MacMahon S, et al. Blood pressure, stroke, and coronary heart disease. Part 2, short-term reductions in blood pressure: overview of randomised drug trials in their epidemiologies context. Lancet. 1990;335:827-838.

203. MacMahon S, Rodgers A. The effects of antihypertensive treatment on vascular disease: reappraisal of the evidence in 1994. J Vasc Med Biol. 993; 4: 265-271.

204. Collins R, MacMahon S. Blood pressure, antihypertensive drug treatment and the risks of stroke and of coronary heart disease. Br Med Bull 1994;50:272-98.

205. Gueyffier F, Boutitie F, Boissel JP, et al. Effect of antihypertensive drug treatment on cardiovascular outcomes in women and men: a meta-analysis of individual patient data from randomised controlled trials. Ann Intern Med. 1997;126:761-67.

206. Psaty B, Smith N, Siscovick D, et al. Health outcomes associated with antihypertensive therapies used as first-line agents: a systematic review and meta-analysis. JAMA. 1997; 277: 739-45.

207. Zanchetti A, Bond MG, Hennig, M, et al. Calcium antagonist lacidipine slows down progression of a symptomate carotid atherosclerosis principal results of the european lacidipine study of artherosclerosis (ELSA), a randomised, double-blind, long-term trial. Circulation. 2002; 106(19):2422-2427.

208. Malacco E, Mancia FG, Rappelli S et al. Treatment of isolated systolic hypertension: the SHELL study results. Blood Pressure. 2003;12:160-167.

209. Lindon MH, Wing MB, Reid CM et al. A comparison of outcomes with angiotensin-converting enzyme-inhibitors and diuretics for hypertension in the elderly. N Engl J Med. 2003; 348:583-592.

210. Black HR, Elliot WJ , Grandits G. Principal results of the controlled onset verapamil investigation of cardiovascular endpoints (CONVINCE) trial. JAMA 2003;289(1G):2073-2082.

211. PREMIER collaborative research group. Effects of comprehensive lifestyle modification on blood pressure control. Main results of the PREMIER clinical trial. JAMA. 2003;289:2083-2093.

212. Bakris Gl, Weir MR, Shanifar S. Effects of blood pressure level on progression of diabetic nephropathy. Results from renal study. Arch Int Med. 2003;163:1555-1565.

213. Chobanian AV, Bakru GL, Black HR, et al. The seventh report of the joint national committee on prevention, detection, evaluation and treatment of high blood pressure. The JNC 7 report. JAMA. 2003;289:2560-2572.

214. The Canadian Hypertension Education Program of the management of hypertension. http://www.chs.md/index2.html

215. Guidelines committee. 2003 European Society of Hypertension, European Society of Cardiology guidelines for the management of arterial hypertension. Hypertension. 2003;21:1011-1053.

216. Douglas JG, Bakris GL, Epotein M, et al. Management of high blood pressure in African Americans. Arch Intern Med. 2003;163:525-541.

217. Hajjar I and Kotchen TA. Trends in prevalance, awareness, treatment and control of hypertension in the United States, 1988-2000. JAMA. 2003; 290:199-206.

218. Laragh JH, Sealey JE. Relevance of the plasma renin hormonal control system that regulates blood pressure and sodium balance for correctly treating hypertension for evaluating ALLHAT. Am J Hypertension. 2003; 16:407-413.

219. Psaty BM, Lumley T, Furberg CD. Health outcomes associated with various antihypertensive therapies used as first-line agents. A network meta-analysis. JAMA. 2003;289:2534-2544.

220. Law MR, Walp NJ., Morris JK, Jordan RE. Value of low dose combination treatment with blood pressure lowering drugs: analysis of 354 randomized trials. BMJ. 2003;326:1427-35

221. Lasaridis AN, Sarafids PA. Diabetic nephropathy and hypertensive treatment: what are the lessons from clinical trials. Am J Hypertension. 2003; 16: 687-697.

A

I

O

P